INTEGRATIVE
Mental Health Care

A THERAPIST'S
HANDBOOK

INTEGRATIVE
Mental Health Care

A THERAPIST'S
HANDBOOK

James Lake

W. W. Norton & Company

New York • London

For information about permission to reproduce selections from this book, write to
Permissions, W. W. Norton & Company, Inc., 500 Fifth Avenue, New York, NY 10110

For information about special discounts for bulk purchases, please contact
W. W. Norton Special Sales at specialsales@wwnorton.com or 800-233-4830

Manufacturing by Quebecor World Fairfield
Book design by Molly Heron
Production manager: Leeann Graham

Library of Congress Cataloging-in-Publication Data

Lake, James, 1956–
Integrative mental health care : a therapist's handbook / James Lake.
p. ; cm.
"A Norton professional book."
Includes bibliographical references and index.
ISBN 978-0-393-70536-2 (hardcover)
1. Mental illness—Alternative treatment—Handbooks, manuals, etc.
2. Integrative medicine—Handbooks, manuals, etc. I. Title.
[DNLM: 1. Mental Disorders—therapy. 2. Integrative Medicine.
3. Mental Disorders—etiology. WM 100 L192i 2009]
RC480.5.L335 2009
616.89'18—dc22
2008055913

ISBN: 978-0-393-70536-2

W. W. Norton & Company, Inc., 500 Fifth Avenue, New York, NY. 10110
www.wwnorton.com

W. W. Norton & Company Ltd., Castle House, 75/76 Wells Street,
London W1T 3QT

1 2 3 4 5 6 7 8 9 0

*For my sons
Daniel and David—
may your journeys on this green planet
be filled with learning, beauty, friendship,
laughter, and love.*

Contents

∼

Preface

⁓

CULTURE, spiritual beliefs, and personal values strongly influence perspectives about the validity of both conventional and nonconventional treatment modalities. Many traditional forms of healing are widely accepted within their parent cultures in the absence of evidence from Western-style research studies. Randomized placebo-controlled trials are regarded as the "gold standard" of evidence in Western culture; however, this requirement is seldom used by other world systems of medicine, including Chinese medicine, Ayurveda, Unani-Tibb, Tibetan medicine, and traditional forms of healing in Africa and Polynesia. Conceptual and practical differences between disparate medical traditions originate in differences in their basic premises about the nature of physical reality, the meaning of causality, and the role of intention in healing. These differences can seldom be bridged by the theories or research methods of contemporary Western science. From my journey as a conventionally trained physician who has sought to go beyond the techniques of clinical therapeutics to deeper matters of healing, I have no doubt that there is profound truth and practical clinical relevance in all ways of knowing about illness. I accept as an obvious truth that many traditional assessment and treatment approaches cannot be translated into the lexicon or concepts of Western science as it exists in the early 21st century. However, if we are open-minded and rigorous, we can learn much that is of value for our clients while adding challenging new dimensions to our professional lives. In writing this book my hope is to stimulate dialogue and debate among Western-trained mental health professionals and healers from all traditions who have devoted their energy to finding new ways to alleviate human suffering.

Acknowledgments

I AM indebted to many friends, colleagues, and teachers along the way for insights and values that influence how I practice medicine and live. My friends and teachers are too often in the position of listening to someone who is impatiently striving for radical transformation of medicine into something that is *more beautiful, more meaningful,* and *more effective* than the orthodox worldview of biomedicine in which I have trained, lived, and worked for decades. I am grateful for their patience, loyalty, and open-mindedness along the way. Important "renegade" colleagues and friends along the path include James Zarcone MD, Scott Shannon MD, Pam Pappas MD, MD(H), Lewis Mehl-Madrona MD, PhD, Jerome Sarris, MHSc(HMed), BHSc (WHMed), Rogier Hoenders MD, Jim Duffy MD, Mark Gilbert MD, Jeannie Achterberg PhD, David Spiegel, MD, Tieraona Low Dog MD, Victoria Maizes MD, Richard Brown MD, Pat Gerbarg MD, and Marlene Freeman MD. As always, I am indebted to Larry Dossey, MD for his vision and tireless devotion to exploring the implications of novel paradigms in health and healing. Fellow psychiatrists who are members of the APA CAM Caucus are too numerous to list by name, but their shared enthusiasm for and professional commitment to alleviating human suffering using non-pharmacological approaches are a constant source of encouragement. I am convinced that the hard work and shared vision of my teachers and colleagues will eventually, *inevitably* result in the evolution of contemporary Western biomedicine into a deeper, more person-centered, and more inclusive way of knowing about the causes and meanings of human suffering, a more rigorous and open-minded medical paradigm, and a more effective and safer assemblage of clinical therapeutics. Sharing the journey with healers of great vision and integrity has made all the difference.

This book was written with the needs of therapists foremost in mind. I want to make special mention of the visionary work of a small group of dedicated therapists in Salem, Oregon, who recently invited me to participate in their important work by presenting a symposium on integrative mental health care. Joan Williamson MA, LPC, Roberta Aronson LCSW, CNT, Nancy Ludwig, MS, RD, LD and colleagues have created a unique non-profit organization committed to promoting the goals of integrative mental health care by educating therapists and promoting patient advocacy at the grassroots level. I believe the work of Integrative Mental Health Care of Oregon provides a compelling model for professional education and community advocacy that will contribute in important ways to mental health care reform at the community level. I hope the work of my colleagues in Salem will inspire others to organize with similar goals across this vast country, where there is urgent need for fundamental reforms in mental health care.

The ideas, opinions, information, and values contained in this book come from years of privileged encounters with people who have sought out my counsel, advice, and empathy in the hope of finding relief from painful experiences of physical, mental, emotional, and spiritual suffering. In some cases insight achieved during therapy has resulted in letting go of suffering. In other cases, clients have benefited because of my familiarity with a particular fact about a conventional drug or an alternative form of treatment. Such "clinical improvements" sometimes stem from technical skill in the context of a consulting relationship in which information is exchanged. However, for the most part, I believe that when a client consistently feels better or functions at a "higher" level, such changes come from insights achieved during their own unique psychological and spiritual journey. At best, the therapist can facilitate this journey with a few well-chosen words or reasonable advice about a medicine or herbal to ingest, a lifestyle change to implement, or a mind–body technique to practice. When a client in my care improves—that is, experiences relief from suffering—I experience gratitude for their good fortune and I then try to understand how this "improvement" was achieved. Sometimes a useful strategy becomes clear in retrospect, but the causes and conditions that manifest as relief of human suffering very often remain a mystery. A clear cause or discernible pattern remains hidden from view because the suffering of every human being is uniquely determined, privately experienced, and not subject to generalization. The same holds true when a client does not "improve" with ongoing treatment in spite of my knowledge, my skill, and my empathy. What remains to me—to the therapist—is a determination to remain compassionate, a profound sense of my ignorance about medicine and the human mind–body–spirit, and humility in the face of suffering, the causes of which can seldom be clearly understood or completely alleviated through careful analysis or the varied therapeutics of the world's great healing traditions. There is no "cure" for human suffering, only more or less skillful means of guiding another person to finding relief from suffering through a new way of experiencing the self or one's relationships, or a different, perhaps more resilient way of being in the world. I am indebted to my patients for their daily teachings in humility, which motivate me to improve my skill as a physician, convince me that I must remain open to learning facts and techniques from many traditions of healing, and help me in my efforts to stay present with an open heart, even when all I have to offer is listening and bearing witness to suffering that I cannot take away.

While the author's ideas determine the broad scope and content of a book, the final form and quality depend on skillful editing. My editors at W. W. Norton, Andrea Costella and Kristen Holt-Browning, have meticulously guided this project from its inception while inviting suggestions for new directions in the writing and accommodating unpredictable changes in my schedule. They have tactfully coached this graying psychiatrist to ensure that central concepts are clearly and concisely expressed, and for this I am grateful.

Finally, there is always an abiding sense of gratitude to my life partner, colleague, and best friend, Nicole Asselborn, MD. Your gentleness and wisdom constantly bring me back to what is most true and important in this life.

Introduction

～

Progress in medicine depends on evolutions in medical theory and research methodology that permit new ways of thinking about illness. Ongoing advances in research will lead to more effective and cost-effective treatments of mental illness. My hope is that the increasing use of integrative approaches in mental health care will reduce costs while improving outcomes. Of course, psychotherapy is fundamentally important for maintaining good mental health as well as for treating a wide variety of mental health problems. The clinical treatment approaches discussed in this book are not intended to replace the need for psychotherapy; rather, they should be implemented in the course of appropriate, supportive, ongoing psychotherapy with clients.

As a founding member and current chair of the American Psychiatric Association Caucus on Complementary and Alternative Medicine, I have long been involved in efforts to facilitate open-minded discussion and debate on the range of nonpharmacological modalities used in mental health care. The principle objective of the caucus is to facilitate open-minded dialogue on complementary and alternative medicine (CAM) and integrative modalities in mental health care and to help psychiatrists and other mental health professionals find reliable information about the safety and efficacy of these nonconventional treatments. The American Psychiatric Association (APA) is the largest professional organization of psychiatrists in the world and, as such, strongly influences the shape of mental health policy not only in this country but in much of the Western world. My hope is that the work that is now taking place within our small caucus and in courses, workshops, and symposia on CAM taught at annual APA conferences will eventually extend to the community of mental health professionals at large and shape future mental health policy here and worldwide.

As a member of the clinical teaching faculty at Stanford Medical School and the Program in Integrative Medicine at the University of Arizona's College of Medicine, and as a frequent presenter at conferences, I am often reminded of how difficult it is to define "complementary and alternative medicine" in a way that reflects shared understandings and captures widely held perspectives about the causes or meanings of mental illness and the essential aspects of different treatment modalities. Perhaps the major reason the professional dialogue on nonconventional therapies has made so little progress after decades of research is that there is still no agreed-on lexicon or broad conceptual framework with which mental health professionals discuss and interpret the diverse understandings and meanings embedded in the world's healing traditions. An important practical consequence of the absence of a universal paradigm of medicine is disagreement on how to define *complementary, alternative*, and *integrative* "best practices" in general and in mental health care specifically.

In the absence of consensus about best practices we are left with the urgent need to summarize what is known about the various nonconventional therapies so that we, as therapists, can understand how to use them skillfully and can then guide our clients to the most available evidence on modalities from the world's diverse healing traditions. Complementary and alternative therapies are already used widely to treat or self-treat mental health problems. Our clients are increasingly using herbal medicines, essential fatty acids, vitamins, and homeopathic remedies. They are receiving treatments from acupuncturists, Ayurvedic physicians, massage therapists, and Reiki masters while often taking prescription medications for depressed mood, anxiety, psychosis, and other mental health problems. The widespread use of nonconventional modalities together with conventional pharmacological treatments means that mental health care in Western countries is de facto integrative, albeit in the absence of communication and coordinated care between alternative medical practitioners, psychologists, and psychiatrists. In my view this fact is reason enough for all mental health care providers to place a priority on understanding the essential concepts and clinical therapeutics underlying the complementary and alternative therapies used to treat or self-treat mental health problems. This book provides a review of the scientific evidence base, safety issues, and specific nonconventional assessment and treatment approaches used in mental health care today.

Is this book for me and how will I benefit from reading it? This book is intended for psychologists, marriage and family therapists (MFTs), clinical social workers, and other nonmedically trained mental health professionals.

Will I be qualified to provide CAM treatments after reading this book? This book will give you the information you need to (1) competently and safely manage your clients' mental health problems using many nonpharmacological therapies, and (2) know when it is appropriate or necessary to refer them to another health care provider for expert consultation. Indeed, *all* mental health professionals should have a solid grasp of both conventional and nonconventional approaches used in the United States to evaluate and treat mental illness in order to be accurately informed about the evidence for available treatment options, know how to best advise clients about treatment options, and know when it is appropriate to refer to mainstream or alternative practitioners. As a therapist approaching your clients from an integrative perspective, your primary focus will continue to be on providing skillful psychotherapy while also advising clients about lifestyle changes involving exercise and nutrition, stress management approaches, mind–body practices, and the appropriate and safe use of certain supplements that may be beneficial for their specific mental health problem and improve their general sense of well-being.

Some psychologists reading this book may reside in states that permit them to prescribe certain psychotropic medications. If you have prescribing privileges, you may (of course) advise clients about the appropriate uses of specific medications, prescribe medications, and give advice about dosing and safety issues. I assume, however, that the majority of psychologists reading this book have no medical training, do not currently prescribe medications, do not intend to undertake the training required to do so, and don't have extensive knowledge of the mechanisms of action and safety problems associated with prescription medications. For therapists who are not medically trained and do not prescribe medications, an important aspect of your work is to know when it is reasonable or medically necessary to refer clients to an emergency room for a problem that warrants urgent care, or to a psychiatrist, family physician, or a nonconventionally trained medical practitioner for a problem that can be adequately addressed through nonurgent medical evaluation and routine treatment. Judgments about when to treat and when to refer should take into account your legal–ethical scope of practice as a therapist, your knowledge of CAM modalities from specialized training you may have received, and the severity of your client's symptoms. Chapters 2 and 3 include discussions of general principles that will help you decide when to manage a client on your own and when to refer to a conventionally trained physician or CAM specialist for evaluation or treatment. The case vignettes in Part II provide in-depth discussions of all phases of history taking, assessment, and formulation and treatment planning.

For which clients is it appropriate to recommend CAM therapies? From this book you will learn how to think integratively when approaching patients with these common mental health problems:

- Moderate and severe depressed mood
- Cyclic mood swings and mania
- Generalized anxiety and panic attacks
- Hyperactivity and distractibility
- Psychotic symptoms and schizophrenia
- Mild cognitive impairment and dementia
- Alcohol and substance abuse
- Insomnia and daytime sleepiness

When should I refer my patients to a CAM specialist? My belief is that it is always in the client's and therapist's best interest to practice medicine in a conservative fashion, avoiding unnecessary risks. This conservative approach applies to considerations of safety and efficacy that must be addressed when both conventional and alternative therapies are being considered. Some patients have tried conventional antidepressants without significant improvement in mood, or they have discontinued antidepressants or antianxiety medications because of adverse effects before they could potentially benefit from them. In such cases it is appropriate to refer patients to a CAM specialist if there is evidence that a particular CAM modality is both safe and beneficial for their specific mental health problem. The scientific evidence supporting the use of various nonconventional modalities is reviewed in Chapter 3. The vignettes in Part II provide examples of circumstances in which it is reasonable to refer clients to CAM specialists for common mental health problems, and they include discussions of the evidence supporting specific CAM treatment recommendations or referrals.

Should I recommend combining CAM treatments with conventional ones? What should I do if my client has a severe mental health problem? When advising a client to use a CAM treatment in combination with a particular conventional treatment, it is important to take into account what is known about the potential benefits and risks of the specific integrative strategy that is being considered before giving specific advice. In keeping with the medical dictum *"primum non nocere"* (first do no harm), I feel strongly that it is always prudent to avoid treatment combinations when there is a known risk of toxicity or potentially serious negative outcomes. Along these lines, the best integrative strategies are those for which clear benefits have been described and no, or negligible, potentially serious risks exist. As a therapist your work with clients centers around psychotherapy, and (unless you are certified to do so) it is not appropriate for you to give specific advice on the use of psychotropic medications or adjunctive strategies involving prescription medications and CAM modalities. However, after reading this book, you will have a basic understanding of when it is appropriate, reasonable, and safe to recommend certain vitamins, essential fatty acids, or trace elements in combination with prescription medications, and you will know how to refer clients to conventionally trained physicians or CAM specialists for consultation and treatment. *Any client who may have a serious medical illness, or who is suicidal, homicidal, or grossly psychotic, should be referred to the nearest emergency room or urgent care facility for sta-*

bilization or psychiatric hospitalization before you schedule regular sessions and offer him or her an integrative care plan.

Is there a specific CAM training course or professional development program that I should take? The annual meeting of the American Psychiatric Association and other large annual conferences now offer continuing education units (CEUs) to psychologists for a wide range of workshops on all aspects of CAM and integrative mental health care. I am not aware of an established training course or certification program in CAM or integrative medicine for psychotherapists. I hope that such a program will emerge out of conversations around this and other books that are now being published on this subject. Until more formal training resources become available, it might be helpful to form study groups on integrative medicine with therapists in your community who share your interest.

My hope is that this book will help you understand the fundamentals of integrative medicine while providing an overview of nonconventional and integrative strategies that can help alleviate human suffering caused by mental illness. May your skill as an integrative therapist grow as you learn from your clients, and may you enjoy a rich network of collaborative relationships with MDs, naturopathic physicians, and other practitioners in your community. Readers interested in a comprehensive medical presentation of the theory and methods of integrative medicine, as well as detailed critical reviews of specific modalities, are referred to my book, *Textbook of Integrative Mental Health Care* (2006, published by Thieme Medical Publishers).

INTEGRATIVE
Mental Health Care

A THERAPIST'S
HANDBOOK

PART I

~

Foundations

People usually fail when they are on the verge of success.
So give as much care to the end as to the beginning;
Then there will be no failure

—*Tao Te Ching*, Lao Tsu, chapter 64

CHAPTER 1

~

The Context of Integrative
Mental Health Care

Iɴ thinking about integrative mental health care, my starting assumption is that every human being is shaped by unique social, cultural, psychological, biological, and spiritual factors that determine his or her physical, psychological, and spiritual health. If this assumption is valid, it naturally follows that standardized biomedical approaches to assessment and treatment cannot potentially address the person-specific, multifactoral, and subtle causes or meanings of symptoms in all individuals. Rather, many assessment methods can be useful in accurately characterizing the various psychological, biological, energetic, and possibly spiritual layers of causation or meaning that contribute to illness, including mental illness, in any single client. Using a variety of assessment tools can result in a more complete and deeper understanding of the nature of a client's illness, the most appropriate and effective treatment plan, and better outcomes. The best treatment plan (1) combines the most effective conventional and nonconventional treatments for a particular symptom (or symptom pattern), (2) is available where clients live, (3) is realistic for their budget, and (4) is congruent with their personal and cultural values.

Ongoing advances in Western medicine and other major world systems of medicine will continue to bring improved understandings of mental illness at the psychological and biological levels, while clarifying the roles of postulated subtle energetic or spiritual factors that directly or indirectly affect human consciousness. Future understanding of normal brain functioning and mental illness will probably incorporate ideas from complexity theory, quantum mechanics, quantum field theory, and other emerging paradigms in science. The result will be a truly *synthetic* approach to understanding and treating human suffering that takes into account the theories of conventional Western medicine, Chinese medicine, homeopathy, and other highly evolved nonbiomedical systems of medicine in the context of cutting-edge science.

DEFINING ALTERNATIVE, COMPLEMENTARY, AND INTEGRATIVE MEDICINE

According to the conventional biomedical model, causes of symptoms that can potentially change the relative activities or brain levels of neurotransmitters include social, familial, or cultural dynamics that result in acute or chronic stress. Thus these dynamics indirectly influence brain functioning by changing levels of stress hormones that affect the synthesis or relative activity levels of neurotransmitters. While this conventional model of causality, which is the core of biomedical psychiatry, probably affords a valid explanation of certain kinds of mental health problems, it cannot adequately explain all mental illness phenomena. Integrative mental health care takes into account classic neurophysiological and psychodynamic understandings of mental illness while being open to other *kinds* of explanations, including emerging concepts in functional medicine and functional brain mapping as well as informational, energetic, and possibly spiritual causes or meanings of mental and emotional distress. According to this eclectic perspective the dynamic causes of mental and emotional symptoms exist at many functional levels in the body, mind, and brain and can be described in terms of relationships between the following domains:

- The central nervous system and the immune system (psychoneuroimmunology)
- The magnetic fields generated by the brain (or relationships between the biomagnetic activity of the brain and the heart)
- Possibly "subtle" energy or information that, according to quantum brain dynamics theory, may be a manifestation of *information* associated with vast arrays of exquisitely coordinated subunits of axons or neuronal cell membranes that correspond to different states or kinds of conscious experience.

Integrative medicine posits that, although symptoms can sometimes be adequately described and evaluated in terms of clearly identifiable "causes," in many cases conventional models of causation do not appear to be operating. In such cases more complete and more clinically useful understandings of symptoms can probably be achieved through an exploration of their underlying *meanings*. In this context meanings can include conventional psychodynamic interpretations as well as familial, social, cultural, or spiritual connotations of distress.

Conventional Western medical treatments of mental illness use synthetic drugs and psychotherapy to achieve the primary goal: diminishing the severity of *particular symptoms*. In contrast, complementary and alternative modalities are generally directed at alleviating suffering or improving functioning of the *whole person*. Nonconventional treatment approaches can be classified as alternative, complementary, or integrative. *Alternative modalities*, such as homeopathy, acupuncture and energy healing, fall outside the conceptual framework of Western medicine—they are generally not endorsed by Western medicine and, in many cases, their underlying principles cannot be demonstrated using Western-style research studies. In contrast, *complementary therapies* are based on theories that are consistent with established Western medical theory, are often supported by considerable evidence, but are nevertheless rejected by many Western-trained physicians for *nonscientific* reasons, including ideological conflicts, high cost, competition with nonphysician health care providers, or problems obtaining insurance coverage. Herbal medicine and electroencephalogram (EEG) biofeedback are examples of complementary therapies. The *integra-*

tive strategies used in mental health care combine conventional drugs or psychotherapy with herbs, vitamins, dietary changes, mind–body therapies, energy healing or other nonconventional approaches in order to more adequately address the complex causes of symptoms than can be achieved using a single conventional, alternative, or complementary modality. Table 1.1 lists representative examples of conventional, alternative, complementary, and integrative approaches used in mental health care.

TABLE 1. Examples of Conventional, Alternative, Complementary, and Integrative Treatment Approaches in Mental Health Care

---

Conventional treatments

- Psychotherapy
- Support groups
- Psychotropic medications
- Electroconvulsive therapy

Alternative therapies

- Acupuncture
- Qigong
- Homeopathy
- Reiki and other energy-based healing approaches

Complementary therapies

- Herbal medicine
- EEG biofeedback
- Omega-3 essential fatty acids
- High-density negative ions

Integrative treatment strategies

- Antidepressants combined with high-potency B-complex for depressed mood
- Antianxiety medications combined with yoga for generalized anxiety
- Bright light exposure, exercise, and lithium for bipolar disorder
- Spiritually oriented support group, dim blue morning light, and kudzu for chronic alcohol abuse

---

When approaching any mental health problem, the most appropriate integrative strategy is that combination of particular conventional and nonconventional treatments that most effectively addresses the root biological or energetic causes or the psychological, social, cultural, and spiritual meanings of the symptoms. Optimal healing is achieved when a therapist skillfully guides his or her client to the most appropriate mainstream and nonconventional medical resources in the context of a psychotherapy grounded in an authentic and compassionate relationship.

BRAIN, MIND, AND MENTAL ILLNESS IN DIFFERENT HEALING TRADITIONS

Disparate healing traditions rest on different assumptions about the causes and meanings of illness. According to conventional Western medicine, physical or mental illness can be completely described in terms of biological causes and current scientific theories. Other traditions, including Chinese medicine, homeopathy, and various schools of "energy" healing, do not share this assumption. In these nonconventional healing traditions, explanations of illness rest on assumptions about fundamental energetic principles that cannot be described in the language of contemporary Western science. Western psychiatry contends that the *mind* is a term used to describe the functions of neurotransmitters in the brain. In contrast, non-Western healing traditions regard consciousness as a primary kind of energy that requires no further explanation in terms of modern brain science. That is, normal as well as abnormal manifestations of consciousness as health and illness cannot be reduced to theories and phenomena accepted by Western science. Integrative medicine takes a more inclusive philosophical position compared to both Western medicine and nonconventional healing traditions. Integrative medicine is based on the premise that human beings are comprised of complex systems of biological, psychological, energetic, and possibly spiritual processes that influence health and illness (Bell, 2002). From this integrative point of view, "meanings" of symptoms can include various psychodynamic or psychoanalytic interpretations in addition to symbolic cultural or spiritual understandings.

Conventional Western medical assessment approaches are based on assumptions about the *kinds* of phenomena that can *potentially cause* symptoms. The dominant paradigm of Western psychiatry—biological psychiatry—posits that the causes of specific symptoms or disorders are dysregulations of specific neurotransmitters or their receptors. However, there is a serious disconnect between this paradigm and the methodology used to characterize and diagnose symptom patterns as discrete "disorders." Conventional psychiatric diagnosis rests largely on standardized interviews and symptom rating scales used to obtain information about the type and severity of symptoms. Although many are available, formal biological assessment tools are seldom used in day-to-day clinical practice. This is probably related to the fact that mental and emotional symptoms are highly subjective and individualized experiences with underlying causes or meanings which can seldom be verified using rigorous empirical analysis or statistical methods. This state of affairs means that (even if they *were used* in clinical settings) contemporary biomedical research methods would often fail to verify that symptoms are "caused" by presumed neurotransmitter "imbalances," and, by extension, that improvements in symptoms are the "effects of" a particular pharmacological or psychotherapeutic intervention. Of course, the same basic conceptual dilemma limits what non-Western systems of medicine can legitimately claim about the nature or causes of mental illness or how their treatments *work*. A consequence of the conceptual gap between medical theory and verified causes of illness is that treatments employed in all healing traditions—whether by Western physicians, Chinese medical practitioners, Ayurvedic physicians, homeopaths, herbalists, or other professionally trained medical practitioners—often continue to be used in the absence of compelling evidence because of entrenched cultural beliefs about their efficacy.

The theory that mental illness is caused by imbalances of neurotransmitters limits the way in which psychiatrists think about and treat mental illness. This position has indirectly restricted the amount of research done on nonconventional healing modalities. Where a multibillion-dollar pharmaceutical industry funds studies on conventional drugs, there is little financial incentive to invest research dollars in natural products that cannot be patented and therefore are not potential sources of future revenues. Since the mid-1990s the National Center for Complementary and Alternative Medicine (NCCAM) of the National Institutes of Health has funded studies on nonconventional treatments, including herbs, acupuncture, yoga, and others. Unfortunately, the research budget of NCCAM is miniscule compared to that of the pharmaceutical industry, and relatively few large quality studies have been conducted on promising nonconventional treatments. A result of this situation is that studies on nonpharmacological treatments of mental illness seldom result in findings that are regarded as conclusive or methodologically sound, and they are therefore frequently dismissed by the Western medical community before they are seriously and objectively reviewed. In addition, there is a strong negative bias in mainstream medical journals against the publication of articles on nonconventional treatments in general (Bender, 2004). Negative bias against nonpharmaceutical modalities in the medical journal literature and academic medicine is taking place in the context of tremendous pressure from the pharmaceutical industry to suppress negative findings and keep drugs of questionable safety and efficacy on the market (Moncrief et al., 2003; Sussman, 2004). Recent disclosures from the Food and Drug Administration (FDA), under the Freedom of Information Act, confirm that many failed drug trials are never published, resulting in erroneous information about the efficacy and safety of many new conventional pharmaceuticals (Bhandari, et al., 2004; Kirsch, 2008). This questionable practice has led to serious widespread concern about the objectivity of industry-sponsored pharmaceutical research, congressional hearings on drug safety, and increased FDA oversight of new drug development efforts.

Limited research progress has therefore been made in identifying the mechanisms of action of herbals, other natural products, mind–body interventions, and spiritual healing practices that are in widespread use (Eskinazi, 1998). The paucity of research into the basic mechanisms of non-conventional modalities will translate into slow progress in the development of treatments that address the biological, mind–body, and postulated *energetic* causes of mental illness in the context of functional medicine, complexity theory, psychoneuroimmunology, and other novel explanatory models of illness (Linde, 2000). In this book I review the evidence for some of the more substantiated nonconventional treatments, and I comment on promising approaches that are being used to treat common mental health problems in the absence of strong research evidence.

THE LIMITATIONS OF CONVENTIONAL MEDICINE AND THE TREND TOWARD CAM

There is a long historical tradition in the United States and other Western countries of using nonconventional treatment modalities in the context of the established dominant paradigm of allopathic medicine. The rapid growth of CAM is being driven by consumer demand for a wide range of treatment choices, growing dissatisfaction with conventional medical care, and increasing openness to new ideas in the institutions of Western medicine (Astin, 1998; Eisenberg et al., 1998). Factors that interfere with the provision of adequate health care by Western medicine include restrictions on the kind and quality of treatments available under managed care, private insurance contracts, and Medicare; concerns over the efficacy and safety of conventional pharmacological treatments; and the increasing cost of medical care in general. It is significant to note that individuals who use nonconventional treatments for any health problem are generally more educated than those who use only conventional treatments (Astin, 1998). Approximately two-thirds of all adults in the United States use various kinds of complementary and alternative approaches for medical or mental health problems (Barnes, 2004). Many individuals who see Western physicians also see Chinese medical practitioners, herbalists, homeopathic physicians, or energy healers for the same problem, and many also self-treat with herbals, supplements, or homeopathic remedies without the advice of a naturopathic physician, conventionally trained M.D., or a mental health professional (Barnes, 2004).

At the same time that patients are demanding more choices in health care, mainstream medicine is becoming more open to change. Courses on complementary and alternative medicine are now offered at most U.S. medical schools, and increasing numbers of physicians are becoming certified to practice Chinese medicine, herbal medicine, homeopathy, or other established world healing traditions. Approximately one-half of U.S. physicians refer patients to acupuncturists, naturopaths, homeopaths, chiropractors, or other nonconventionally trained practitioners because they believe that these approaches are safe and effective. Together these trends are stimulating an evolution in U.S. medical care toward an eclectic network of perspectives, skills, and services that address the patient's body, mind, and spirit.

Western medicine is based on a particular conceptual framework or paradigm that has led to major breakthroughs in the understanding and treatment of mental illness. However, like all systems of medicine, Western biomedicine is limited in scope because it accepts only certain kinds of evidence about the causes of illness (Hahn, 1995). By extension, it is unlikely that conventional biomedical psychiatry will be able to adequately explain the myriad causes of mental illness (Hahn, 1995). Future research studies will probably confirm some theories of mental illness resulting in novel assessment and treatment approaches, while refuting others (Margolin, 1998; Verhoef, 2000). Using a variety of assessment approaches to explore the biological or energetic nature of illness will help clinicians understand symptoms in new ways and ultimately lead to *more complete* theories of the psychological, social, cultural, biological, and energetic causes of mental illness. An example is the combined use of electroencephalographic (EEG) and electrocardiographic (EKG) monitoring to help explain relationships between the brain and the heart in normal states of consciousness as well as mental illness. In addition to such high-tech assessment approaches, methods borrowed from Chinese medicine and other ancient healing traditions will lead to new understandings about energetic "imbalances" that may cause cognitive or emotional symptoms or interfere with treatment response.

RESEARCH IN COMPLEMENTARY AND ALTERNATIVE MEDICINE: IMPLICATIONS AND EVIDENCE

Widely used treatments in conventional mental health care include certain types of psychotherapy, hypnosis, numerous prescription medications, and other approaches that have not been substantiated by strong evidence from placebo-controlled double-blind research studies and thus do not meet the rigorous "gold standard" requirements for medical evidence established by Western medicine (Geddes et al., 1996). In spite of the absence of compelling evidence, many conventional modalities are widely used because they are endorsed by expert consensus. Evidence-based medicine (EBM) has been defined as "the conscientious, explicit and judicious use of current best evidence in making decisions about the care of individual patients" (Sackett et al., 1996). Clinical care standards of EBM are largely based on the findings of systematic reviews of several well-designed placebo-controlled randomized studies that are believed to provide the best evidence for claims of efficacy. The widespread endorsement of EBM in Western countries is setting higher standards for uniformity and rigor in medical research with the goal of reconciling best medical practices with the most rigorous kind of evidence. EBM is already playing an important role in shaping revised practice guidelines in various medical specialties that are more in line with the best available medical evidence.

EBM has been criticized because it assigns lower priority to evidence from research studies that do not conform to its standards (i.e., double-blind, randomized, placebo-controlled trials) and are therefore not subject to consideration in systematic reviews. Along these lines, many CAM modalities are difficult to evaluate using Western-style research studies. Nevertheless, it has been estimated that over 100 complementary and alternative modalities are now widely used in Western countries, side by side with more established conventional medical practices (Ernst, 1997). Future studies will probably confirm the efficacy claims of certain conventional and CAM modalities, while disproving others, resulting in the gradual transformation of orthodox Western medicine into an eclectic paradigm that incorporates modalities from a variety of healing traditions that are validated by strong evidence (Verhoef, 2000). Western medicine is continuously reevaluating its basic assumptions as new theories emerge, such as complexity theory, psychoneuroimmunology, and quantum field theory that challenge its basic tenets (Turner, 1998). As the conceptual framework and clinical therapeutics of Western medicine change and expand, novel research methods will be developed, permitting rigorous investigation of CAM modalities that are not amenable to randomized controlled protocols. Likewise, conventional psychiatry will necessarily change, too, as it incorporates new ways of conceptualizing, diagnosing, and treating the causes of mental illness.

THE INCREASING USE OF CAM IN MENTAL HEALTH CARE

Approximately 72 million Americans—fully one-third of the adult population—use at least one complementary or alternative therapy annually (Tindle et al., 2005). Likewise, more and more people are using nonconventional and integrative therapies to treat or self-treat mental health problems (Eisenberg et al., 1998). It has been estimated that as many as 10% of U.S. adults take conventional drugs for depression, anxiety, schizophrenia, or other mental health problems. At the same time, approximately 10% of U.S. adults who visited an alternative medical practitioner in the previous year had a psychiatric diagnosis, and half of those had sought care specifically for a mental health problem (Druss & Rosenheck, 2000). A survey of naturopathic physicians, acupuncturists, chiropractors, and massage therapists found that 11% of visits focused on mental health problems (Simon et al., 2004). It is significant that the majority of individuals who see alternative medical practitioners for a mental health problem are self-referred and do not disclose their use of nonconventional therapies to their family physician, psychiatrist, or therapist. A large survey of U.S. adults found that over 50% of individuals diagnosed with an anxiety disorder and 60% of individuals diagnosed with a mood disorder use a nonconventional modality, but few disclose this information to their family physician or psychiatrist (Kessler et al. 2001). The majority of individuals who use nonconventional therapies see a conventionally trained physician for the same health problem. Among individuals hospitalized for a severe mental health problem, almost two-thirds had used a nonconventional modality within the past year, and fully 80% had not disclosed this information to their psychiatrist (Elkins et al., 2005). Severe depressed mood is the strongest predictor of CAM use in psychiatrically hospitalized individuals (Unutzer et al., 2000). The majority of people who use both conventional and nonconventional treatments for anxiety and severe depression believe that they are equally effective, in the absence of convincing scientific evidence, in many cases

(Barnes, 2004). The increasing rate of self-treatment in combination with nondisclosure raises significant safety issues because the use of vitamins, herbs, or other natural substances in combination with prescription medications may result in serious toxic interactions.

Recent systematic reviews of controlled trials on antidepressants noted that adverse effects may exceed their beneficial effects (Kirsch, 2008; Montcrief, 2004). Although millions benefit from new treatments of mental illness, there are also serious safety issues, including weight gain and the risk of diabetes when taking many of the newer antipsychotics, and concerns about an increased risk of suicide among children and adolescents taking antidepressants (Gibbons, 2005). These concerns are complicated by the high costs of many new drugs that make them unaffordable to large segments of the population (Moran, 2004). Constraints of outpatient mental health care under health maintenance organizations, managed care, and Medicare translate into brief impersonal encounters with psychiatrists, psychiatric nurses, and other mental health professionals. In parallel with these trends accumulating research evidence is supporting claims that many nonconventional approaches used to treat mental health care are safe, effective, and affordable.

THE FUTURE OF THE DSM: NEW CONCEPTS IN THE DIAGNOSIS AND CLASSIFICATION OF PSYCHIATRIC DISORDERS

There is a great deal of controversy over the validity of the concept of "disorder" in mainstream psychiatry, and this disagreement will almost certainly result in basic changes in methods and criteria used to diagnose and classify mental illness in future editions of the *Diagnostic and Statistical Manual of Mental Disorders* (DSM). The fourth edition, text revised (DSM-IV-TR), is currently under review and a fifth edition is scheduled for publication in 2012. An important argument against current methods used to classify and diagnose psychiatric disorders is that relatively few "discrete," unchanging symptom patterns (i.e., "disorders) have been found that actually fulfill DSM requirements for symptom type, severity, and duration. In fact, findings of numerous large epidemiological studies show that symptoms of mental and emotional distress are experienced in ways that are highly variable in populations diagnosed with the same DSM-IV "disorder." Furthermore, the pattern of symptoms experienced by an individual diagnosed with a particular disorder often changes over time in ways that are difficult to describe, explain, or predict using the DSM.

It has been suggested that a more valid way to conceptualize mental illness would be based on the idea of a *continuum* of disparate symptoms or symptom *patterns* that change over time in relation to other symptoms (or symptom patterns). The DSM-V will hopefully bring significant advances to the diagnosis and classification of mental illness. Unfortunately, however, this explanatory model of mental illness will continue to reflect entrenched Western philosophical assumptions about the causes of symptoms and will likely exclude discussion of other (i.e., non-Western) valid explanatory models.

SAFELY ISSUES IN CAM AND INTEGRATIVE MEDICINE

Because relatively few studies have examined specific combinations of conventional and nonconventional treatments, safety problems in integrative mental health care are not well understood at present. In some cases synergistic benefits achieved by combining two or more treatments can be inferred on the basis of what is known about their respective mechanisms of action. For example, folate can be safely combined with selective serotonin reuptake inhibitors (SSRIs) or S-adenosyimethionine (SAMe; a widely used nonconventional treatment of depression) and is known to boost the antidepressant effect of both treatments. The good news is that few serious safety problems have been documented to occur with herbs and other natural products that are widely used to treat mental and emotional symptoms. However, when considering an integrative strategy for your client's mental health problem, a good rule of thumb is to assume that adverse effects caused by interactions can take place when two or more biologically active substances are used, including medicinal herbs, amino acids, hormones, essential fatty acids, vitamins, and of course conventional medications. A review of research on herbal safety concluded that all patients should be warned about potential risks when taking any biologically active natural product together with a medication (Izzo, 2001). In addition, it is always essential to advise your clients to *avoid* using particular combinations of drugs and herbs or other natural products that are known to result in serious safety problems. Examples of such combinations include St. John's wort (*Hypericum perforatum*) and immunosuppressive agents, and *Ginkgo biloba* and blood-thinning medications such as warfarin.

Understanding the causes of adverse effects or toxicities associated with a particular treatment or combination of modalities requires extensive medical training. While I'm aware that courses on psychopharmacology are now available to psychologists, as preciously noted I am assuming that most readers have little or no formal training in medicine or psychopharmacology. Giving medical advice about about the benefits and risks of specific pharmacological treatments should be the responsibility of physicians and psychologists who are certified in their respective states to prescribe medications. By the same token, detailed advice about the relative advantages and risks of specific complementary and alternative modalities should be the domain of nonconventionally trained medical practitioners who specialize in a particular system of medicine (e.g.) naturopaths, Chinese medical practitioners, homeopaths). Clients will likely ask you about the potential benefits and safety issues associated with a range of conventional and CAM therapies. When a client asks a question about possible safety issues associated with a specific herb or medication, your responsibility is not to give specific medical advice (i.e., unless you are qualified to do so after taking an advanced course on a specific CAM modality) but to provide a general framework for thinking about safety and refer him or her to an appropriate health care provider, whether physician, psychiatrist, naturopathic physician, or appropriate CAM specialist. If your client does not have an existing relationship with a health care provider, or has already approached their family physician, naturopathic physician, herbalist or other healthcare provider but has not been able to find satisfactory answers to questions about safety, it is appropriate to provide specific information from reliable references or web sites and to guide him or her in making prudent decisions. Fortunately, there are excellent resources available on the safety of natural products. You may want to purchase a copy of the *CRC Press*

Botanical Safety Handbook (McGruffin et al., 1997) or *Mosby's Handbook of Drug–Herb and Drug–Supplement Interactions* (Harkness & Bratman, 2003) for your office. I also encourage you to make use of excellent web-based resources for the most up-to-date information about safety issues associated with herbals and other natural products, in addition to herb–drug interactions (see Appendix B).

In addition to the biological therapies, potential safety issues must be considered when discussing somatic, mind–body, and energy therapies with your clients. For example, although massage and chiropractic are generally done in a way that avoids injury, cases of serious injury have been reported with these somatic therapies. Obviously, it is important to refer clients to chiropractors, massage therapists, and other body therapists who are respected in your community and are not facing malpractice suits. Yoga and tai chi chuan are highly evolved mind–body practices that are among the safest therapeutic approaches for anxious individuals, although rare case of psychosis have been reported following the *unskilled* practice of Qigong by people with schizophrenia or borderline personality disorder. Clients who have chronic pain or other serious medical conditions should talk with their physician before engaging in any mind–body practice or receiving chiropractic or other body-centered therapies. Scientifically validated energy therapies, including bright light exposure, sound therapy, and microcurrent electrical stimulation, can be used safely in conjunction with conventional pharmacological therapies. Common adverse effects associated with herbals and other natural substances, as well as somatic, mind–body approaches, and energy therapies used to treat mental health problems, are discussed in the vignettes in Part II.

LEGAL AND ETHICAL ISSUES IN USING CAM IN MENTAL HEALTH CARE

The use of nonconventional approaches in mental health care has stimulated discussion on scope-of-practice issues, the importance of obtaining informed consent, and the ethical and legal issues that come into play when referring clients to alternative medical practitioners. These issues are of concern to both psychiatrists and psychologists. When thinking through complicated ethical and legal issues, most clinicians do not have the benefit of competent legal advice, partly because there is no consensus among psychiatrists and psychologists regarding ethical and legal guidelines or constraints pertaining to scope of practice or making referrals to nonconventional modalities. In this section I briefly summarize what I believe are reasonable starting points for thinking about ethical and legal issues that often arise when working with clients interested in exploring nonconventional treatments and in considering when and where to refer clients for consultation.

Malpractice is defined as failure to use the agreed-on standard of care when treating a patient, resulting in harm to the patient. Practitioners trained in different conventional and nonconventional traditions are ethically and legally obliged to follow disparate standards of care dictated by their respective professional associations. As a therapist, the standard-of-care norms that you are expected to follow are defined by the state professional board that licenses you to practice. These norms are in flux at this time because of the trend toward granting prescribing privileges for psychologists in several states. If you live in a state where psychologists may legally prescribe medications and you are certified to do so, then you may of course choose to provide this service to your clients. However, I strongly encourage you to first contact your malpractice insurance carrier to confirm that your understanding of your right to prescribe is correct under state law, and also that you are adequately covered in the event of a negative outcome.

When a court renders a judgment that failure to follow the state-mandated standard of care has resulted in harm to a client and that malpractice has been committed, the relevant professional board may impose penalties on the therapist or physician, including suspending or revoking the therapist's license to practice psychotherapy. General guidelines have been put forward for U.S. physicians who practice (or recommend) certain nonconventional therapies; however, there are significant differences with regard to "scope of practice" between states. In the context of medical care, "fraud" is considered to take place when a physician, therapist, or other health care provider deliberately conveys false or misleading information to a patient, potentially resulting in harm. The ethical and legal responsibilities of therapists to their clients are determined by the therapeutic interventions offered and the specific goals of treatment. When a client enters into treatment, an implicit contract exists between the therapist and client in which the therapist *agrees* to treat the client and the client willingly *consents* to receive treatment. This relationship may continue over a period of months or years or be limited to a few brief sessions.

A contract between a psychotherapist and a client usually emphasizes conventional psychotherapy, although other modalities may be used in the context of ongoing therapy. For example, therapists are increasingly teaching clients about healthy lifestyle changes that encompass exercise, good nutrition, and stress management. Increasing numbers of psychologists are taking courses on targeted amino acid therapy (TAAT) and other nonconventional modalities and providing specific recommendations to clients in efforts to address neurotransmitter "imbalances" or other causes of dysfunction at a psychosomatic level. Even though you may be knowledgable about, or have training in, one or more CAM modalities, it is advisible to consult with your professional organization or malpractice insurance carrier to determine specific requirements of your state prior to administering any nonconventional treatment. By the same token, when a client has severe symptoms that will probably not respond to psychotherapy, improved nutrition, supplements, or lifestyle changes, you are ethically obliged to offer referrals to appropriate medical care in a timely manner. For example, a client who is suicidal, grossly psychotic, or experiencing narcotic-induced auditory hallucinations (i.e., clients who meet criteria for being placed on a 72-hour hold) should be referred immediately to the nearest emergency room for stabilization and possible psychiatric hospitalization.

From a legal–ethical perspective the goals of a contract between a patient and a client are implied by the kinds of therapeutic modalities employed or recommended during therapy. Regardless of the modalities employed, the therapist must provide competent professional care, and the client is ethically responsible for adhering to treatment recommendations or informing the therapist if he or she disagrees with those recommendations—including choosing to not follow through with a referral and discontinuing treatment. *Liability for malpractice can extend to a referral to an alternative medical practitioner that results in harm to your client.* In practical terms, this liability translates into a need to become familiar with the qualifications and reputations of alternative medical practitioners in your area before making specific referrals.

All mental health care providers should learn about the legal and ethical norms of their profession when treating or referring clients. Laws pertaining to the practice of nonconventional forms of therapies are being debated in state legislatures, but at present there is no clearly established legal regulatory framework to guide practitioners. Michael Cohen's (2003) book is an excellent and comprehensive resource on the complex legal–ethical considerations involved in the practice or recommendation of complementary and alternative medicine.

~

CHAPTER 2

Evaluating a Client from an Integrative Perspective:

The Intake Interview, Assessment, and Formulation

THIS chapter provides a broad overview of the intake interview, assessment, and formulation processes, including specific nonconventional approaches, used in an integrative assessment of mental health problems. Nonconventional assessment approaches include novel biological tests (e.g., emerging functional brain imaging technologies, and approaches from Chinese medicine and other healing traditions based on analysis of energetic imbalances). Understanding the theory and appropriate uses of available conventional and nonconventional assessment approaches will help guide you in knowing when it is appropriate to refer a client to a conventional or alternative medical practitioner for specialized assessment.

THE INTAKE INTERVIEW IN INTEGRATIVE MENTAL HEALTH CARE

The first encounter with any new client begins with a structured clinical interview and rapidly progresses to assessment, formulation, and treatment planning. In the real world of day-to-day clinical practice these steps often take place in parallel. The mini-mental status exam (MMSE) takes little time to administer and often provides useful information about the new client's general mental and emotional state. During the course of the interview with a new client, pertinent social, psychological, and medical histories are elicited, and the client's cultural background and religious or spiritual beliefs are explored with the goal of determining how diverse factors may be causing or exacerbating symptoms or interfering with treatment. At the beginning of the intake interview I often tell new clients about the kinds of services I provide in broad outline. It is also important for them to know that I am interested in more than just their family history, a description of their symptoms, and the names of the medications they are taking. My intention is to invite clients to talk about what matters most to them and not just provide rote answers to standardized questions they may assume I will ask based on their previous work with psychiatrists. The following remarks and questions are offered as a practical framework for structuring the integrative intake interview.

Start with brief comments about your integrative practice, for example: "In my practice I do psychotherapy and teach my clients about [e.g., nutrition, mind–body work, stress management skills]. I have specialized training in [e.g., EEG biofeedback, hypnotherapy, amino acid therapy], and I sometimes refer clients to [e.g., doctors, neurologists, naturopathic physicians, energy healers]."

Begin with Open-Ended Questions

In the first part of the intake interview your chief goal is to invite clients to tell you their stories in their own words. Open-ended questions are often helpful for eliciting broad themes that lead to more specific inquiries later in the interview.

"It is important for me to understand what you are experiencing. Can you tell me about that in your own words?" The goal here is to avoid having clients repeat diagnostic labels they may have received and for you to obtain as clear an understanding as possible of their subjective experiences of symptoms that are causing them distress or impairing their functioning.

"What do you think is causing your problem(s)?" If clients have more than one problem, it is important to find out what they think underlies all of their mental health problems. For example, your client may feel strongly that all of his or her symptoms and distress are being caused by a particular medical disorder, chronic work stress, a cultural or spiritual issue, etc. Depending on the direction the interview takes, follow-up questions can be asked about medical, social, family or spiritual/religious factors.

"**Can you tell me about any medical or mental health problems in your family, including problems like yours?**" You are gathering pertinent family history, including information about relatives with medical disorders, mental illness, and substance abuse problems.

"**What is the most important thing I need to know about you to best understand your problem?**" Here the goal of the inquiry is to find out as much as you can about your client's beliefs and perceptions regarding the nature or cause(s) of his or her problem. The client's answers will probably provide important clues about core symptoms, any ongoing medical problems (or beliefs about medical problems), and closely held social, cultural, or spiritual values.

Move from Generalities to Specifics

Once central themes of your client's life and "story" are clear, the focus of the intake interview can shift from a general conversation to a more focused exchange of questions and answers. At this stage the goal is to follow leads provided in the broad brush strokes of your client's story by asking specific questions to gather the information that will be necessary for completing an integrative formulation. It is important to find out about the specifics of all (conventional and CAM) modalities your client has previously tried for the same problem, including doses (or durations of treatment for acupuncture, chiropractic manipulation, healing touch, or other procedures), whether the treatment worked, problems with adverse effects or toxicities, and concerns about the cost or convenience of receiving the treatment. Following are examples of useful questions for soliciting pertinent clinical information from your client's story.

"**If [specify treatment] worked for the same problem before, why did you decide to stop the treatment?**" Here you are probing for specific factors that may interfere with clients' response to the same treatment if it is resumed to treat the same problem. They may have hoped that they no longer needed the treatment to function, or the treatment may have cost too much for their budget. They may have "forgotten" to continue the treatment (find out what "forgetting" means), or they may have experienced adverse effects about which they are uncomfortable talking (e.g., sexual side effects).

"Tell me about your nutrition." I believe it is fundamentally important to ask new clients about nutrition because of well-described relationships between nutrition and both physical and mental health. The way your clients talk about nutrition will give you a general sense of whether nutritional deficiencies are playing a role in their mental health problem(s).

"Tell me what you do for exercise [or for physical activity]." Your clients' levels of physical activity will probably be related to their general energy level, as well as their general state of physical and psychological well-being. Significantly reduced or absent physical activity is often associated with depressed or anxious mood, as well as syndromes of chronic fatigue and chronic pain.

"Has alcohol or drug use ever been a problem for you?" I ask every new client about alcohol and drug abuse. Finding out about ongoing or previous substance abuse is an important part of gathering history. Failure to ask directly about substance abuse and make appropriate and timely interventions can significantly interfere with the broader treatment goals, delay or diminish treatment response, and put you in the position of enabling a chronic alcoholic or narcotic abuser by avoiding talking about a serious problem. Furthermore, ongoing abuse will almost certainly interfere with the beneficial effects of any form of treatment, be it conventional, alternative, or integrative. Substance abuse is highly prevalent in people with mental health problems and plays a significant role in both physical and mental health. (Of course, it is important to reassure clients that all information about substance abuse will remain strictly confidential.)

"Do you have problems sleeping?" Sleep problems—including difficulty falling asleep, frequent waking, and oversleeping—frequently accompany mental health problems, increase feelings of distress and loss of control in the face of mental illness, cause chronic daytime fatigue, and diminish resilience and capacity to cope with illness. The specific pattern of disturbed sleep can provide valuable clues about factors that are related to clients' physical and mental health, including drinking habits, adverse medication effects, and medical disorders that may be interfering with sleep.

"How do you handle stress?" Everyone experiences stress in work, relationships, and school, and there is always a relationship between a person's awareness of and capacity to cope with stress and his or her degree of mental health. Some individuals are aware of the physical and psychological effects of stress in their lives, whereas others are apparently oblivious. Answers to this question will help you gauge your clients' degree of insight into the kinds of stresses that are causing or contributing to their mental health problems. It will also provide an introduction to a later conversation about useful stress management strategies.

"Tell me a little about your most important relationship." Everyone has various types of relationships with other humans and animals. The capacity to function in relationships is a general indicator of mental health. Your clients' answers will provide information about their chief relationship, if any, and also give you a sense of the relative importance of relationships in their lives. A client who has no (human) friends and describes her bond with her cat as the most important relationship in her life signals a need to rule out social phobia, schizoid personality disorder, and perhaps obsessive–compulsive disorder and certain psychotic disorders, whereas a client who talks about having a different lover every month suggests the need to explore other possibilities.

"Is your mental health problem caused by, or causing, difficulties at work?" Many people who have mental health problems believe that their problems are causing, or are caused by, work-related stress. Of course, many clients find themselves caught in a vicious circle in which work causes stress and its symptoms, and the symptoms then interfere with their ability to work (which makes the symptoms worse). It is important to know about the relationship between work stress and symptoms, as well as clients' perceptions and beliefs in this area, in order to suggest the most appropriate and effective strategies for stress management.

"Have any tests been done to find out what is causing your problem(s)?" Has your client been medically evaluated, using conventional diagnostic laboratory tests of blood, urine, etc., in efforts to determine a possible biological cause of their symptoms? If so, what tests have been done and what are the results and their significance? Is your client being followed on a regular basis for ongoing assessment of the problem with appropriate laboratory tests or diagnostic imaging studies? Has your client been evaluated using any nonconventional tests—for example, functional tests of the urine or blood for amino acid levels or neurotransmitter metabolites, or "energetic" assessment by a Chinese medical practitioner or energy healer? If so, what are the findings, their significance, and are they being appropriately followed for any needed ongoing evaluation?

"Do you have any medical problems? If so, are they currently being treated?" A complete list of any medical problems is an important part of your client's history. It is also important to know whether your client is being treated for a medical problem, what that treatment is, and whether it is effective. Depressed mood, anxiety, sleep disturbances, fatigue, and other common mental health problems are frequently related to an underlying medical disorder, but can also be caused by the adverse effects of conventional pharmacological treatmen).

"It is important for me to have a complete list of all medications, supplements, vitamins, herbals, or homeopathic remedies you may be taking, including doses and times of day they are taken." In the interest of time, when scheduling an intake with new clients, I ask them to make this list and bring it to the first session. Establishing exactly what your client takes for medical or mental health problems is an essential part of the history. I make notes about durations, any adverse effects, concerns about cost, etc., during the intake interview and attach the list to the chart for future reference. If you have some knowledge of prescription medications, vitamins, amino acids, herbals, etc., it is appropriate to ask questions about effective dosing, specific adverse effects, or suspected toxic interactions.

However, as most readers are psychotherapists and not certified in psychopharmacology, concerns about safe or effective dosing or potentially toxic drug–drug or drug–supplement interactions should be addressed through consultation with a physician.

"Are you currently being treated by an alternative medical practitioner for any medical or mental health problem?" It is helpful to mention a few examples of CAM practitioners—for example, Chinese medical practitioners, chiropractors, massage therapists, and energy healers. Write down the name of the CAM practitioner, the goals of the treatment, how long they've been receiving treatment, and what their experience has been so far. In describing specialized therapies they are receiving from a CAM practitioner, clients often recall additional supplements or herbals they are taking in the context of that therapy. You can then add these to your list for completeness.

"Do you have any cultural, religious, or spiritual issues or problems that might be important for me to know about?" Most clients, especially in the early stages of therapy, do not bring up this area unless you ask them explicitly. Obtaining this information at the outset will give you valuable clinical insights into possible relationships between clients' cultural identity and religious or spiritual beliefs and their emotional and psychological well-being. In my clinical practice I have found that focusing on cultural or spiritual concerns in psychotherapy can be an effective strategic approach when working with individuals who are struggling with existential issues, such as the absence of meaning in their personal, professional, or social lives.

Of course, many other general and specific questions can be asked, depending on your client's issues and history. By the end of the intake interview you should have a basic understanding of core symptoms, pertinent family and medical histories, important relationships, any substance abuse problems, and distress related to cultural identity or spiritual beliefs. You should have a complete list of all medications and supplements, including doses, times taken, any associated adverse effects, and how long they have been taken. You should also know whether clients are being treated by conventionally trained or alternative medical practitioners for any medical or mental health problem, what the treatment consists of, how long they have been in treatment, and whether they are responding to treatment. Ideally, by the end of the intake interview, you will have enough information to make some initial recommendations about psychotherapy, lifestyle changes (e.g., nutrition, exercise), stress management, mind–body work, and select supplements. Depending on the complexity of clients' medical history and any ongoing medical problem, you may have a sense of whether it is appropriate to to refer them to a family physician, psychiatrist, or naturopathic physician for consultation. If you are certified to prescribe medications in your state, it may be appropriate at this early stage in your relationship with new clients to mention conventional pharmacological treatment choices or, if they are already taking a medication, to comment on the possible need for changes in medications or doses (i.e., if they are not responding to medications or experiencing adverse effects). However, I believe it is generally preferable to first consult with the prescribing physician before giving specific medication advice to any client, even if you are qualified to do so. For medical–ethical reasons it is important to obtain a signed release from clients to exchange information with the nurse or physician responsible for prescribing their medications before giving any specific advice about changes in medications or doses.

AFTER THE INTAKE INTERVIEW: URGENT VERSUS ROUTINE REFERRALS

If clients report a history or symptoms that warrant urgent concern over a possibly emergent medical problem—including severe headaches, a history of untreated head injury, changes in the level of consciousness or other severe new-onset changes in mental functioning, nausea, vomiting, or other serious, rapidly evolving physical complaints—they should be referred to an urgent care facility or emergency room *immediately*. For example, a client who reports progressive memory loss or symptoms that may be caused by near-stroke episodes should be referred to a neurologist for consultation and appropriate diagnostic tests. If clients become acutely medically ill while being treated by nonconventionally trained practitioners, it is important to refer them immediately to their primary care physician or to the nearest emergency room in order to ensure that they are evaluated and treated as rapidly as possible using mainstream medical approaches.

If a client discloses a plan to commit suicide or is gravely disabled because of severe psychotic symptoms or acute alcohol or drug intoxication, it is imperative to arrange for an urgent psychiatric evaluation at the nearest hospital emergency room. If that option is not available or your client refuses your advice, you may have to call 911 to request advice and assistance from the local police department.

If clients have symptoms that may be related to a previously diagnosed medical disorder, it is prudent to refer them to their primary care physician or the conventional medical specialist who is already managing their care. Some clients may talk about vague symptoms such as unusual feelings in their bodies that are difficult to describe, or they may not be able to provide a clear or complete history, making it difficult to know whether they are psychotic, severely depressed, experiencing dissociative symptoms, or under the influence of narcotics. If your client is very depressed, overweight, has heart disease, and is preoccupied with intense spiritual concerns about dying, for example, reasonable recommendations include an appointment with a primary care physician to check the status of his or her heart disease; possibly starting the client on an appropriate conventional or nonconventional treatment for depressed mood, including improved nutrition and exercise, combined with supportive and insight-oriented psychotherapy; and helping the client find a spiritual practice that addresses his or her fear of dying. Heart disease is an example of a medical problem that is commonly seen together with depression. Relationships between depression and heart disease exist on many psychological and biological levels. If a client with a history of heart disease reports acute episodes of chest pain (i.e., angina), you should *refer him or her immediately to the nearest emergency room or urgent care center*. The chief responsibility of a conventionally trained physician is to rule out medical illness on the basis of the patient's self-reported history, collateral information, and any assessment findings. In cases where a medical problem has already been diagnosed and is being treated, but there is no recent worsening or progression of symptoms, there is probably no need to refer the client back to the physician for further assessment.

ASSESSMENT IN INTEGRATIVE MENTAL HEALTH CARE: GETTING STARTED

At the end of the initial interview it is important to share your clinical impression with the client and to mention any concerns that suggest the need, if any, for specialized assessment. If you believe more formal assessment will help clarify the causes of your client's distress, it is helpful to explain why you think he or she should be evaluated, briefly describe the test or tests you think will be helpful, and, ideally, refer your client to a reputable physician or alternative medical practitioner whom you *know* and *trust*. Depending on your familiarity with the range of treatment choices, it may also be appropriate at this early stage to to make some initial recommendations or appropriate referrals. In many cases, the clinician to whom you refer a client for specialized assessment will also provide treatment, but in other cases assessment findings may point to surprising or unexpected causes of symptoms and suggest a referral to a clinician with a completely different perspective. In the real day-to-day practice of mental health care, assessment and treatment are parallel threads of effective integrative management and thus often take place in tandem.

Types of Information Used in Psychiatric Assessment

In determining which treatment to recommend, conventionally trained physicians as well as practitioners trained in non-Western systems of medicine take into account both qualitative and quantitative information. Qualitative information is gathered during routine sessions and includes observations about the client's general state of mind, behavior, attitude toward treatment, and general feelings of well-being (or lack thereof) before and after treatment. Strictly quantitative information is seldom the mainstay of psychiatric evaluation in any healing tradition because subjective symptoms are inherently difficult to "reduce" to discrete causes, and because reliable quantitative data describing postulated biological or energetic causes (and confirming their links to symptoms) are often difficult to obtain. In Western medicine quantitative information is obtained from specific laboratory tests and brain imaging studies. Quantitative methods used in conventional biomedical psychiatry to identify the causes of mental and emotional symptoms include laboratory analysis of the blood (including complete blood count and iron), thyroid hormones, other hormones, and brain scans showing both structure and function (e.g., CT, MRI, fMRI, QEEG, SPECT, and PET). Although abnormal findings regarding electrical brain wave activity, electrolytes, blood cell count, thyroid function, kidney function, or genetic markers are often present with mental and emotional symptoms, the relationships between genetic abnormalities, medical illness or neurotransmitter imbalances, and mental illness are complex and subtle, and it is often difficult to demonstrate that a specific abnormal biological finding is the cause of a particular mental health problem. In other words, quantitative assessment approaches generally yield *nonspecific* information about a person's brain structure and function or general state of health. The often ambiguous clinical information available from conventional Western psychiatric assessment generally fails to point to definitive conclusions about the biological causes of mental or emotional symptoms at the level of molecules, neurons, or brain circuits, much less cultural, spiritual, or postulated energetic or spiritual factors that may contribute to the formation or evolution of symptoms.

The best way to think about how to evaluate clients from an integrative perspective is to review the evidence for different conventional and nonconventional approaches used to assess their core symptom(s) and, if indicated, make referrals for specialized assessment that might yield information that can inform treatment choices. I am assuming that readers are already familiar with established conventional assessment approaches, and so comment only briefly on them. Mainstream assessment approaches evaluate the underlying causes of mental illness in the context of widely accepted psychological and biological theories. These approaches include structured clinical interviews, specialized neuropsychological tests, structural and functional brain imaging studies, and laboratory tests of the blood and urine. Table 2.1 lists assessment approaches used in conventional Western psychiatry to evaluate mental illness.

TABLE 2.1 Representative Conventional Psychiatric Assessment Approaches

Structured clinical interviews

Hamilton Depression Inventory (Ham-D)
Hamilton Anxiety Inventory (Ham-A)
Beck Depression Inventory (BDI)
Brief Psychiatric Rating Scale (BPRS)
Yale–Brown Obsessive–Compulsive Scale (YBOCS)

Neuropsychological testing

Thematic Aperception Test (TAT)
Bender–Gestalt Test
Wechsler Adult Intelligence Scale
Wisconsin card sorting test

Biological assays

Complete blood count
Serum iron levels
Fasting glucose
Urinalysis
Electrolytes
Thyroid (and other hormone) serum levels

Brain imaging studies

Computerized tomography (CT) scan
Magnetic resonance imaging (MRI) showing brain structure
Functional magnetic resonance imaging (fMRI) showing both
    structure and function
Single photon emission computerized tomography (SPECT) showing
    regional blood flow in brain
Positron emission tomography (PET) showing regional metabolic
    brain activity

THE LIMITATIONS OF CONVENTIONAL PSYCHIATRIC ASSESSMENT

Western medicine and other systems of medicine use objective methods to gather information that can be verified by empirical tests, whereas other systems of medicine rely on a combination of objective findings and the clinician's intuition. Contemporary Western medical theory is based on chemistry and biology, in contrast to most non-Western systems of medicine, which base their understandings of the nature of illness and healing on deeply rooted philosophical or spiritual beliefs. In conventional Western psychiatry there is no single dominant explanatory model of mental illness, only an eclectic assortment of psychological, genetic, and neurobiological theories. Like conventional pharmacological treatments of mental illness, mainstream approaches used to evaluate the underlying causes of symptoms are often helpful but also have inherent limitations (Berrios, 2002). Although standardized symptom rating scales and laboratory tests can elucidate the psychological and social *meanings* and biological *causes* of certain symptoms, many conventional assessment tools have limited accuracy and reliability and do not examine numerous possible causes of mental illness in the context of the latest scientific advances in brain research and medicine.

The inherent limitations of contemporary Western psychiatric theory as an explanatory model of mental illness have resulted in the classification of psychiatric disorders (i.e., according to the DSM) on the basis of *phenomenological similarities between symptoms* and not presumed biological abnormalities at the level of hormones, immune function, neurotransmitters, or brain circuits. After decades of research the mechanisms of action of many psychotropic drugs are still poorly understood, and many drugs in widespread use are supported by equivocal evidence for a postulated mechanism of action at the level of changes in specific neurotransmitter systems believed to manifest as improvements in depression, anxiety, psychosis, memory loss, and other mental health problems. This equivocal evidence suggests that Western medical theory, in its current form, cannot adequately explain the causes of mental illness. In fact, recent studies on non-Western healing traditions, including Chinese medicine and homeopathy, point to *nonclassical* causes of both physical and mental illness that may be consistent with the predictions of complexity theory, quantum field theory, or other emerging paradigms in mainstream Western science. My own journey as a conventionally trained physician and a student of Chinese medicine, mind–body practices, herbal medicine, and other non-Western healing traditions has led me to believe that disparate systems of medicine embody different but valid *ways of knowing* about the nature and causes of illness and different but valid *ways of creating or facilitating* the conditions that lead to beneficial responses and ideally, in some cases, permit "healing" to take place.

Thinking about these broad conceptual problems in the context of my day-to-day experiences as a clinician is consistent with the view that an adequate explanatory model of mental illness cannot rely on one single idea or theory, but must include a broader understanding of the nature of human consciousness. This model should take into account the dynamic nature of *symptom patterns* as they reflect unique social and cultural circumstances and biological, psychological, energetic, and spiritual factors that impact human consciousness and behavior. Such a model would not reduce human suffering to the statistically "averaged" distributions of symptoms (and their presumed correspondences to neurotransmitter imbalances) that are conceptualized as discrete *disorders* in the DSM. Approaching clients from the eclectic perspective of integrative medicine generally results in deeper understandings of the causes or meanings of symptoms, more inclusive and clinically useful formulations, more thorough and more *client-centered* treatment planning, improved relationships between therapists and their clients, and, in many cases, better outcomes.

Nonconventional Assessment Approaches

Like Western-trained physicians, many nonconventionally trained medical practitioners also use quantitative assessment approaches to evaluate mental illness. Quantitative assessment approaches not presently accepted by mainstream Western psychiatry include so-called "functional medicine" tests of the urine or blood for byproducts of serotonin, GABA, and other neurotransmitters; specialized functional brain mapping techniques; and analysis of the vascular autonomic signal (VAS). Quantitative electroencephalography

(QEEG) brain mapping is a specialized kind of electroencephalography (EEG) that in some cases can provide a *picture* of abnormal brain electrical activity that can help distinguish symptoms that are similar at a phenomenological level but are probably "caused" by different kinds of functional abnormalities in the brain. Because this approach can sometimes distinguish subtle differences in electrical activity underlying different kinds of symptoms, QEEG brain mapping can help identify the most efficacious conventional or nonconventional treatment for a specific kind of abnormal electrical brain activity. The history, together with relevant qualitative and quantitative information obtained from a formal medical or neuropsychological evaluation, are integrated in a systematic formulation of the causes, conditions, or meanings of the client's symptoms. Appropriate biological, somatic, mind–body, energy, or spiritual treatment choices are then considered, depending on the type and severity of symptoms and their underlying causes or meanings.

It is important for every mental health professional to be familiar with the evidence for nonconventional assessment approaches before recommending a particular one to a client. Whereas some nonorthodox assessment approaches have been validated by significant research evidence, others remain essentially untested by Western-style research studies. Iridology, hair analysis, radionics, psychic diagnosis, and electroacupuncture are examples of unverified assessment tools that probably do not provide reliable information (Ernst, 1995). In my opinion, it is unreasonable to suggest these approaches to clients in the absence of solid research evidence supporting their claims. In fact, suggesting that your client try one of these unproven approaches may delay both diagnosis and treatment.

Functional Medicine Assessment

A functional medicine assessment evaluates relationships between nutritional status, neurotransmitters, endocrine and immune function, and symptoms of depression, anxiety, psychosis, and other symptoms (Delgado & Moreno, 2000). Functional tests include serum and urinary assays of neurotransmitters and their metabolites, vitamins, minerals, amino acids and their metabolites, hormones, fatty acids, and immunological factors and molecules (called *interleukins*) that mediate the body's inflammatory response. Research findings suggest that immunological dysregulation plays a significant role in the pathogenesis of mood disorders, schizophrenia, Alzheimer's disease, as well as other degenerative neurological disorders (Sperner-Unterweger, 2005). Relationships between immunity and mental illness are poorly understood, and the same immunological dysregulation is sometimes found in individuals with disparate symptoms (Irwin, 2008). Studies done to date have not found correlations between specific immunological markers and particular psychiatric symptoms or disorders (Dantzer et al., 1999; Castanon et al., 2002). Nevertheless, chronic depressed mood is often associated with suppression of certain immunological factors, including natural killer cell activity, and excess activity of other factors; however, these relationship are inconsistent. Depressed patients who do not respond to conventional pharmacological treatment may have increased cell-mediated immunity (Kulmatycki & Jamali, 2006). Abnormal elevation of a specific molecule that mediates inflammation (i.e., a pro-inflammatory cytokine) is often present in individuals diagnosed with schizophrenia, mania, and PTSD. Recent studies suggest that nonspecific overactivation of the immune system involving helper T cells takes place in subgroups of schizophrenics (Strous & Shoenfeld, 2006). The immune-mediated dysregulation of both dopamine and glutamate neurotransmission has also been implicated in the pathogenesis of schizophrenia (Muller, 2006). In response to these findings, anti-inflammatory and immune-modulating therapies are being investigated as promising future treatments of mood disorders and schizophrenia.

Horrobin (1996,1998) has proposed a "membrane phosopholipid" model of schizophrenia, which argues that abnormal metabolism of phosopholipids, resulting from genetic and environmental factors, manifests as a chronic severe constellation of symptoms typically diagnosed as a variant of schizophrenia or schizoaffective disorder. The membrane phospholipid hypothesis posits that a spectrum of psychiatric disorders is associated with abnormalities in neuronal membranes, and that the kind and severity of symptoms are functions of the magnitude and specific type of metabolic errors resulting in abnormal phospholipid metabolism.

If clients' histories suggest that functional testing might help clarify underlying causes of their mental health problem at the level of immune or neurotransmitter functioning, you may wish to refer them to a local family physician, psychiatrist, or naturopathic physician who is familiar with functional medicine. If clinicians in your area are not familiar with functional medicine testing, the official web site of the Institute of Functional Medicine (*www.FunctionalMedicine.org*) is an excellent place to find out more about this rapidly evolving field of medicine and identify resources for making referrals.

Quantitative Electroencephalography and Heart Rate Variability Analysis

QEEG analysis is currently used as a research tool to evaluate abnormalities in brain electrical activity underlying a range of mental health problems. In the coming years this assessment method will probably emerge as a significant adjunct to conventional psychiatric assessment. Research studies have established that specific kinds of abnormal EEG activity are associated with different core symptoms or disorders (Hughes & Roy, 1999). Abnormal EEG findings occur in up to 40% of depressed patients, and "small, sharp spikes" are often present in severely depressed suicidal patients (Small, 1993). QEEG analysis of unipolar depressed patients often reveals increased alpha or theta power and decreased interhemispheric coherence (Nieber & Schlegel, 1992). Decreases in prefrontal cordance, a combined measure of absolute and relative EEG power, may predict response of previously treatment-resistant depressed patients to conventional antidepressants (Bares et al., 2007). Cordance may also be a useful indicator when planning treatment for cocaine addiction. Cocaine abusers who had high cordance measures were much more likely to complete treatment programs, compared to matched patients with low cordance (Venneman, 2006). QEEG analysis can be used to distinguish mildly demented depressed individuals from depressed individuals who complain of cognitive impairments (Deslandes, 2004).

Although there are no specific QEEG markers for different mood disorders, reduced alpha activity and increased beta power increase the likelihood of bipolar disorder over unipolar depression (John & Princhep, 1993). In contrast, a finding of increased alpha or theta power suggests that the most likely diagnosis is unipolar depression, and appropriate treatment can be started. Global disturbances in EEG synchronization are similar in schizophrenia and bipolar disorder; however, in contrast to patient with schizophrenia, bipolar patients *do not* show disorganization in the superior temporal lobes. In schizophrenia EEG activity can be categorized into discrete patterns that may prove to be more specific indicators of diagnostic subtypes than specific positive or negative symptoms of psychosis (John et al., 2007). Specific abnormal QEEG findings in individuals diagnosed with a mood disorder, schizophrenia, or obsessive in compulsive disorder (OCD) may predict differential response rates to different classes of conventional medications (Small, 1999; John & Princhep, 1993). Information obtained using QEEG brain mapping may be as specific and clinically relevant as data obtained using advanced functional brain imaging studies such as fMRI, PET, and SPECT, and it may offer a more cost-effective alternative for evaluating neurobiological abnormalities associated with a broad range of mental health problems. If you think a client may benefit from having a QEEG, you should find a neurologist in your community who knows how to do this procedure. Some QEEG technicians come to outpatient settings to make recordings. Findings are subsequently returned with a report explaining their clinical significance and suggesting novel treatment strategies.

Stress caused by intense emotional states is associated with autonomic arousal that can significantly affect subtle aspects of heart rhythm, the so-called "heart rate variability." Research studies suggest that HRV may correlate with measures of regional cerebral blood flow as measured by PET (Lane et al., 2008). One study found that individuals diagnosed with panic disorder and decreases in normal HRV, experienced desirable increases in HRV in response to cognitive–behavioral therapy but not to a conventional pharmacological treatment (Garakani et al., 2008). HRV monitoring will eventually emerge as a practical clinical approach for evaluating relationships between physiological stress, as measured by subtle changes in heart rate, and emotional and cognitive stress associated with intensely experienced emotions in both healthy and mentally ill populations.

Methods Used to Evaluate Postulated "Subtle" Energies

Some assessment approaches used in non-Western healing trada-tions claim to detect "subtle" energetic clues about the causes of mental illness. Highly refined diagnostic skills, grounded in ancient traditions of Chinese medicine and Hindu Ayurveda, as well as modern technological approaches are being used in outpatient clin-ical settings to evaluate responses to acupuncture and qigong. Skilled Chinese medical practitioners obtain empirical and intu-itive information about the balance between the complementary energetic principles of yin and yang, the two postulated forms of "*qi*," or energy, that contribute to health and illness. Subtle ener-gies described in Chinese medicine and other non-Western systems of medicine may be consistent with the observation that all living organisms emit ultra-weak photons. Under certain conditions these biophotons are emitted as highly ordered or "coherent" light (Schwabl, 2005). Findings of studies on biophoton emissions from the human body have led to speculation about the possible pres-ence of "light channels" that regulate energy and information trans-fer within the body, biological rhythms associated with the intensity and patterns of biophoton emissions, and diseases related to ener-getic "asymmetries" between the left and right sides of the body (Wijk & Wijk, 2005). Subtle differences in the wavelength and coherence of biophoton emissions associated with certain acupuncture points ("acupoints") may correspond to energetic imbalances in yin and yang that manifest as discrete neurological or psychiatric disorders (Yang et al., 2004). The findings of a double-blind study suggest that skilled Chinese medical practition-ers are able to reliably estimate changes in yin and yang energy fol-lowing treatment (Langevin, 2004). More studies are needed to determine whether clinicians who claim to intuitively measure sub-tle energies are somehow able to detect ultra-weak biophotons, electromagnetic fields, or other classically described energies asso-ciated with living organisms.

Measuring electrodermal potentials at acupoints following qigong treatment may provide useful information about changes in the quality of bioelectrical activity following acupuncture or qigong therapy (Sancier, 2003; Zhang, 2002). Clinical methods used to detect subtle characteristics of the human pulse have been refined over millennia in Western, Chinese, Ayurvedic, and Tibetan systems of medicine. Case reports suggest that certain pulse characteristics described in Chinese, Ayurvedic, and Tibetan medical assessment correspond to energetic imbalances manifesting as particular cognitive or affective symptoms (Hammer, 2001). For example, mild to moderate symptoms of anxiety, depressed mood, or irritability are often associated with a "tight" or rapid rate when the pulse is taken at the pericardium position and "smooth vibration" over the entire pulse at all depths. In contrast, severe psychiatric symptoms are more often associated with a "rough vibration" over the entire pulse, and "slipperiness" in certain aspects of the pulse. The most severe symptoms are often associated with the most erratic or abnormal energetic qualities of the pulse, resulting in a "pulse picture" that is "overwhelmed" by "chaos in the circulation" (Hammer, 2001).

Analysis of the vascular autonomic signal (VAS) is an emerging technology-based approach that complements assessment methods used in traditional Chinese medicine. The VAS is a postulated reflex that brings the endocrine, immune, and autonomic nervous systems into optimum energetic balance in response to external and internal physiological and energetic stressors. Acupuncturists use the VAS reflex to assess the energetic imbalances associated with medical and psychiatric disorders. Findings of Doppler imaging studies suggest that subtle changes in arterial wall tone consistent with the hypothesized VAS reflex may occur almost instantaneously in response to *energetic* stimuli that affect the physical and psychological state of the body but *do not* enter into conscious awareness (Ackerman, 2001). According to the theory, particular substances induce specific resonance patterns that trigger changes in autonomic arousal. More studies are needed to determine whether the VAS reflex can be used to determine optimum acupuncture or conventional treatments for energetic imbalances associated with specific psychiatric disorders.

Over time, some of the above assessment approaches will probably become accepted by mainstream Western psychiatry, while others will remain the exclusive domain of alternative medical practitioners. Table 2.2 lists functional medicine, imaging, and energetic assessment approaches not presently endorsed by orthodox

Western psychiatry but in widespread use by alternative medical practitioners to evaluate depression, anxiety, psychosis, cognitive impairment, and the other mental and emotional problems covered in this book. The table can be used as a general guide for recommending specialized assessment or making appropriate referrals to conventionally trained or alternative medical practitioners once core symptoms have been identified. Please note that when I recommend making a referral to a naturopathic physician, I mean a doctor of naturopathy (ND) who has completed a rigorous 4-year training program and is licensed to practice medicine by a governing state medical board. Many individuals who call themselves naturopaths have not completed a rigorous medical training program, are not doctors of naturopathy (NDs), have widely varying training and skill levels, and are not regulated by a state medical board. For your client's best interest in making a referral to the most qualified practitioner, and your interest in minimizing liability risk, I would advise against consulting with practitioners who represent themselves as naturopaths but who have not completed training at a credentialed program at the doctoral level. Although family physicians and NDs have differences in medical outlook and training, the day-to-day clinical work done by both is often quite similar. In my experience, when formal biological testing is needed, including analysis of blood and urine to determine nutritional status, etc., it is reasonable (and legally defensible) to refer clients to either a family physician or an ND.*

---

* Many states do not allow NDs to practice medicine. In these states, of course, it is neither reasonable nor legally defensible (i.e., in the event of malpractice allegations to refer a client to an ND.

TABLE 2.2 Nonconventional Approaches Used to Assess Common Mental Health Problems

Core symptom for which assessment approach results in useful information	Description of assessment approach	Clinical significance of findings	Planning treatment based on assessment	Arranging appropriate referrals for assessment findings
Depression	Check serum folate, B-12, omega-3 fatty acid levels	Low levels of B vitamins and omega-3 fatty acids often correspond to more severe symptoms	Improved response to antidepressants with supplemental folate, B-12, and omega-3s	Write note to family physician or N.D.
	Measure serum cholesterol level	Low serum cholesterol levels may predict severe depression and high suicide risk drugs may improve mood	Dietary changes or changes in doses of cholesterol-lowering	Write note to family physician or N.D.
	QEEG analysis of brain wave activity	Specific QEEG findings correspond to different subtypes of depression or bipolar disorder and may predict differential response to medications	QEEG findings may be useful in identifying the most effective treatment	Write note to family physician suggesting secondary referral to neurologist

TABLE 2.2 *Continued*

Mood swings	Check blood folate levels	Low red blood cell folate levels (but *normal* serum levels) frequent in mania	Improved response to mood stabilizers with folate supplementation	Write note to family physician or N.D.
	QEEG analysis of brain wave activity	Bipolar patients have distinctive abnormalities	QEEG findings may be useful in planning most effective treatment	Write note to family physician suggesting secondary referral to neurologist
	Analysis of the VAS	Rapidly cycling bipolar patients may have a specific energetic pattern	VAS findings may help identify most effective medication or acupuncture treatment	Refer patient to Chinese medical practitioner
Anxiety and panic	QEEG analysis of brain wave activity	Findings may correspond to specific anxiety symptoms	QEEG analysis may be useful guide to optimizing treatment, especially in OCD	Write note to family physician suggesting secondary referral to neurologist
	Check serum cholesterol level	Total cholesterol is often *elevated* (in contrast to depressed patients, in whom cholesterol is abnormally *low*)	Cholesterol levels return to normal with symptomatic improvement following treatment	Write note to family physician or N.D.

TABLE 2.2 *Continued*

	EDST (Electrodermal Skin Testing)	Energetic changes in certain meridians may provide useful diagnostic information	Specific findings helpful in identifying most effective conventional or energetic therapy	Refer to healing touch practitioner familiar with EDST
Hyperactivity and distractibility	Serum zinc level	Abnormal low zinc levels may interfere with normal brain function, manifesting as symptoms of ADHD	Zinc supplementation may result in symptomatic improvement	Refer to naturopathic physician or M.D. trained in integrative medicine
	Serum ferritin level	Nonanemic children diagnosed with ADHD may have abnormal low serum iron levels	Oral iron supplementation may result in symptomatic improvement	Refer to naturopathic physician or M.D. trained in integrative medicine
	QEEG brain mapping	Abnormal EEG activity often present in individuals diagnosed with ADHD	Specific EEG abnormality may provide clues to most efficacious treatment	Refer to neurologist who can arrange for QEEG

TABLE 2.2 *Continued*

Schizophrenia and psychotic symptoms	Check red blood cell fatty acid levels; check serum DHEA level	Levels of arachadonic acid and DHA often abnormally low	Symptomatic improvement with fatty acid supplementation	Write note to family physician, N.D., or psychiatrist
	Niacin challenge test	Low levels common in schizophrenia; reduced flushing in schizophrenics	Improvement with supplementation, especially *negative* symptoms; helps distinguish between different psychotic disorders	Write note to family physician, N.D., or psychiatrist
Memory loss and other types of cognitive impairment	QEEG analysis of brain wave activity	Specific abnormalities in different stages or types of dementia and following stroke	Helps clarify diagnosis and identify most effective medication or EEG biofeedback treatment	Write note to family physician suggesting secondary referral to neurologist
	Serum zinc and magnesium levels	Low levels of these minerals may increase risk of Alzheimer's disease	Findings are inconsistent and poorly understood; supplementation may *not* improve symptoms	Write note to family physician or N.D.

Appendix B)

TABLE 2.2 *Continued*

	Virtual reality testing	Cognitive testing in a virtual reality environment reveals cognitive performance deficits	Permits earlier identification of type and severity of degenerative disorders	Provide client with resources on VR therapy centers (see Appendix B)
Substance abuse and dependence	In alcoholics check serum levels of vitamins A, C, B (several), and essential fatty acids	General malnutrition caused by chronic alcohol abuse often associated with vitamin deficiencies	Supplementation can improve general health but little benefit if client continues to abuse alcohol	Write note to family physician or N.D.
	QEEG analysis of brain wave activity	Different abnormalities in alcoholics and cocaine abusers	Specific findings useful in planning effective EEG biofeedback program to reduce relapse risk	Refer to therapist trained in EEG biofeedback (see Appendix B)
	Analysis of the VAS	Abnormal energetic pattern often seen in alcoholics or narcotics abusers	VAS findings help identify most effective conventional or nonconventional (i.e., acupuncture) therapy	Refer to Chinese medical practitioner or other clinician with training in VAS analysis (see Appendix B)

TABLE 2.2 *Continued*

Insomnia and fatigue	Check serum levels of vitamins C, folic acid, B-12, and E	Abnormal low levels often seen with insomnia and daytime sleepiness	Supplementation sometimes improves sleep and daytime energy	Write note to family physician or N.D.
	Check for food allergies	Dairy and wheat allergies sometimes cause daytime sleepiness	Eliminating dairy and wheat products from diet sometimes improves energy level	Write note to family physician or N.D.
	Check for hypoglycemia	Hypoglycemia often associated with daytime sleepiness	Dietary changes that correct hypoglycemia often improve overall energy level	Write note to family physician or N.D.

QEEG—quantitative electroencephalogram
VAS—vascular autonomic signal
OCD—obsessive–compulsive disorder
N.D.—doctor of neuropathy
EDST—Electrodermal skin testing
ADHD—attention-deficit/hyperactivity disorder.

Using certain nonconventional approaches together with established Western medical assessment methods can sometimes result in more reliable or complete information about the physiological, mind–body, or energetic causes of mental illness. For example, obtaining a serum homocysteine level in a client who is depressed, after using the Ham-D to evaluate the severity and characteristics of his or her symptoms, will help determine whether a biological problem is interfering with normal synthesis of neurotransmitters involved in mood regulation. The finding of an abnormally high homocysteine level would then suggest certain "targeted amino acid" modalities. The judicious use of both conventional and nonconventional assessment and treatment approaches can help clarify the complex causes of symptoms and provide clues to more specific and more effective treatments than might be suggested if only one kind of assessment approach is utilized. The vignettes in Part II are offered as examples of realistic clinical situations in which useful information is obtained using diverse assessment approaches at different phases of the therapist–client relationship.

Choosing the Most Appropriate Assessment Strategy

Certain assessment methods are more useful than others for clarifying the causes of a particular symptom. Determination of the *optimum* assessment approach when evaluating a target symptom (or symptom pattern) begins with a review of the evidence supporting the use of both conventional and nonconventional approaches. Conventional and nonconventional assessment approaches in relation to many common mental or emotional symptoms are summarized in Table 2.2 and reviewed in greater detail in the clinical case discussions in Part II. The same reasoning is used whether you are considering referring a client for assessment using a conventional or nonconventional approach. The most important initial question to ask is *"What kind of information should I look for to clarify my client's problem and lead to the best treatment?"* In other words, what factors or phenomena are pertinent to an accurate and complete understanding of the causes, course, conditions, or meanings of a particular symptom or symptom pattern? This inquiry includes considerations of the phenomenal basis of the formation or worsening of mental and emotional symptoms at all levels: social, psychological, biological, "energetic," and possibly also spiritual processes. When evaluating symptoms, it is often useful to think in terms of different hierarchical levels in a web-like structure in which disparate causes and meanings are interrelated and interact in direct or indirect ways to keep symptoms active. Productive and relevant assessment strategies are those that accurately identify *core* causes or meanings of the symptom pattern in question. There are multiple possible connections between the levels at which psychological, biological, informational, or energetic causes or meanings of symptoms exist, and, by extension, disparate treatments address the various *kinds* and *levels* of these underlying causes or meanings with various degrees of effectiveness. For example, a finding on QEEG analysis of abnormal left frontotemporal lobe activity in the mid-alpha frequency range (10–12 Hz) in a patient who complains of impairment in attention following a closed head injury suggests that treatments directed at "renormalizing" frontotemporal brain electrical activity in the mid-alpha range would probably result in improved attention. Reasonable treatment choices would then include certain EEG-biofeedback protocols, binaural sound, mind–body practices, certain natural products or synthetic drugs, and possibly also virtual reality graded exposure therapy (VRGET). The logic of integrative treatment planning is explored in detail in the following chapter.

When to Refer to a CAM Practitioner for Specialized Assessment

Only after clients have been evaluated and successfully treated for a serious medical or psychological problem is it prudent and appropriate to refer them to a nonconventionally trained medical practitioner for further evaluation and ongoing management of persistent mental and emotional symptoms. When history and symptoms do not suggest the presence of a rapidly worsening medical problem, or in cases where a primary medical illness was previously suspected but has been ruled out by a Western physician, and your client prefers to work primarily with an acupuncturist, herbalist, or other alternative practitioner, it is reasonable for him or her to do so if there is good evidence that the nonconventional treatment being used is both safe and effective for the mental health problem (see Chapter 3). When considering making a referral for assessment by a nonconventional practitioner, you should review the evidence for the approach you have in mind and explain why you think specialized assessment could yield useful information. As a conventionally trained Western physician, it is my strong belief that the evidence supporting both conventional and nonconventional assessment approaches should be carefully discussed with clients before any referrals are made. In general, referring a client to a particular nonconventional practitioner for assessment should be considered after conventional assessment has failed to yield specific useful information about possible medical causes of their symptoms. Recommending a specific nonconventional assessment approach is prudent when there is a significant probability of obtaining clinically relevant information that will clarify underlying causes of symptoms and guide treatment planning. Table 2.2 provides a general overview of nonconventional assessment approaches that can yield useful clinical information about common mental health problems.

As I have already mentioned, in cases where reliable information has been obtained from the history and a multidimensional formulation has led to an effective treatment strategy, there is probably no need for more formal assessment. However, in cases where clinically useful information has not been obtained from the initial assessment, it is important to carefully review your client's symptoms and history to search for salient facts that may have been missed during the intake interview. (By "clinically useful" information I mean assessment findings that give you a better understanding of the cause[s] of your client's mental health problem and influence your judgment about appropriate treatment or referrals). It is important to talk openly with your client about options for specialized assessment or treatment, address questions about practical issues such as cost and any stress associated with a referral, and then refer your client to a physician or alternative medical practitioner who will be able to competently perform the most appropriate, affordable, and realistic kind of assessment. A complete assessment may involve only one referral to a particular clinician in the community for a specific test, or several referrals over a period of weeks or months to both conventionally trained physicians and alternative medical practitioners. You should continue to refer clients for assessment, as needed, until emerging findings provide a clear picture of the causes or meanings of their primary symptoms, and they are responding to ongoing treatment.

Although Chinese medicine and many other non-Western healing traditions are frequently effective for chronic problems, they are seldom helpful when treating medical emergencies. Possessing a general knowledge of the evidence for conventional and nonconventional assessment approaches when evaluating a client with a particular mental health problem will help you know when it is appropriate to refer clients for more formal diagnostic assessment. Emerging assessment approaches such as the approaches discussed above are currently not used in conventional Western mental health clinics but will eventually help distinguish incipient dementia from other neurodegenerative disorders, identify specific functional or electromagnetic abnormalities associated with a specific client's depressed or anxious mood, and clarify the nature of other kinds of biological or energetic factors associated with mental illness that are not amenable to mainstream biomedical assessment. In sum, potential benefits of assessment using nonconventional approaches when evaluating mental illness include:

• Clarifying underlying causes of symptoms when the diagnosis remains unclear in cases where the complete history is difficult to obtain or conventional assessment approaches have not resulted in clinically useful information.
• Obtaining specific diagnostic information pointing to possible underlying biological causes of symptoms provides clues about the most appropriate and effective integrative treatment plan.
• Referring clients to Chinese medical practitioners, homeopaths, energy healers, or nonconventional practitioners for formal assessment of "energetic imbalances" may help clarify important energetic causes of symptoms that are not addressed by mainstream Western medicine.

Evaluating the causes of symptoms will lead to information that will help guide you thinking about the most effective or appropriate treatment. Of course, any symptom or complex symptom pattern can have numerous possible causes or symbolic meanings for the person experiencing it. In some cases the history alone may provide enough clinical information to formulate the primary causes or meanings of a client's distress and begin treatment. For example, a client who is moderately depressed and is having relationship problems, does not drink or use drugs, and has no significant family or medical history can safely be diagnosed and treated for depression in the absence of more formal assessment. In other cases it may be appropriate to refer a client for evaluation using one of several conventional or nonconventional assessment approaches that can help identify possible underlying causes of their symptoms at a psychological, biological, or energetic level. For example, in the case of a severely depressed client with liver disease caused by hepatitis C and a strong family history of bipolar disorder, who has not improved with conventional antidepressants or psychotherapy, certain nonconventional assessment approaches may yield clinically useful information suggesting more effective conventional or nonconventional treatment choices.

Referring clients to other clinicians will broaden your network of peers and professional colleagues and also foster collaborative treatment planning. In deciding whether and how to refer a client for assessment, there are always two basic choices: the use of one assessment approach or the use of two or more approaches in parallel. Most therapists recommend that their clients try one assessment approach at a time because of practical constraints on cost and availability. In my experience, it is usually better to recommend one assessment approach at a time to avoid confusion and unnecessary costs. Disparate assessment approaches used in different traditions of medicine may yield contradictory or inconsistent findings. Thus, recommending only one assessment approach at a time avoids the risk of confusing your client or confounding the diagnostic picture. However, recommending single assessment approaches in succession may delay formulation and effective treatment planning. It is always best to recommend a referral to a conventionally trained physician or alternative medical practitioner who can evaluate your client using approaches that will most likely yield reliable clinical information about causes or meanings of core symptom(s). Of course, the formal assessment approach that has the highest degree of clinical utility depends on the core symptom(s) being evaluated and the patient's history. In one case the most useful assessment approach might be a test of the urine or blood levels of specific vitamins. In another case the most appropriate assessment approach might be QEEG analysis of brain activity, or analysis of the energetic status of your client by a Chinese medical practitioner or homeopath. Of course, as a psychotherapist, you are superbly qualified to work with clients when addressing familial, social, psychological, or cultural meanings that may be keeping symptoms active or interfering with response to treatment. If you are trained in psychopharmacology and certified to prescribe medications in your state, you may also elect to advise your clients about appropriate and safe uses of psychotropic medications in the context of an integrative care plan.

The vignettes in Part II show how to assess and formulate the steps involved in recommending assessment and treatment for several common mental health problems. They also provide examples of appropriate referrals to conventionally trained or CAM specialists for cases involving serious or complex medical or psychiatric problems.

Complicated Cases Call for Specialized Assessment and Referral

In cases where the history is extremely complicated (or unreliable) and there are known medical problems or reasons to suspect an undiagnosed medical or neurological problem, formal assessment is often necessary to characterize the biological or energetic causes or the psychological or spiritual meanings of symptoms. In such cases the most appropriate assessment approach depends on the core mental or emotional symptom(s) that is the focus of attention (i.e., the symptom that is causing the greatest amount of distress or interfering with normal functioning) and the specific medical or neurological problems that are being ruled out. Assessment priority is often clear when a single symptom pattern has been identified as the primary cause of distress or impairment. However, at the time of the initial interview or during the course of treatment, a client may report many apparently unrelated symptoms, changes in symptom severity, changes in kinds of symptoms, and so forth. In such cases the clinician must decide whether to focus on one primary symptom or two or more core symptoms at the same time. For example, many clients who come to treatment for depressed mood have significant anxiety problems, or vice versa. By the same token, individuals who are struggling with depression or alcohol abuse often experience moderate or severe symptoms of cognitive impairment. When evaluating a client, you need to decide whether the causes or meanings of disparate symptoms are directly or indirectly related to one another or are following separate but overlapping trajectories. Your major goal when evaluating such individuals is to prioritize assessment or treatment choices for different kinds of symptoms on the basis of their relative severity and the degree to which they are related or exist independently of one another. In my clinical practice I have observed that although most clients complain of vague or nonspecific symptoms, they typically also report *one principal symptom or symptom pattern* associated with severe distress or progressive impairment in social, intellectual, or occupational functioning. In such cases, the initial priorities of assessment and treatment planning are relatively clear.

When a thorough history reveals two or more principal symptoms associated with significant distress or impairment, it is important to ask which specific conventional or nonconventional assessment approaches will most likely provide clinically useful, accurate, and *reliable* information about the underlying causes or meanings of a symptom. (In my own clinical experience as a psychiatrist treating or consulting on thousands of patients in private practice, outpatient managed care environments, inpatient psychiatric units, emergency rooms, hospital intensive care units, and inpatient medical-surgical services, I have encountered relatively few patients who complain of more than two primary *unrelated* mental or emotional symptoms.) The vignettes in Part II illustrate simple cases involving one primary or core symptom and more complex cases involving two or more core symptoms and suggest appropriate referrals for assessment and treatment. In some cases you will need to decide whether to recommend that a client be evaluated using two or more assessment approaches at the same time in order to obtain a *symptom picture* that is more accurate or complete than can be obtained using only one assessment approach.

I have enormous respect for the world's great healing traditions. My circle of professional colleagues and peers includes Chinese medical practitioners, Ayurvedic physicians, doctors of homeopathy, naturo-pathic physicians, chiropractors, massage therapists, Reiki masters, medical qigong healers, as well as psychiatrists trained in one or more of these non-Western healing traditions. In this context my own experience as a clinical psychiatrist has given me a conservative bias when it comes to talking with clients about conventional phar-macological treatments. My view on this subject is that in compli-cated cases, recommendations pertaining to the use of conventional medications or other Western therapies should be made only by con-ventionally trained medical doctors. As is true of Chinese medicine and other established world systems of medicine, the science and art of Western medicine require mastery of an enormous amount of technical information, following years of study of the so-called "basic sciences" and further years of supervised clinical training. By the same token, just as a Western trained M.D. who has a superficial familiarity with Chinese medicine is not qualified to suggest specific herbal or acupuncture treatments to a patient, Chinese medical practitioners, Ayurvedic physicians, homeopathic physicians, and other nonconventionally trained medical practitioners who have a rudimentary knowledge of Western medicine are not qualified to rec-ommend specific conventional treatments to patients because they lack the depth of knowledge and clinical experience to do so compe-tently and safely. If, after interviewing a new client, you believe that you do not have a clear understanding of the nature or severity of his or her mental or emotional symptoms, it is prudent to obtain super-vision from a more experienced therapist who can guide you in ask-ing questions that will clarify important aspects of history, help you develop a more adequate formulation of the case, or suggest produc-tive directions for referrals to provide more formal assessment.

The use of two or more assessment approaches in parallel is rea-sonable in cases where the core symptom has not improved or has worsened during the course of treatment, or the clinical picture is complicated by newly emerging symptoms. These circumstances suggest that important information was overlooked in the initial interview, the initial assessment and treatment plan did not ade-quately characterize or address the core symptom(s), or other psychi-atric or medical problems may be contributing to your client's distress or interfering with response to treatment. In such cases there is some urgency in accurately identifying the underlying causes or meanings of the client's distress. First, go over the client's history and current symptoms in detail to ensure that pertinent medical, psychological, spiritual, or other problems have not been overlooked. Then, consider which assessment approaches are likely to provide findings that will help clarify the nature of the persisting symptoms. For example, referring a client with severe anxiety and palpitations who has not improved with appropriate treatment to both a cardiologist for conventional tests and to a Chinese medical practitioner for energetic assessment, possibly including analysis of the VAS, will help determine whether the anxiety is primarily physiological or energetic in nature. It is important to *always clearly document* in clients' charts that they understand and agree to your reasons for recommending referral to another clinician for formal assessment. Of course, it is fundamentally important to take your client's cultural values and religious or spiritual beliefs (if any) into account when recommending any assessment or treatment approach.

When a client is not improving with ongoing treatment, useful assessment approaches are those that will most reliably yield accurate and specific information about the cause(s) of a symptom or symptom pattern resulting in unresolving distress or interfering with normal functioning. The case vignettes in Part II provide realistic examples of appropriate referrals for specialized assessment when a client does not improve with treatment and the underlying causes of symptoms remain unclear.

FORMULATION IN INTEGRATIVE MENTAL HEALTH CARE

Obtaining useful information about the underlying causes or meanings of a mental health problem sometimes takes as few as one or two sessions. In other cases, however, it may take months to establish a therapeutic alliance with a client through which the nature of the problem gradually becomes clear. When the history is complete and the initial assessment has been conducted, the next step is to formulate all pertinent issues in the case, including both quantitative and qualitative information pertaining to the social, cultural, psychological, biological, or energetic causes or meanings of your client's symptom(s). In conventional Western medicine agreement on which circumstances and symptoms are *most significant* leads to priorities about treatments that address the *presumed* underlying causes of those particular target symptoms. In the tradition of Western biomedicine, when a biological cause cannot be verified, the client's symptom is often regarded as a psychosomatic manifestations of distress and the search for other possible causes or meanings of the symptom ends. In contrast, formulation in integrative medicine takes into account the range of possible biological, mind–body, energetic, or spiritual causes or meanings of symptoms. As in conventional mental health care, making an integrative formulation will help you organize pertinent information before going on to the step of planning treatment. For example, the finding of an abnormally low level of a serotonin metabolite in the urine of a depressed client suggests that treatment strategies directed at increasing brain serotonin levels would be beneficial.

Ideally, assessment comes before formulation and treatment planning. However, for practical purposes treatment is usually started in parallel with any appropriate assessment, and emerging findings lead to commensurate changes in the formulation and treatment plan on an ongoing basis. History, symptoms, and any pertinent assessment findings are woven into a multidimensional formulation of the causes or meanings of core symptoms—which frequently change in light of new history or assessment findings.

Depending on a client's history, general health, severity of symptoms, a review of treatments that have already been tried, preferences, and financial constraints, the formulation will suggest appropriate treatment recommendations possibly including exercise, dietary changes, conventional antidepressants, and supplementation with certain amino acids and vitamins. Your hypothesis about the causes or meanings of your client's distress is probably correct when the treatment plan based on the formulation results in sustained clinical improvement. However, in some cases your initial formulation and recommendations for specialized assessment will fail to yield useful information about the psychological, biological, or energetic causes of your client's medical or mental health problem. At such times remember that future sessions will give you ample time to gather additional information that will help you know when to recommend other assessment approaches that may yield more useful information and point to the need for a particular therapy or referral to a family physician, naturopathic physician, or alternative medical practitioner. All vignettes in Part II include detailed formulations that essentially link the history and pertinent assessment findings to appropriate treatments or referrals.

In cases where the history is straightforward or symptoms are of moderate severity, the MMSE and a structured clinical interview may provide enough information to narrow down your client's history and symptoms to a concise formulation of salient biological, psychological, social, spiritual, or possibly energetic factors that subsequently become the basis of an effective integrative treatment plan. In more complicated cases, in which history is complex or unclear or symptoms are severe, determining the biological or energetic *causes* or the psychological or spiritual *meanings* (e.g., a relationship problem or spiritual conflict that is manifesting as despair or anxiety) of symptoms may require the use one or more conventional or nonconventional assessment approache to achieve an accurate and complete formulation and to plan an appropriate and adequate treatment strategy. Specialized symptom rating scales can often provide useful information about the severity of mood, anxiety, or cognitive symptoms when interviewing new clients. More formal neuropsychological assessment can provide additional information in cases where history is not clearly established or symptoms are vague.

Symptoms—Not Disorders—Provide the Foundations of A Good Formulation

Psychiatrists, psychologists, and other mental health professionals are trained to diagnose clients from the perspective of the *Diagnostic and Statistical Manual of Mental Disorders* (DSM), now in its fourth revised version. However, in the day-to-day work of mental health care, discrete symptoms—not disorders—are usually the focus of clinical attention. Information obtained from the history together with any formal assessment findings contribute to a multidimensional understanding of the causes and meanings of symptoms. Therefore, in practical terms, mental health professionals formulate their client's distress in terms of their emotional, cognitive, and behavioral symptoms. For example, a particular client may have sustained euphoric or irritable mood but may not have the other symptoms required for a diagnosis of bipolar disorder using DSM criteria. Likewise, a client may be depressed or anxious, but the range and severity of the symptoms may not qualify as "major depressive disorder," "generalized anxiety disorder," or another DSM disorder. In fact, symptoms that are *not* included under the umbrella of a DSM disorder may be the focus of attention in a clinical encounter. Furthermore, symptoms that reflect a mental health problem are uniquely configured in different individuals and generally continue to change throughout clients' lifetimes in response to changing stresses in their environment and new psychological, biological, and spiritual problems. Important aspects of formulation and treatment planning will expectably change in parallel with such changes.

As this book is being written, there is a great deal of debate over the validity of many DSM-IV "disorders" and disagreement over the most appropriate methodology to use when "constructing" complex definitions of psychiatric disorders in terms of biological, social, cultural, and other causes. In fact, the next version of the DSM, scheduled for completion in 2012, as noted previously, will probably introduce many radical conceptual changes in ways to "think about" mental illness. Integrative mental health care, the subject of this book, employs a range of assessment tools in order to examine the unique causes of symptoms of *individual* clients.

CHAPTER 3

~~~~~

Recommending Treatment and Making Referrals

GROWING use of nonconventional treatments in mental health care is taking place in the context of increasing awareness of the limitations of conventional pharmacological and other conventional treatments. Research in the neurosciences will certainly continue to yield important advances that include novel pharmacological treatments and innovative clinical applications of electricity and magnetic fields. Many neurotransmitters that are now poorly understood will probably provide important future clues about both normal and abnormal mental and emotional states. Unfortunately, there is an enormous discrepancy between the sophisticated conceptual models of mental illness, grounded in the latest brain research, and the availability of new classes of drugs based on cutting-edge science. During the past few years relatively few new drugs targeting psychiatric disorders have been developed and successfully brought to market. At the same time new drug development costs continue to soar. Although pharmaceutical companies invest heavily in new drug development, recent legislation has mandated stringent new FDA requirements for safety and efficacy that have increased costs and increased the steps needed to get a new drug to market. Increasing development costs of new drugs are then passed on to patients, health management organizations (HMOs), and insurance companies. The ever-escalating cost of pharmacological treatments can be seen as an invitation to examine the range of nonconventional modalities that hold promise for the treatment of depression, anxiety, schizophrenia, alcohol and drug abuse, and other major mental health problems.

In addition to the increasing cost of conventional pharmacological therapies, drug safety has recently become a major public concern. It has been estimated that in the United States alone over 100,000 hospitalized patients die annually from medications administered for appropriate reasons at indicated doses. Many prescription-related fatalities are caused by drug–drug interactions or interactions between a synthetic drug and a natural product being used to self-treat a medical or psychiatric problem. The magnitude of this problem is difficult to estimate but is likely very high, as the majority of individuals who have a mental illness use two treatments at the same time and seldom disclose their use of nonconventional therapies to their psychiatrist or primary care physician. This safety issue is of particular concern in the elderly population because roughly half of hospitalized elderly patients take seven or more prescription medications, resulting in increased risk of serious, sometimes fatal, drug–drug interactions. It has been estimated that approximately half of individuals who take conventional medications for a mental health problem experience little or no improvement in symptoms. The problem of "treatment resistance" has eluded well-funded research programs aimed at elucidating the neurobiological causes of mental illness and developing more efficacious treatments for depression and other psychiatric disorders. Poor response to conventional pharmacological treatment is related to many factors, including the limited efficacy of some drugs, and high rates of patient noncompliance due to adverse effects (e.g., weight gain, loss of sexual drive) in the context of brief impersonal "medication management" sessions that omit psychotherapy.

VARIETIES OF NONCONVENTIONAL MODALITIES

When asked about complementary and alternative therapies, most people cite vitamin C, a few other vitamin supplements, ginko biloba, and perhaps St. John's wort. While these biological substances are important nonconventional treatments, significant research advances are also taking place in somatic, mind–body, and energy-based therapies used to treat mental health problems. Many of these therapies have been used to treat a range of medical and mental health problems for hundreds, and in some cases thousands, of years; however, relatively few of them have been rigorously examined by Western-style research studies. In spite of the relative paucity of evidence for most treatments that are not part of conventional Western medicine, it has been argued that therapies used in Chinese medicine, Ayurveda homeopathy and other established world systems of medicine rest on fundamentally valid principles that cannot be verified by the empirical methods of Western science (Carlston, 2004; Richardson, 2002). Furthermore, many nonconventional therapies are difficult to evaluate using Western-style research studies, and so the evidence for them accumulates at a very gradual pace. Nonconventional modalities also receive limited coverage in mainstream medical journals (Bender, 2004). This limited coverage means that individuals who search Medline (or other established medical databases) often cannot find useful information about nonconventional therapies (Beckner & Berman, 2003). The lack of exposure hampers therapists' and patients' efforts to make reasonable choices about the most appropriate non-pharmacological treatment for their problem.

It is possible to conceptualize any nonconventional treatment modality as belonging to one of five categories:

- *Biological treatments* achieve therapeutic effects through a discrete biological mechanism of action at the molecular, cellular, or organ level (e.g., conventional medications, vitamins, minerals, medicinal herbs, amino acids, omega-3 fatty acids).
- *Somatic treatments* foster general feelings of well-being, affect the body as a whole (e.g., exercise, chiropractic treatment, massage), but do not operate through a discrete biological mechanism of action.
- *Mind–body practices* combine a particular mental technique with physical training with the goal of optimizing mind–body functioning and alleviating symptoms (e.g., yoga, tai-chi).

• *Scientifically validated forms of energy and information* include electromagnetic fields, bright light, and sound and microcurrent electrical stimulation. Specific therapeutic applications use different durations, frequencies, and power characteristics of these established forms of energy and information to achieve beneficial effects.

• *Postulated "subtle" energy therapies* have not been validated by Western science (e.g., shamanic healing, Reiki, qigong, prayer, healing touch, therapeutic touch, and techniques used in energy psychology).

TABLE 3.1 Representative Nonconventional Therapies

Biological	Somatic	Mind–Body	Validated Energy Therapies	Not Validated Subtle Energy Therapies
Improved nutrition	Exercise	Yoga	Biofeedback (including EMG, EEG, others)	Acupuncture
St. John's wort	Massage	Tai chi		Qigong
Valerian	Chiropractic	Meditation	Light therapy	Healing touch
Natural supplements (e.g., vitamins, minerals, SAMe, Omega-3 fatty acids)	Dance therapy and other expressive movement therapies	Mindfulness-based stress reduction	Binaural sound	Reiki
			Music therapy	Energy psychology
			Virtual reality exposure therapy	

SAMe - S-adenosylmethionine; EMG - electromyogram; EEG - electroencephalogram.

With the exception of postulated subtle energy therapies, rigorous scientific studies have elucidated the mechanisms of action of treatment modalities in each category, and some modalities are supported by considerable research evidence. However, as is true for many conventional pharmacological treatments of mental illness, many CAM modalities remain in use on the basis of professional consensus in the absence of strong evidence. Treatments supported by limited evidence are not reviewed here. However, it is important to note that new research findings are continually coming to light. Future research studies will probably confirm the effectiveness of certain approaches while refuting others.

In view of how little we understand about the causes of mental illness, it is reasonable to speculate that the effectiveness of certain conventional and nonconventional treatments may be related to subtle biological, energetic, or informational mechanisms of action that have not (yet) been clearly elucidated by science and may even lie outside the purview of orthodox Western medicine. Most nonconventional therapies that have been rigorously evaluated in Western-style research studies involve a well-described biological mechanism of action. Examples of scientifically validated nonconventional *biological* treatments of depressed mood include St. John's wort (*Hypericum perforatum*), S-adenosylmethionine (SAMe), 5-hydroxytryptophan (5-HTP), and folic acid. In contrast to therapies whose beneficial effects are the result of an established biological mechanism of action, most mind–body therapies and nonconventional therapies involving light, electricity, sound, or subtle energies have not yet been evaluated in rigorously designed scientific studies. Mind–body therapies that are seen as clinically (as opposed to scientifically) beneficial for the prevention or treatment of mental illness include meditation, tai chi, and yoga. Reiki, qigong, and homeopathy, which are based on postulated subtle energies, are widely used to treat mental and emotional symptoms but have not been verified by Western science. In spite of the absence of compelling evidence from research studies, mind–body therapies as well as homeopathy, qigong, Reiki, and other "energy" healing practices are widely embraced in popular U.S. culture and Western Europe and are gaining acceptance among psychiatrists, family physicians, and psychologists because they have general beneficial effects on health and well-being and do not pose risks or increase practitioner liability. Readers interested in a more comprehensive review of the evidence for the broad range of nonconventional and integrative treatments are referred to Lake (2006).

NONCONVENTIONAL BIOLOGICAL TREATMENTS

Dietary Modifications

Malnourishment is frequently associated with mental illness. Increasing the amount and quality of protein in the diet, reducing amounts of refined sugar and caffeine, and moderating alcohol consumption often result in improved overall mental health. Highly restrictive diets probably reduce the distractibility and hyperactivity in some children diagnosed with ADHD; however, findings of studies done to date are inconsistent (Rojas & Chan, 2005). Foods rich in the B-vitamins, folate, pyridoxine (B-6), and methyl-cobalamin (B-12) are beneficial for general mental health because the vitamins function as essential cofactors in the synthesis of serotonin, dopamine, and norepinephrine (Bourre, 2006; Agency for Healthcare Research and Quality Publication, 2005; Werbach, 1999). Evidence from epidemiological studies suggests that increased consumption of fish high in omega-3 essential fatty acids may be protective against depressed mood (Tiemeier, 2003; Silvers, 2002). Diets high in fish may also reduce the risk of developing Alzheimer's disease and other forms of dementia (Kalmijn, 1997). Specific dietary interventions for common mental health problems are reviewed in more detail in Part II.

Natural Products

Like conventional pharmaceuticals, nonconventional biological therapies have beneficial effects when they change brain function in specific ways. Mechanisms of action of herbals, amino acids, and other natural products include increasing brain levels of particular neurotransmitters, "rebalancing" postulated dysregulations between two or more neurotransmitters, and indirectly addressing mental and emotional symptoms by changing the general activity of parts of the brain involved in mood regulation, higher cognitive functioning, memory, alcohol or drug craving, sleep and wakefulness, and so forth. In North and South America as well as Europe and Australia vitamins, minerals, amino acids, essential fatty acids, hormones, and herbs are widely used to treat, or self-treat, mental illness.

Most herbs used to treat mental illness in the United States and other Western countries are known to us from the tradition of naturopathic herbal medicine. Certain herbals are supported by strong evidence, whereas others have little or no evidence (Sarris, 2007; Mischoulon, 2007). A systematic review of placebo-controlled trials on St. John's wort for moderately depressed mood identified several studies that showed superior efficacy compared to placebo; however, many studies had inconsistent outcomes and were limited by design problems (Linde et al., 1996). Ginkgo biloba is probably beneficial in some cases of Alzheimer's disease and age-related memory loss, but the findings of controlled trials are inconsistent (Ernst, 1999; Birks & Grimley, 2004). Kava is beneficial for generalized anxiety but not panic attacks (Pittler & Ernst, 2004). In a recent systematic review of controlled studies, Krystal and Ressler (2002) concluded that valerian root extract is a safe and effective treatment for situational insomnia. Golden root (*Rhodiola rosea*), introduced to Western Europe and the United States from Russia, is proving to be beneficial for depressed mood and as a cognitive enhancer, and preliminary findings suggest that this herb may be especially beneficial for mood changes related to menopause (Brown & Gerbarg, 2004). More studies are needed to confirm the safety and efficacy of golden root before it can be widely recommended for the treatment of depressed mood. Compared to widely used Western herbs, relatively little research has been conducted on compound herbal formulas from non-Western healing traditions. Whereas Western herbal remedies are generally based on a single plant or plant part, compound herbal formulas consisting of a dozen or more separate plants are used in Chinese, Ayurveda, and Tibetan systems of medicine.

In addition to herbals, many other kinds of natural products are being used in the United States, Canada, and Western Europe to treat mental and emotional symptoms. The use of omega-3 essential fatty acids for depression, bipolar mood swings, and attention-deficit disorder (ADD) is supported by growing but still inconclusive evidence (Ross et al., 2007). Dehydroepiandrosterone (DHEA), a precursor of testosterone, has been shown to reduce the severity of depressed mood and may also be beneficial in some cases of schizophrenia characterized by predominantly negative symptoms (Schmidt et al., 2005; Strous et al., 2003).

Functional medicine is an evolving paradigm that views illness phenomena as *informational changes* in intercellular communication processes manifesting as pathology at the level of cell and organ networks (Bland, 1999). Functional medicine argues that mental illness is the result of interactions between biological factors, lifestyle, diet, and environmental influences that cause changes in genetic expression manifesting as mental and emotional symptoms.

Serotonin syndrome is a potentially life-threatening situation resulting from excessive levels of the neurotransmitter serotonin in the central nervous system. The syndrome can result from high doses of drugs that affect brain serotonin level, including SSRIs and other antidepressants. It can also be a consequence of interactions between medications and supplements that affect brain serotonin levels, including 5-HTP. Symptoms of serotonin syndrome range from mild agitation, dilated pupils, elevated heart rate, and perspiration to potentially life-threatening symptoms such as hyperthermia (body temperature above 104), acute confusion, delirium, muscular rigidity, seizures, renal failure, coma, and death. Any client with symptoms that may reflect an on-going serotonin syndrome should be advised to seek immediate medical care.

Functional medicine approaches used to treat mental illness include targeted amino acid therapy (TAAT) and high-dose supplementation with certain vitamins and minerals. It has been suggested that taking large doses of specific amino acids, which are required building blocks of neurotransmitters, can correct imbalances in neurotransmitters and improve symptoms of mental illness. In fact, research studies show that specific amino acids are beneficial for individuals with depression, anxiety, insomnia, and ADD. Amino acids are often used in combination with conventional drugs but can also be beneficial when taken alone. A commonly used integrative treatment strategy for depressed mood is combining 5-HTP, the immediate precursor or serotonin, with a conventional antidepressant (Shaw et al., 2004; Sargent et al., 1998). This combination can result in significant improvement in mood at relatively lower doses of conventional antidepressants, compared to antidepressants alone. However, because of the risk of serotonin syndrome, safety issues must be taken into account when considering recommending this strategy. In addition to specific herbals, amino acids, vitamins, and essential fatty acids, multi-ingredient nutrient formulas are increasingly being used to treat mental health problems including depressed mood, bipolar disorder and others. Table 3.2 lists nonconventional biological therapies that have been shown to be efficacious for depression, anxiety, cyclic mood changes, psychosis, and the other common mental health problems discussed in this book. More detailed reviews of the evidence for modalities used to treat specific mental health problems are provided in Part II.

Certain nonconventional biological modalities can be used safely with antidepressants, antipsychotics, or antianxiety drugs to increase their efficacy, reduce adverse effects, or both, whereas others should not be combined with drugs because of potential toxic interactions. Integrative strategies that are both safe and effective are reviewed in Part II. General safety issues involved in considering the use of non-conventional therapies and specific safety problems associated with specific combinations of nonconventional biological modalities and medications are discussed below. The vignettes in Part II cover (1) the reasoning process involved in identifying evidence-based non-conventional and integrative treatment strategies that address a particular client's core symptom(s), (2) formulating an adequate treatment plan, (3) if needed, recommending treatment, and (4) if indicated, making appropriate referrals for consultation and treatment by a conventionally trained or alternative medical practitioner.

As is true for many conventional pharmacological treatments, the safety and effectiveness of some nonconventional biological treatments have been verified by controlled, double-blind studies and rigorous systematic reviews of those studies. For example, combining specific vitamins, essential fatty acids, amino acids, or other natural products with a conventional drug can add to, and in some cases accelerate, the effect of the drug on depression, anxiety, psychosis, or insomnia (Coppen & Bailey, 2000; Jazayeri et al., 2008). Supplementing the diet with certain vitamins can result in significant improvements in mood and cognitive functioning and a reduction in anxiety. Validated nonconventional biological treatments of depressed mood include St. John's wort, SAMe, 5-HTP, folic acid (a B-vitamin), and ecosapentanoic acid (EPA), an omega-3 essential fatty acid (Thachil et al., 2007). Folate, especially in the form of methylfolinic acid, has beneficial antidepressant effects when taken alone and acts synergistically when combined with a conventional antidepressant (Kelly et al., 2004). Other B-vitamins, including B-6 and B-12, are sometimes beneficial against depression. Less robust

TABLE 3.2 Representative Nonconventional Biological Therapies for Mental Health Problems

	Herbs	Vitamins and minerals	Amino acids	Essential fatty acids	Hormones
Depression	St. John's wort, golden root	Folate, B-6, B-12, C, D, and E; possibly selenium	SAMe, also 5-HTP, acetyl-L-carnitine; possibly L-tyrosine and L-phenylalanine	Omega-3s (especially EPA)	DHEA
Anxiety	Kava; ashwagondha; passion flower extract; essential oils of lavender and rosemary (applied to skin)	Niacin for general calming; Phosphorous for panic attacks; magnesium for GAD	L-theanine; 5-HTP and L-tryptophan		DHEA for PTSD
Hyperactivity and distractibility	Extract of the bark of the French maritime pine, *Bacopa monnieri* ("Brahmi")	Zinc supplementation primarily for hyperactivity; iron (for children who are iron-deficient)	Acetyl-L-carnitine	High-dose omega-3 essential fatty acids	None
Cyclic mood changes and bipolar disorder	St. John's wort possibly effective for SAD	Folate plus lithium may improve response in manic phase; monthly B-12 injections; magnesium supplementation	L-tryptophan Acute tyrosine depletion	Omega-3s Choline plus lithium may improve response	None

TABLE 3.2 *Continued*

	Herbs	Vitamins and minerals	Amino acids	Essential fatty acids	Hormones
Psychotic symptoms and schizophrenia	Certain Ayurvedic herbals; ginkgo biloba may augment conventional antipsychotics	Niacin, folate, and thiamin may augment antipsychotics	Glycine may augment antipsychotics	High doses of omega-3s (especially EPA), especially in early acute phase of illness	DHEA plus antipsychotic especially for negative sx estrogen for postpartum psychosis
Mild cognitive impairment and dementia	Ginkgo biloba (all dementias) kami-untan-to (a compound herbal formula)	B-12 and thiamin; taking C and E together may reduce Alzheimer's risk	Acetyl-L-carnitine for mild dementia	Phosphatidyl serine	DHEA may slow decline vascular dementia; testosterone may slow decline in XXX
Alcohol and substance abuse	Ashwagondha in narcotics abuse and withdrawal; valerian for benzodiazepine withdrawal	B-vitamins (especially thiamin); antioxidants may reduce hangover severity; magnesium, zinc may improve cognitive confusion	Taurine may reduce alcohol withdrawal severity; SAMe may reduce alcohol craving	Omega-3s may reduce alcohol withdrawal severity	None

TABLE 3.2 *Continued*

	Herbs	Vitamins and minerals	Amino acids	Essential fatty acids	Hormones
Insomnia and fatigue	Valerian extract; ginkgo biloba (with antidepressant) may increase sleep quality; ashwagondha	Folate, thiamin, and magnesium	5-HTP and L-tryptophan	None	Melatonin; DHEA may increase REM sleep

SAMe - S-adenosylmethionine; 5-HTP - 5-hydroxytryptophan; EPA - ecosapentantoic acid; DHEA - dehydroepiandrosterone; GAD - generalized anxiety disorder; PTSD - posttraumatic stress disorder; SAD - seasonal affective disorder; REM - rapid eye movement.

evidence exists for antidepressant effects of the amino acid acetyl-L-carnitine and the prohormone DHEA but reports of improved mood are often associated with regular use of these natural products also. High doses of niacin are used to treat psychotic symptoms in people with schizophrenia, sometimes with dramatically positive results. In addition to these integrative approaches, regular exercise, changes in nutrition, bright light exposure, and somatic and mind–body techniques can be safely combined with conventional pharmacological therapies.

When certain biological modalities are combined, their beneficial synergistic effects may translate into lower effective doses of conventional medications (i.e., compared to the use of medications alone), a reduced incidence of adverse effects, greater adherence to medications, faster response to treatment, and reduced risk of relapse. Numerous studies have confirmed that certain vitamins and amino acids can be safely combined with conventional antidepressants, antipsychotics, and antianxiety drugs. Examples of integrative treatment strategies known to have beneficial synergistic effects include combinations of folate, B-12, and SAMe with a synthetic antidepressant. Folate and B-12 are essential cofactors in the synthesis of SAMe and are centrally involved in the synthesis of neurotransmitters from this amino acid.

In contrast to natural products that produce beneficial clinical effects, certain herbals and supplements are probably no more effective than placebos. However, the placebo effect also plays a significant role when conventional medical treatments achieve beneficial outcomes (Dixon & Sweeney, 2000). For example, meta-analyses suggest that many conventional drugs used to treat depressed mood and other mental illnesses are probably no more effective than placebos (Kirsch et al., 2002; Thase, 2002; Sussman, 2004; Kirsch, 2008). How placebos alleviate symptoms is poorly understood, and there is still no adequate explanatory theory of this phenomenon.

NONCONVENTIONAL NONBIOLOGICAL MODALITIES

In addition to vitamins, herbals and other nonconventional biological modalities, different kinds of somatic, mind–body, and energy-information modalities are used to treat or self-treat mental health problems. The following sections are intended to provide a broad overview of these treatment categories. Part II contains more detailed reviews of the research evidence for specific somatic, mind–body, and energy-information modalities as treatments of depression, anxiety, psychosis, and other other common mental health problems. Table 3.3 lists representative somatic, mind–body, and energy-information modalities in relation to the core symptoms for which these therapies may be efficacious.

TABLE 3.3 Representative Somatic, Mind–Body, and Energy-Information Therapies

	Somatic Therapies	Mind–Body Therapies	Energy-Information Modalities Validated	Not Validated Subtle Energy-Information Modalities
Depression	Exercise Partial sleep deprivation Chiropractic	Yoga	Bright light exposure High-density negative ions Dim green, blue, or red light Music	Reiki Homeopathy Religious and spiritual beliefs Healing touch Qigong
Anxiety	Massage Exercise Dance therapy and other expressive movement therapies	Mindfulness-based stress reduction; other forms of meditation Guided imagery Yoga	EEG biofeedback and heart rate variability (HRV) biofeedback (other biofeedback approaches) Music Virtual reality graded exposure therapy (VRGET)	Acupuncture Qigong Healing touch Reiki Homeopathy Religious or spiritual beliefs Energy psychology
Hyperactivity and distractibility	Massage	Yoga Meditation	EEG biofeedback	Homeopathy
Cyclic mood changes and mania	Exercise	Mindfulness training Meditation Yoga	Early morning bright light exposure	None
Psychosis	None	Yoga Spiritually oriented group therapy	None	Religious or spiritual beliefs Laser acupuncture Qigong

TABLE 3.3 *Continued*

	Somatic Therapies	Mind–Body Therapies	Energy-Information Modalities Validated	Not Validated Subtle Energy-Information Modalities
Dementia and cognitive decline	Exercise Massage	None	Transcranial electrical stimulation Music Bright light exposure EEG biofeedback	Healing touch
Substance abuse	Exercise	Mindfulness training Meditation Spiritually focused groups Yoga	EEG biofeedback Virtual reality graded exposure therapy (VRGET) Dim morning light	Qigong
Insomnia and fatigue	Exercise Passive body heating	Yoga Bright light exposure EEG biofeedback Cranioelectrotherapy stimulation		Acupuncture

SOMATIC AND MIND–BODY APPROACHES

Numerous studies have found that exercise has beneficial effects on depressed mood and anxiety in adults; however, there is less evidence of the benefits of exercise in children and adolescents (Ströhle, 2008; Larun et al., 2006). Regular aerobic or strengthening exercise results in increased CNS levels of dopamine, norepinephrine, and serotonin, which are known to reduce the severity of depressed mood. The mood-enhancing effects of regular exercise may be comparable to those of cognitive therapy and conventional antidepressants. Regular therapeutic massages are known to be beneficial for moderately severe symptoms of anxiety (Kim et al., 2002). Numerous studies show that the regular practice of yoga helps to alleviate symptoms of depression, anxiety, insomnia, and substance abuse (Shannahoff-Khalsa, 2003). Practicing yoga also reduces the severity of obsessions and compulsions (Chaudhary et al., 1988; Shannahoff-Khalsa et al., 1999). Findings of randomized controlled trials comparing chiropractic spinal manipulation with sham spinal manipulation suggest that symptoms of moderate depressed mood, generalized anxiety, and overall psychological functioning improve with regular treatment (Middleton & Pollard, 2005). Dance movement therapy and other expressive movement therapies probably improve mood and overall emotional functioning in depressed individuals; however, most evidence for these approaches comes from case studies (Ritter, 1996).

Scientifically Validated Energy-Information Therapies

Scientifically validated energy-information modalities are based on classically described forms of energy or information found in light, sound, and electricity and are believed to alter functioning of the brain or body in beneficial ways. Specific applications include the use of light, high-density negative ions, cranio-electrotherapy stimulation musical tones, biofeedback, and virtual reality exposure therapy.

Light Exposure Therapy

Many studies have investigated bright light exposure as a treatment for depression and insomnia. It is well established that full-spectrum bright light simulating early morning sunlight causes suppression of melatonin production by the pineal gland, resulting in improved mood in those suffering from seasonal affective disorder (SAD). A systematic review and meta-analysis of controlled studies concluded that regular exposure to artificial or natural bright light in the early morning is as effective as conventional antidepressants for both seasonal and nonseasonal depressed mood (Golden et al., 2005). A separate systematic review concluded that early morning full-spectrum bright light exposure is only "modestly" effective for the treatment of people with unipolar depressed mood (Tuunainen et al., 2004). The most recent systematic review of studies on bright light exposure for nonseasonal depressed mood found that combining bright light exposure with conventional antidepressants improved outcomes, but bright light alone was ineffective (Even et al., 2008). Exposure to dim morning blue or red light might be as effective as bright light for individuals who experience seasonal depressed mood (Wileman et al., 2001). Depressed individuals exposed to low-intensity artificial light 2 hours before sunrise ("dawn simulation") may achieve an accelerated response to antidepressants (Benedetti et al., 2003). Extensive research has also validated early morning bright light exposure therapy as an effective treatment of insomnia related to disturbances of normal circadian rhythms caused by shift work or jet lag. However, clients should be cautioned that bright light exposure late in the day can *worsen* symptoms of insomnia (Campbell et al., 1995). When bright light exposure is used to treat a circadian sleep disturbance, taking melatonin before bedtime sometimes results in more rapid improvement (Kayumov et al., 2001). Clients who use bright light to treat depression, fatigue, or insomnia should be warned to avoid sun lamps that emit harmful ultraviolet rays. In addition to its established effects on melatonin, bright light exposure may facilitate subtle *energetic* or *informational* changes in the biomagnetic field activity of the brain, resulting in beneficial changes in depressed mood and other symptoms (Curtis, 2004).

High-Density Negative Ions
Non-ionizing negative ions are a promising emerging treatment for depression. Several controlled studies have concluded that regular exposure to high-density negative ions has beneficial effects on seasonal depressed mood and is probably as effective as bright light exposure in this population (Terman & Terman, 1995). In one randomized sham-controlled study, almost two-thirds of depressed individuals exposed to high-density negative ions reported significant improvements in mood, compared to only 15% of individuals exposed to low-density negative ions. In another study, depressed individuals randomized to bright light exposure versus high-density negative ions experienced equivalent improvements in mood (Terman et al., 1998).

Cranioelectrotherapy Stimulation

Cranioelectrotherapy stimulation (CES) is a kind of electromagnetic energy therapy used to treat chronic pain, anxiety, and insomnia. This treatment is based on the application of an extremely weak electrical current to the head or neck, using electrodes. It has been suggested that micro-current stimulation of the brain causes changes in brain-wave characteristics that result in symptom reduction. A meta-analysis of double-blind controlled trials on CES for generalized anxiety concluded that this approach results in short-term improvement of symptom severity (DeFelice, 1997). Research findings on CES for insomnia are highly inconsistent; the sleep-inducing benefits of very weak electrical currents probably depend on current strength, frequency, and treatment duration.

Music and Sound

Music has been used historically in many world healing traditions to foster relaxation and as a form of treatment for anxiety and depression. Research findings suggest that certain musical tones probably have beneficial effects on depressed mood, anxiety, and poor concentration. Listening to relaxing music may be more effective than cognitive therapy in generally anxious patients (Kerr, et al., 2001). Certain musical tones or tonal progressions probably have general beneficial effects on mental health. It has been established that listening to music increases brain endorphin levels, which may result in improved mood (Drohan, 1999). Sounds in certain frequency ranges delivered to the ears at slightly different times (i.e., "binaural sound") may improve symptoms of depressed mood and generalized anxiety (Milligan & Wald Koetter, 2000; Atwater, 1999).

Biofeedback Training

Numerous studies confirm that many forms of biofeedback, using information obtained from EEG, galvanic skin response (GSR) or EMG recordings, reduce symptoms of anxiety, inattention, and depressed mood (Vanathy et al., 1998; Gruzelier & Egner, 2005; Monastra et al., 2005). EEG biofeedback training may be as effective as conventional medications for the treatment of generalized anxiety (Sarkar et al., 1999), and certain EEG biofeedback protocols have been found to reduce the severity of depressed mood (Baehr &

Rosenfeld, 2003). Regular weekly biofeedback training and conventional antianxiety medications probably have comparable efficacy in treating chronic generalized anxiety. Measures of heart rate variability (HRV), used in a form of biofeedback aimed at changing the brain's general level of arousal, may reduce the severity of depressed mood (McCraty et al., 2001). There is evidence that subtle aspects of the heart's rhythm become synchronized with certain characteristics of the brain's electrical activity and that the "dance" between the heart and the brain is involved in the regulation of emotions (Schwartz & Russek, 1996; McCraty et al., 2001). Emerging biofeedback approaches aimed at improving depressed mood will probably combine HRV and EEG biofeedback.

Virtual Reality Graded Exposure Therapy
Virtual reality graded exposure therapy (VRGET) is an emerging computer-enhanced exposure therapy that combines advanced computer technologies to create realistic virtual environments that provide visual, auditory, tactile, vestibular, and olfactory cues to patients in the context of cognitive–behavioral therapy. The goal of VRGET is to evoke a deep sense of immersion in the reality of a simulated world that provides graded levels of exposure to a feared circumstance or object, resulting in rapid desensitization (Wiederhold & Wiederhold, 2000). During VRGET the therapist tracks the client's arousal level by monitoring heart rate and respiration while providing verbal cues about breathing and other relaxation strategies.

Energy-Information Therapies Not Validated by Western Science
This category includes therapies based on so-called "subtle" energies that have not been validated by Western-style research studies. Chinese, Ayurvedic, and Tibetan systems of medicine employ a variety of energy therapies to restore balance in the body. Prayer, healing touch, qigong, reiki, and emerging techniques used in energy psychology also fall into the category of subtle energy therapies. Acupuncture and energetic treatment modalities employed in Chinese, Ayurvedic, and Tibetan medicine, as well as in indigenous shamanic healing rituals and other traditional systems of medicine, are based on "qi," "prana," and other postulated subtle energies

believed to have beneficial effects on general well-being (i.e., improvements in physical and mental health; Engebretson & Wardell, 2007). Acupuncture is used in both Chinese and Tibetan forms of medicine, but not in Ayurveda. Many studies have rigorously evaluated the therapeutic claims of acupuncture for the treatment of depressed mood, anxiety, insomnia, psychosis, substance abuse, and other mental health problems (Birch, 2004; Pilkington et al., 2007). Although certain acupuncture techniques are probably more effective than others for specific mental health problems, research findings to date are highly inconsistent (see next section) (British Acupuncture Council, 2002). In this context it is important to comment that research on acupuncture and other energetic modalities is constrained by basic differences in the conceptual foundations of Western and non-Western systems of medicine.

Qigong and therapeutic touch probably help reduce symptoms of anxiety and improve feelings of well-being. Reiki, a form of energy healing from Japan, may be beneficial in some cases of depressed mood and anxiety. Serious studies on prayer and other forms of "directed intention" as treatments for mental illness are only beginning to take place. Group expectation effects probably result in reports of beneficial outcomes associated with prayer and energy healing; however, emerging research findings suggest that directed human intention can influence brain functioning and possibly also affect the health and well-being of other persons, even at a distance (Achterberg et al., 2005). A more complete understanding of therapeutic outcomes associated with acupuncture and other subtle energy therapies may come from research progress in the neurosciences, complexity theory, and quantum field theory, resulting in novel paradigms that take into account putative non-local effects of consciousness in healing (Dossey, 1997; Shang, 2001; Hankey, 2004).

Acupuncture

Beneficial effects of acupuncture are probably related to established neurophysiological mechanisms as well as energy-based principles that have not been elucidated by Western science. The cumulative case report and research literature on the use of acupuncture in the treatment of mental health is vast and cannot be adequately summarized here (Flaws & Lake, 2001). Systematic reviews of sham-controlled studies on manual acupuncture, electroacupuncture, and laser acupuncture for depressed mood report inconsistent findings (Mukaino et al., 2005; Smith & Hay, 2005; Leo & Ligot, 2007; Wang et al., 2008). It is significant that the only systematic review that included studies published in Chinese-language journals found evidence of beneficial effects of acupuncture on general emotional well-being (Wang et al., 2008). Findings from studies on acupuncture as a treatment for anxiety, substance abuse, psychosis, and insomnia are also inconsistent. Findings of a pilot study suggest that stimulation of certain acupuncture points improves symptoms of post-traumatic stress disorder (PTSD) (Hollifield, Sinclair-Lian & Hammerschlag 2007). There is still no consensus on what constitutes "sham" treatment in studies on acupuncture, and it has been suggested that there can be no sham acupuncture protocol because, according to Chinese medical theory, stimulation of virtually any point on the body can potentially result in beneficial effects. Other factors that have interfered with efforts to rigorously evaluate acupuncture using Western-style research studies include differences between Western and Chinese medicine in the diagnostic criteria used to define study populations, the small sizes of most published studies, lack of randomization to true acupuncture versus "sham" acupuncture, differences in type of acupuncture used, specific needling technique, duration of treatment, intervals between treatment, and total number of sessions (Leo & Ligot, 2007). Large studies based on standard treatment protocols are needed to determine whether acupuncture results in general improvement in emotional well-being or has therapeutic effects on specific mental health problems, including depressed mood and anxiety.

Homeopathy

Homeopathy is a kind of subtle energy healing technique based on the concept of treating the symptom with minute doses of . . . the symptom. Homeopathic remedies may mediate beneficial changes through subtle changes in energy or information in the immune system and brain that may not be explainable in the context of Western science. There is a widely shared perception in the Western medical community that beneficial outcomes in response to homeopathic remedies are due to placebo effects (Ernst & Resch, 1996). However, some researchers contend that conventional medical research methods lack the means to evaluate the mechanism of action of homeopathic remedies, which has been described as a special kind of vital energy. It has been suggested, for example, that the mechanism of action of homeopathy and so-called energy healing methods may be consistent with large-scale quantum field effects or other kinds of energy or information that operate at subtle levels in the body and brain and cannot be reduced to electromagnetic waves, molecular interactions, or other well described mechanisms of action underlying conventional treatments (Smith 2004). Homeopathic remedies are best administered by a skilled homeopathic physician after the unique energetic "constitutional type" of the client has been determined.

The Role of Religious Affiliation and Spiritual Beliefs in Mental Health

The majority of ill people believe that their religious or spiritual beliefs have beneficial effects on their health (Larson & Milano, 1996). Many studies show that religious involvement or spiritual practice is associated with generally better mental health compared to individuals who are not engaged in religious or spiritual activities (Tsuang et al., 2002; Gartner et al., 1991; Koenig & Futterman, 1995).

Prayer and Distant Healing Intention

It is estimated that approximately 30% of U.S. adults use prayer in efforts to improve their health (McCaffrey et al., 2004). A physician survey found that 40% of family physicians pray with their patients, and most believe that prayer has therapeutic effects on their patients' medical problems (Anderson et al., 1993). A systematic review found that beneficial effects on medical and mental health problems were reported in 60% of studies of prayer and healing intention (Astin et al., 2000). A rigorous examination of the effects of prayer and healing intention on mental health is difficult to achieve because of basic differences between patients' and healers' belief systems and problems controlling for subjective variables that may interfere with study designs or influence outcomes (Abbott, 2000). Extensive case reports suggest that prayer and other forms of healing intention frequently result in beneficial effects on physical and mental health (Benor, 2002). It has been suggested that a widely shared belief in the efficacy of prayer and healing intention significantly influences positive outcomes when prayer is used for self-healing (Palmer et al., 2004). A review of the research literature on prayer and other forms of healing intention suggests that spiritual healing approaches may have subtle effects on the physiology and energetic constitution of complex living systems including the human body and brain (Zahourek, 2004). Small controlled trials have found above-chance correlations between EEG activity and brain metabolic activity, suggesting that healing intention may affect the brain functioning of other persons at a distance (Standish et al., 2003; Radin, 2004; Achterberg et al., 2005). The beneficial effects of prayer and other forms of healing intention cannot be adequately explained by contemporary Western scientific theories, and their elucidation probably will require fundamental advances in science.

Reiki

Reiki is an energy-based healing practice that was introduced to the West from Japan in the 19th century. In this form of energy healing direct contact between the Reiki practitioner and the patient is not considered necessary. Claims of beneficial effects from Reiki are based on the belief that skillfully directed intention can result in improved physical or psychological functioning. Reiki treatments are administered directly to the patient or across considerable distances. Preliminary research findings suggest that depressed or anxious individuals who receive regular Reiki treatments experience reductions in the severity of their symptoms (Shore, 2004). Therapeutic effects of Reiki on mental health may be associated with changes in brain electrical activity and autonomic arousal level (Mackay et al., 2004).

Healing Touch and Therapeutic Touch

Healing touch is another form of subtle energy healing used to treat both physical and emotional symptoms. Specific healing touch techniques include "charka spreading," "mind clearing," and "stopping." Healing touch practitioners claim that "energetic" contact between the practitioner and patient has beneficial effects on physical and emotional well-being. Like Reiki, healing touch does not employ direct touch; rather, the practitioner positions his or her hands over the patient's body to achieve certain kinds of beneficial energetic effects. In contrast to healing touch and Reiki, therapeutic touch practitioners use gentle physical touch on specific parts of the patient's body. Benor (2002) published a comprehensive review of studies on healing touch and therapeutic touch.

Energy Psychology

Energy psychology is a relatively new development that purports to manipulate the energetic characteristics of the same meridians conceptualized in Chinese medicine with the goal of improving mental health (Gallo, 1999). Thought field therapy and emotional freedom technique are specific energy psychology methods that have become popular in recent years in spite of limited evidence supporting their efficacy. Few studies have tested the claims of energy psychology, and existing findings have been negative or inconclusive.

STEPS IN PLANNING INTEGRATIVE MENTAL HEALTH CARE

The first step in planning an appropriate integrative treatment plan involves identifying specific modalities supported by the strongest evidence of efficacy for a particular symptom. The vignettes in Part II emphasize modalities supported by good research evidence for the treatment of common mental health problems. The formulation often suggests reasonable treatment choices addressing the biological, somatic, or mind–body *causes* or psychological or spiritual *meanings* of symptoms (see Chapter 2).

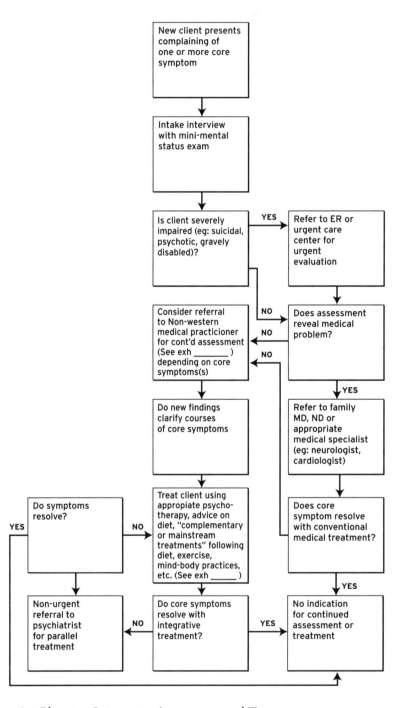

Figure 3.1 Planning Integrative Assessment and Treatment

Any conventional and nonconventional treatment modality can be classified according to the level of evidence that supports its use for a particular mental health problem. *Well-substantiated* treatments are supported by compelling evidence of efficacy when used to treat a particular symptom. *Provisional* treatments are widely used to treat a particular problem but may be supported by limited evidence from well-designed studies. At the lowest tier of evidence, many conventional and nonconventional modalities are used to treat or self-treat mental illness in the absence of supporting evidence or the presence of clear negative findings confirming that they do not work as claimed. Western biomedicine regards *empirically validated* modalities as the most substantiated kinds of treatment, yet relatively few pharmacological treatments are substantiated by consistent positive findings of large, double-blind studies or meta-analyses of well-designed studies. Many conventional and nonconventional treatments or procedures are supported by provisional or limited evidence but continue to be used on the basis of consensus among the physicians or alternative medical practitioners who prescribe or perform them.

In cases when you have offered everything you can within your scope of practice—and psychotherapy has either not provided relief or has been declined, and advice on nutrition, exercise, stress management, and certain natural supplements has not been beneficial—it is reasonable, legally defensible, and ethically responsible to refer the client to a psychiatrist, family physician, naturopathic physician, or appropriate alternative medical practitioner for consultation. If you are concerned that an undiagnosed, untreated, or inadequately treated medical problem may be affecting your client's mental health or safety, you should refer him or her to a physician or—if the client does not have a family physician or N.D.—to an urgent care center. Just as you would want to know about the training background, experience, and reputation of a psychiatrist, naturopathic physician, or family physician before recommending a conventionally trained Western physician, you should likewise try to find out about the professional qualifications and reputations of nonconventional practitioners before making specific referrals for treatment. When considering recommending a particular treatment approach or making a referral to a psychiatrist, naturopathic physician, family physician, or alternative medical practitioner for treatment using a particular conventional or nonconventional therapy, it is important to keep the following questions in mind:

- Does research evidence support the use of the treatment being considered for your client's mental health problem(s)? What is the strength of the evidence?
- What are reasonable conventional and nonconventional treatment modalities?
- What risks are associated with the preferred modality, including known adverse effects and interactions with any conventional medications or natural products your client is taking?
- How has your client previously responded to other conventional and nonconventional treatments, including the treatment you are recommending?
- Is a qualified practitioner of the therapy under consideration available in your community and affordable to your client?

Table 3.4 lists the logical steps involved in assessment, formulation, treatment recommendations depending on your client's mental health problem(s), and referral recommendations (knowing when and how to refer clients depending on the type and severity of their symptoms, pertinent psychiatric, family and medical history, treatments that have already been tried, and practical issues of cost, insurance coverage, and availability of qualified clinicians). Ideally, treatment recommendations and referrals should be based on (1) the strength of evidence that a specific conventional or nonconventional modality will alleviate a particular symptom (or complex symptom pattern), (2) your familiarity with the modality from formal training or clinical experience, and (3) issues of cost, availability, and patient preferences.

TABLE 3.4 Treatment Planning in Integrative Mental Health Care

Initial Sessions

1. Review the evidence for appropriate conventional and nonconventional treatment approaches directed at factors identified in the formulation. Identify appropriate treatment modalities, starting with those that are most substantiated by research evidence, and advise client accordingly. Initiate treatment consistent with your training or clinical experience.

2. If consultation with a conventionally trained or CAM practitioner is indicated, refer client to practitioner.

3. In cases where more substantiated treatments have been tried previously without benefit, review history to confirm that client followed directions and treatment was appropriately administered at therapeutic dose or duration by qualified practitioner.

4. Work closely with client to develop an integrative treatment plan that is realistic, taking into account personal values and preferences, financial constraints, and availability of qualified conventional or nonconventional practitioner in your area.

5. For moderate symptoms emphasize the importance of commitment to healthy lifestyle changes, improved nutrition, mind–body practices, exercise, and an appropriate use of supplements.

6. For more severe symptoms emphasize the importance of commitment to biological treatments recommended by yourself, an M.D., N.D., or alternative medical practitioner, including conventional medications and nonconventional biological modalities, and encourage regular follow-up with the medical practitioner managing the client's care.

6. If you are a psychologist certified in psychopharmacology in your state, you may elect to prescribe medications and give advice on changing medications or doses and managing side effects. Before giving specific advice about dosing or prescribing new medications, it may be in your client's best interest (and help you limit unnecessary liability) to first consult with the conventional medical practitioner who originally prescribed the psychotropic medications.

8. Offer appropriate ongoing psychotherapy, depending on your client's level of insight and motivation.

9. Identify and answer questions about safety issues associated with recommended conventional or nonconventional treatments and provide detailed safety information or recommend resources your client can use to obtain reliable safety information (p. 29 Appendix A for useful books on safety). When addressing questions about medication safety issues, it is often helpful to refer clients to the prescribing nurse or physician. For questions about nonconventional treatments, refer clients to the alternative medical practitioner who is treating them.

10. Discuss realistic expectations of treatment course and clinical improvement.

Follow-Up Sessions

---

1. Review changes in core symptom(s) and address problems that may be interfering with adherence to treatment plan.

2. If your client is also being seen by a psychiatrist, family physician, naturopathic physician, or other Western medical or alternative practitioner, leave phone message after appointment summarizing significant new information from history, changes in treatment, adverse effects, etc. Make comments and suggestions for specialized assessment or changes in treatment plan.

3. If indicated, recommend referrals to specific conventionally trained or alternative medical practitioners for specialized assessment of symptomatic changes or newly emerging symptoms.

4. Explain to your client the significance of pertinent laboratory data from psychiatrist or other Western or alternative medical practitioner.

5. Discuss appropriate new directions in integrative management (if any) based on new assessment findings or changes in symptoms. Make appropriate recommendations or referrals as indicated.

Psychotherapy should always be offered as a core treatment of any mental health problem, including schizophrenia and other psychotic disorders. Even when conventional medications or nonconventional treatments are successful, psychodynamic issues are almost always present. Conventional pharmacological treatments and the range of nonconventional treatments discussed in this book are not intended as substitutes for psychotherapy. Clients who have the capacity for insight should be encouraged to consider participating in psychotherapy on an ongoing basis. Of course, the type of psychotherapy and frequency of visits will depend on the kind and severity of symptoms and your client's preferences and financial factors.

Regular follow-up appointments are used for reviewing client progress, continuing appropriate psychotherapy, and consulting with any conventional or alternative medical practitioners who are also treating your client. Follow-up appointments can take place at intervals of days or weeks, depending on the severity of symptoms and need for ongoing psychotherapy. I have found that patients generally improve more rapidly when engaged in supportive psychotherapy or cognitive–behavioral therapy when receiving conventional or nonconventional treatment for a mental health problem. For mild or moderate symptoms it is reasonable to schedule regular sessions every 2–4 weeks, unless, of course, your client is strongly motivated to pursue psychotherapy on a more frequent basis. Severe symptoms warrant closer supervision and thus more frequent appointments. In cases where your client's mental health problem does not improve with good adherence to an appropriate treatment plan, it is reasonable to discuss alternative treatment choices and to refer your client to qualified conventional or nonconventional practitioners who can administer those treatments.

THE INTEGRATIVE MANAGEMENT OF MILD AND MODERATE SYMPTOMS

Clients who are interested in conventional or nonconventional biological treatments for mild or moderate symptoms should be encouraged to try approaches that can be self-administered before starting a conventional pharmacological treatment, targeted amino acid therapy, or other nonconventional biological therapy that requires monitoring by a skilled clinician. Modalities that are often beneficial when symptoms are mild or moderate include dietary changes, increased exercise, guided imagery or other forms of relaxation, the use of certain vitamins and other supplements, as well as the practice of yoga, tai chi, qigong, or other mind–body modality. These self-administered approaches are often as effective as conventional medications or high-potency natural products for mild or moderate symptoms of depressed mood, anxiety, insomnia, and other common mental health problems. This approach also avoids potential problems with the adverse effects that are frequently encountered with conventional medications and high-potency natural products. If your client has worked on improving nutrition and physical activity and tried other appropriate lifestyle changes (above) but continues to experience symptoms of moderate severity, it is prudent to consider prescription medications or a specialized regimen of amino acid therapy or herbals. If you are not certified to prescribe medications, you should make a referral to a psychiatrist, naturopathic physician, or family physician for consultation. If you do not have training in targeted amino acid therapy or the use of specific herbals and other natural products, it is generally safer to refer your client to an appropriate CAM practitioner (after first going over the evidence for the various nonconventional treatment modalities in the context of your client's preferences and local availability of skilled practitioners).

Even when a client has been referred to a conventionally trained or alternative medical practitioner for specialized treatment, ongoing supportive psychotherapy or cognitive–behavioral therapy should be encouraged. Cognitive–behavioral therapy is often helpful for moderate symptoms of anxiety and depression, and supportive psychotherapy is always appropriate when a client has insight and is motivated to explore dynamic or interpersonal issues that bear on his or her symptoms. I often encourage my clients to keep a journal in order to monitor progress and record any problems that arise in the course of treatment. It is prudent to refer a client to a psychiatrist, naturopathic physician, or family physician when symptoms of mild or moderate severity remain unchanged or become worse following 1 month of consistently self-administered approaches, including vitamins, exercise, stress management, dietary changes, a regular mind–body practice, etc. Certain natural products that are known to be efficacious for mild or moderate symptoms are synergistic with conventional medications and may be safely combined with them. These include the B-vitamins (folate, thiamin, and B-12), the amino acid 5-HTP, and the omega-3 fatty acid EPA (ecosapentanoic acid). Combining these and other natural products with established pharmacological treatments can significantly improve response compared to conventional medications alone. Furthermore, successful integrative treatment strategies may allow your client to reduce the effective dose of a conventional medication, thereby reducing the risk of adverse effects.

THE INTEGRATIVE MANAGEMENT OF SEVERE SYMPTOMS

In contrast to the integrative management of mild or moderate symptoms, reasonable strategies addressing severe symptoms almost always include a pharmacological agent or a nonconventional biological treatment supported by compelling evidence. In some cases it is appropriate to recommend changes in diet, exercise, a regular stress reduction program, certain vitamin or other supplements, psychotherapy, or a mind–body practice. However, severely symptomatic individuals are often profoundly impaired and cannot be expected to consistently follow recommendations for lifestyle changes; therefore such advice is often of limited benefit.

When working with a client who is profoundly depressed, anxious, or psychotic, the most important task is to make an urgent referral to the emergency room of a local hospital or an appropriate Western physician who can evaluate your client within 24 hours. As noted above, determining whether your new client with severe symptoms is suicidal, homicidal, or gravely disabled (i.e., unable to care for his or her basic needs of food, clothing, and shelter) is your single most important responsibility. Anyone who is suicidal, homicidal, or grossly psychotic should be transported by a close friend or relative or by ambulance to the nearest emergency room or urgent care center for immediate evaluation, treatment, and possible hospitalization. Clients who are not suicidal, homicidal, or acutely psychotic but report severe symptoms of anxiety, depressed mood, cognitive impairment, psychosis, or disturbed sleep or chronic fatigue, should be referred to a psychiatrist, naturopathic physician, or primary care physician for prompt evaluation and consideration of conventional medication management. Of course, if you are certified to practice psychopharmacology, you may elect to manage this part of your client's treatment. As when evaluating mild or moderate symptoms, the first appointment with a severely symptomatic client includes a complete medical, social (including alcohol and substance abuse), cultural, and psychiatric history and prompt referral to a psychiatrist, N.D., or family physician for appropriate assessment to help determine whether there is an underlying biological cause of your client's symptoms (e.g., thyroid studies, electrolytes and complete blood count [CBC], brain scan). Thyroid hormones are commonly too low or too high in cases of severe depression and anxiety, a problem that can be effectively managed with thyroid hormone supplementation. Severe mental and emotional symptoms often accompany anemias, disturbances in electrolytes, and abnormally low or high serum cholesterol levels. Severe symptoms often remit when an underlying medical problem is correctly diagnosed and effectively treated. Alcohol and drug abuse are often associated with severe mental and emotional symptoms, including mood swings, anxiety, insomnia, and psychosis. It is always prudent to refer clients who chronically abuse alcohol or drugs to an appropriate rehabilitation program.

When primary medical causes of severe symptoms have been evaluated, treated, or excluded by a Western physician and the client has been started on an appropriate course of treatment, appointments for ongoing psychotherapy should be scheduled. The frequency of sessions will of course depend on how rapidly your client responds to treatment as well as his or her motivation and capacity to do challenging psychological work. In some cases, including clients suffering from acute symptoms of psychosis or PTSD, it is prudent to avoid the stress of insight-oriented psychotherapy or other psychotherapies (e.g., Gestalt therapy or cognitive-behavioral therapy) that can potentially destabilize an already fragile client. When a severely symptomatic client complains of two or more core symptoms, it is important to decide whether to treat both symptoms at the same time or one following the other. In my experience severely symptomatic clients generally have a specific problem that is the most important issue to address. In all cases the severely symptomatic client should be encouraged to try only those conventional, nonconventional, or combined treatments that are supported by the strongest evidence. When working with a client who has severe or acute symptoms, your primary task is *not to recommend* a specific treatment plan (unless you are certified to prescribe psychotropic medications), but to review reasonable choices in general and refer your client to an appropriate conventionally trained physician or alternative medical practitioner who is qualified to prescribe medications and monitor your client's progress.

Severe symptoms are often difficult to treat even using psychotherapy as well as the range of conventional and nonconventional therapies. Psychological issues that frequently result in poor outcomes include primitive or self-defeating defense mechanisms. However, your client may also have an undiagnosed medical problem (e.g., hypothyroidism, other endocrinological disorder, a progressive degenerative neurological disorder, cancer), be surreptitiously abusing alcohol or drugs, or have an energetic imbalance or spiritual problem that is interfering with the beneficial effects of psychotherapy and other treatments.

Designing a Practical Integrative Care Plan

In some cases there will be relatively little difference between the level of evidence supporting conventional and nonconventional treatments that constitute reasonable choices for a particular client. When this is the case, it is important to select modalities that have a high probability of success, taking into account treatments that have already been tried in the context of your client's personal preferences and financial constraints. Certain conventional or nonconventional therapies may not be available where you live and so should not be recommended, unless your client has the financial means to travel. For example, although emerging evidence supports many treatments used in Ayurvedic medicine, relatively few Ayurvedic physicians practice in the United States at present. Finding an Ayurvedic physician who specializes in mental health problems might thus prove quite complicated and time-consuming. Other modalities might be locally available through skilled medical practitioners but too expensive for your client or unacceptable for cultural reasons. Although there is emerging evidence for acupuncture as a treatment for anxiety and depression, many clients express doubts or anxiety about "having someone stick needles in me to make me feel better." Along the same lines, it is not prudent to emphasize conventional antianxiety medications for a moderately anxious client who has previously experienced serious adverse effects from similar medications. It is unlikely that your client would follow through with your recommendation to see a psychiatrist to begin such treatment, and he or she may not return to you for psychotherapy. A key point here is the fact that dietary changes, regular exercise and relaxation, a mind–body practice, and certain supplements are often as effective for moderate symptoms as conventional pharmacological treatments. You will encounter clients who regularly claim to "forget" to use a recommended treatment and do not improve. In such cases it is helpful to examine possible psychodynamic meanings or neurobiological causes of "forgetting." For example, forgetting may reflect unconscious conflicts about getting well. On the other hand, a client who forgets and has word-finding difficulties or other symptoms suggesting a more general problem with memory or judgment may be in the early stages of dementia or have an undiagnosed neurological problem.

TERMINATION

As is true when working with all clients in the context of psychotherapy, you and your client will eventually address issues of ongoing therapy versus termination. Some clients elect to terminate treatment when their symptoms have improved significantly, they have achieved important insights through psychotherapy, and healthy lifestyle changes and (if needed) medications or supplements have become a routine part of life. Of course, following termination clients may continue taking a particular conventional or nonconventional treatment to address a specific mental health problem, and with your encouragement they will hopefully also continue exercising, practicing yoga, engaging in guided imagery exercises, using bright light exposure, or doing a variety of other activities that will probably contribute to sustained improvements in their mental health.

SOME FINAL WORDS ON SAFETY

When considering treatment choices from different healing traditions, it is important to keep in mind how little is currently understood about potential toxicities resulting from combinations of specific herbals and synthetic drugs. For this reason it is generally prudent for your clients to use potent biological therapies from a particular healing tradition unless their medical care is being managed by someone who is qualified to treat them using both Western medications and biologically active therapies from another system of medicine (e.g., Chinese medicine, Ayurvedic medicine, homeopathy). Although most of you are not in a position to recommend specific combinations of potent biological treatments, it is nonetheless appropriate to caution your clients about unknown risks when biological treatments from disparate medical traditions are used at the same time.

As I noted previously, a central part of every physician's training is to "first do no harm." As a physician, I am liable for untoward medical consequences that result from the treatments I prescribe or recommend and the advice I give my patients. Because of the oath of ethical conduct I have sworn to uphold and the legal context in which all physicians practice medicine, my perspective is to do whatever is necessary to avoid undue risk. In practical terms this translates into a routine of confirming acceptable risk—preferably including the absence of reports of serious adverse effects or potentially toxic interactions—before recommending the combined use of two or more specific medications or other biological treatments from nonallopathic systems of medicine. In some cases there is explicit research evidence for synergistic effects when two biological therapies are used together.

However, there are many more anecdotal reports of *apparent* safety concerns than conclusive findings of formal studies. It is not your responsibility to verify that treatments recommended by your client's physician, naturopath, or Chinese medical practitioner are safe in combination. You can and *should*, however, encourage clients to talk with their physician if you suspect that they are using potent biological therapies associated with potential safety problems. Excellent resources on safety are included in Appendix for your use in cautioning clients about potential risks associated with herbals and other natural products in combination with conventional medications. My conservative view as a physician is that it is always prudent and legally defensible to consider recommending two or more specific biological therapies—including conventional medications, herbals, amino acids, and others—in combination *only* when there is documentation of little or no risk of toxicities and *only* when there is clear evidence for beneficial synergistic effects of the specific combination.

PART II

Clinical Problem Solving

Introduction

∽

THE balance of this book is devoted to discussion of practical clinical applications of nonconventional and integrative assessment and treatment strategies for the following:

- Moderate and severe depressed mood
- Cyclic mood swings and mania
- Generalized anxiety, panic attacks, obsessions and compulsions
- Hyperactivity and distractibility
- Psychotic symptoms and schizophrenia
- Mild cognitive impairment and dementia
- Alcohol and substance abuse
- Insomnia and daytime sleepiness

Chapters begin with concise reviews of both mainstream and nonconventional approaches used to evaluate and treat a particular core symptom. As you know from your training and clinical experience, depressed mood, anxiety, psychosis, cognitive impairment, insomnia, and other symptoms occur across a range of psychiatric disorders. On this basis, principles of assessment and treatment used in the vignettes are developed in the context of core symptoms rather than the diagnostic categories used in DSM-IV. The vignettes are composite stories derived from actual patient encounters over 15 years of my own clinical practice. They are intended as tools for psychologists and other nonmedically trained mental health professionals interested in learning how to think integratively when addressing common mental health problems in an outpatient setting. In constructing the vignettes I have assumed that clinicians who use this book work in a collegial environment with psychiatrists, naturopathic physicians, family physicians, and alternative medical practitioners, and both make and receive referrals for treatment.

Each chapter includes two vignettes that provide realistic examples of integrative management of the eight core symptom patterns discussed in this book. The first vignette in each chapter illustrates the integrative management of a client with moderate symptoms. The second vignette illustrates the management of more severe or complex cases of the core symptom pattern being addressed. The narratives illustrate the multitiered patient-centered approach that is the basis of integrative mental health care starting with the initial interview and progressing through formulation, assessment, treatment, and follow-up. The course of a therapist's relationship with a client is followed until the often subtle or complex causes or meanings of symptoms have been clearly elucidated and an effective and realistic treatment plan is in place. Included are discussions of appropriate indications for referral for urgent or routine evaluation to an emergency room, urgent care center, or a conventionally trained physician. The vignettes also provide examples of appropriate referrals to Chinese medical practitioners, naturopathic physicians, and other alternative medical practitioners. As in actual clinical practice, many vignettes involve more than one social, psychiatric, medical, energetic, or spiritual problem and show the interplay between these factors and the client's distress. The vignettes conclude with a summary of the most salient aspects of integrative management developed in the vignette.

~

CHAPTER 4

Moderate and Severe Depressed Mood

Psychiatrists and psychologists use structured interviews such as the Beck Depression Inventory to gather pertinent familial, social, and medical history and to rate the severity of the depressed mood. However, recent findings suggest that standardized rating scales used to measure outcomes are not reliable (Babgy et al., 2004). Furthermore, most psychiatrists do not rely on rigorous criteria for evaluating changes in depressed mood when assessing treatment outcomes.

Psychiatrists and family physicians sometimes order laboratory studies to determine whether an underlying medical problem may be causing a patient's depression. Frequently ordered screening tests include thyroid hormone levels, complete blood count, and blood electrolytes. (An antidepressant is often recommended before results of laboratory tests are even known.) Medical treatment is started when laboratory findings point to a medical problem (e.g., hypothyroidism). In addition, all practitioners should be aware that alcohol and drug abuse often manifest as depressed mood, and all clients who report mood changes should be asked about these issues.

Emerging research findings suggest that depressed mood is associated with abnormally low blood levels of the B-vitamin folate (Bottiglieri, 1996) and cholesterol (Bocchetta et al., 2001). In contrast, higher than normal levels of homocysteine may be associated with an increased likelihood of depressed mood (Folstein et al., 2007). The fatty acid content of red blood cells may be a useful predictor of outcomes when both conventional drugs and natural supplements are used to treat depression (Tiemeier et al., 2003). Analysis of the urine for metabolites of certain neurotransmitters can sometimes provide information about the biochemical nature of a client's depressed mood. To date, however, findings do not point to consistent correlations between urinary metabolite levels and brain neurotransmitter levels (personal communication, Kellerman, 2005). As noted previously, a specialized kind of electroencephalography called QEEG is being studied as a tool for predicting response to antidepressants and will probably become a standard assessment tool when evaluating difficult-to-treat cases of depression (Thatcher, 1998; Gallinat et al., 2000). Homeopathic physicians claim that individuals with certain energetic constitutional types are predisposed to depressed mood and are more likely to respond to specific homeopathic remedies (Gaylord & Davidson, 1998). Analysis of the VAS reflex, an approached based on Chinese medical pulse diagnosis, may help to identify conventional and nonconventional treatments that are most likely to be efficacious in the treatment of depressed mood (Ackerman, 1989).

TREATMENT

Conventional Treatments

Many different conventional antidepressants are available for the treatment of depressed mood. Various medications belong to different drug "classes," work in different ways in the brain, and have different adverse effects. Certain antidepressants are sedating and generally taken before sleep, whereas others can cause subjective feelings of activation and are most often used in the morning. In general, more recently introduced antidepressants, including the SSRIs, have fewer serious adverse effects compared to tricyclic antidepressants and other classes of antidepressants. Electroconvulsive therapy

(ECT) is sometimes used when a patient with severe depressed mood fails to respond to multiple trials of antidepressants. Transcranial magnetic stimulation is a new treatment approach that may ultimately replace ECT, but its efficacy has not yet been substantiated by research findings (Martin et al., 2004). Many studies show that psychotherapy and conventional antidepressants have equivalent efficacy as treatments of depressed mood (Casacalenda et al., 2002). Patients who engage in psychotherapy while taking an antidepressant generally have better outcomes than individuals who use either conventional approach alone (Pampallona et al., 2004).

Nonconventional Treatments

Research findings suggest that outcomes improve when conventional antidepressants are combined with certain natural products, including folate and omega-3 essential fatty acids. However, studies on omega-3s as a stand-alone therapy in depressed mood have yielded inconsistent findings (Thachil et al., 2007). St. John's wort (*Hypericum perforatum*) is widely used to treat depressed mood. A systematic review of double-blind controlled trials of St. John's wort for depressed mood concluded that the herbal is superior to placebo for moderate depressed mood but ineffective for more severe depressed mood (Linde & Mulrow, 2004). Most studies comparing St. John's wort and conventional antidepressants for moderate depressed mood show equivalent efficacy (Davidson, 2002; Szegedi et al., 2005). A systematic review of controlled trials on folate supplementation in depressed individuals taking conventional antidepressants concluded that folate (1 mg/day) supplementation resulted in relatively greater improvement in mood compared to individuals taking only antidepressants (Taylor et al., 2004). Taking supplemental folate should be recommended to anyone who is depressed because this B-vitamin is a required cofactor for the synthesis of neurotransmitters that are believed to be deficient in depressed individuals.

Relatively few controlled studies have been done on omega-3 essential fatty acids for depressed mood; however, results to date are promising. As noted, the omega-3 called EPA, in particular, may have beneficial effects against depressed mood when taken alone or in combination with conventional antidepressants. A recent study found that EPA (1 gm/day) and fluoxetine (Prozac) were equally effective against depressed mood, and the group taking both improved more than individuals taking either treatment alone (Jazayeri et al., 2008). Meta-analyses of studies on omega-3s in depressed mood report consistent beneficial effects when they are used adjunctively with conventional antidepressants, but inconsistent effects when used as a stand-alone therapy (Parker et al., 2006; Freeman et al., 2006; Lin & Su, 2007). The optimal dose of omega-3s for depressed mood has not been established; however, studies published to date suggest that lower doses (e.g., 2 g/day) may be more efficacious than higher doses (up to 4 g/day (Mischoulon et al., 2008). Rare cases of hypomania have been reported by depressed individuals who take large doses of EPA. Clients who take this natural substance should be warned about this possibility and be under the medical supervision of their family physician or psychiatrist.

Extensive research has been done on the amino acid S-adenosyl-methionine (SAMe) for depressed mood. A meta-analysis of placebo-controlled trials concluded that SAMe has equal or superior efficacy to conventional antidepressants for moderate to severe symptoms of depressed mood (Agency for Healthcare Research, 2002). Combining SAMe with conventional antidepressants may result in improved outcomes, compared to patients who take antidepressants alone (Papakostas et al., 2004). However, this integrative approach should be tried only under medical supervision because of the risk of a potentially serious adverse effect known as "serotonin syndrome." Several cases of mild, but not severe serotonin syndrome have been reported when SSRIs and other antidepressants that affect serotonin in the brain are combined with SAMe.

Compared to SAMe there is relatively less evidence for 5-hydroxytryptophan (5-HTP) as a treatment of depression when used alone or in combination with conventional antidepressants. A systematic review of controlled trials on 5-HTP and L-tryptophan in depressed mood concluded that 5-HTP is more effective than placebo for moderately depressed mood (Shaw et al., 2004). 5-HTP is a naturally occurring amino acid found in many foods and is the immediate precursor of serotonin. To date there have been no reports of serotonin syndrome when 5-HTP is combined with a SSRI antidepressant; however, individuals who use this integrative approach should be cautioned about the possibility of serotonin syndrome. Acetyl-L-carnitine is another amino acid that may have antidepressant effects. However, few studies have been conducted on it, and therefore this naturally occurring substance should not be recommended as a first-line treatment of depression (Pettegrew et al., 2000).

There is considerable evidence for the robust antidepressant effect of regular exercise (Lawlor & Hopker, 2001). Exercise, cognitive therapy, and conventional antidepressants may have equivalent efficacy for the treatment of moderate depressed mood (Tkachuk & Martin, 1999; Blumenthal et al., 1999). Early morning bright light exposure often reduces the severity of depressive mood symptoms regardless of whether mood changes follow a seasonal pattern (Golden et al., 2005). When depressed individuals are exposed to dim blue or green light 2 hours before waking, they respond faster to conventional antidepressants than individuals who are not exposed to "dawn simulation" (Benedetti et al., 2003). Depressed individuals who exercise or use bright light therapy while taking an antidepressant may also improve faster and stay well longer than those who use either approach alone (Partonen et al., 1998).

Emerging research findings suggest that exposure to high-density negative ions may have equal efficacy to full-spectrum bright light exposure for treatment of seasonal depressed mood (Goel et al., 2005). Listening to music may have beneficial effects on emotional well-being and mood (Drohan, 1999). Sounds of certain frequencies perceived at slightly different times on the left and right side of the brain (i.e., "binaural sound") may help improve mood in depressed alcoholics (Milligan & Waldkoetter, 2000).

A novel form of biofeedback based on the brain's electrical activity, called EEG biofeedback (or "neurotherapy"), is probably beneficial in some cases of depression; however, more studies are needed to confirm strong or consistent beneficial effects (Baehr et al., 2001; Baehr & Rosenfeld, 2003). There is mixed evidence for acupuncture as a treatment for depression, and certain needling techniques are probably more effective than others (Wang et al., 2008; Smith & Hay, 2005; Leo & Ligot, 2007. Preliminary findings suggest that applying tiny electrical currents to acupuncture needles may be more beneficial than standard acupuncture (Hechun et al., 1995). In addition, the regular practice of yoga results in significant reductions in the severity of both moderate and severe depressed mood (Woolery et al., 2004; Janakiramaiah et al., 2000).

Regular meditation practice or mindfulness-based stress reduction (MBSR) may improve the antidepressant effects of cognitive therapy in moderately depressed individuals (Mason & Hargreaves, 2001). Religious beliefs and spiritual practice are associated with lower rates of depressed mood (Kendler et al., 2003). Few studies have explored the effects of prayer and energy healing techniques, such as Reiki, qigong, and healing touch, as treatments of depression. Findings of a small open study suggest that healing touch may have general beneficial effects in moderate depressed and bereaved individuals (Bradway, 2003; Robinson, 1996). A small sham-controlled trial found that Reiki treatment resulted in improved mood in moderately depressed stressed individuals (Shore, 2004). Table 4.1 lists nonconventional and integrative modalities used to treat depression.

TABLE 4.1 Nonconventional and Integrative Treatments of Depressed Mood

More substantiated:

- SAMe alone or combined with antidepressant
- St. John's wort (for moderate depressed mood)
- Folate plus antidepressant
- Omega-3 essential fatty acids alone or plus antidepressants
- Regular exercise
- Bright light exposure therapy

Less substantiated:

- Early morning "dawn simulation"
- Music and binaural sound
- 5-hydroxytryptophan
- Acetyl-L-carnitine
- EEG biofeedback
- Yoga
- Meditation and mindfulness-based stress reduction (MBSR)
- Acupuncture (including electroacupuncture)

- High-density negative ions
- Religious beliefs and spiritual practices
- Healing touch, Reiki, energy psychology, and other energy healing approaches

---

CASE VIGNETTES

Moderate depressed mood

Intake

Nancy is 49 years old, divorced, and works as an accountant in a large brokerage firm. She last dated someone 5 years ago. Her adult children live on the East Coast and she has only a few close friends with whom she seldom socializes. She has experienced "small bouts of depression" since her early 40s. She started having panic attacks at about the same time, prior to a "big family trip" to Europe with her sisters and mother. Her panic attacks were so severe that she had to cancel the trip. Soon afterward her family physician started her on the SSRI antidepressant paroxetine (Paxil). She reported: "I felt great in a few weeks and the panic attacks were gone." After 3 months she had returned to her previous good mood, and she experienced no recurring panic episodes. With the guidance of her family physician she was gradually "weaning off" paroxetine, but her mood "soon bottomed out," and she began to experience feelings of "terrible anxiety" as she was about to discontinue the medication. At that point her family physician started her on an antidepressant called mirtazepine (Remeron), which she took at bedtime because of its sedating side effects.

Nancy's mood improved somewhat over the ensuing weeks, but she remained depressed, constantly craved sweets, and often woke up in the middle of the night and proceeded to eat chocolate or ice cream. She felt fatigued most of the day because of "the mirtazepine haze," and she continued to have occasional uncued panic attacks of moderate intensity lasting about 3 minutes. She began to feel uneasy, "like I was randomly walking through the maze of antidepressants" without a clear strategy. A close friend told Nancy about Dr. Reynolds, a family physician who had completed an advanced fellowship training in integrative medicine and used both conventional and alternative therapies in his medical practice. Nancy's friend had seen Dr. Reynolds for a headache problem and assured her that she would find his style refreshing: "He listens to you first and doesn't just talk at you and give you pills." The idea of working with an integrative physician was very appealing to Nancy. Medication side effects were interfering with her ability to concentrate at work, and as a Christian Scientist, Nancy's goal was to avoid taking all medications and to rely on prayer alone to take care of both her medical and mental health problems.

Intake

At her first session with Dr. Reynolds, Nancy briefly reviewed her history. She denied new or severe stresses and described work as "the same old thing." She confirmed significant morning grogginess since beginning the mirtazepine. She seldom exercises but recently had started to practice yoga. She had gotten into a habit of eating fast food for lunch, and often for dinner, and craves chocolate. Nancy described her weight as "going up and down" over the years. Her most recent panic attack had occurred the day before a scheduled meeting with her supervisor, "but there was no real reason for it . . . my boss and I have a cordial relationship." Her panic attacks generally last a few minutes, and are associated with dizziness, shortness of breath, and tightness in the chest but no chest pain or radiating pain or numbness. She is not aware of a relationship between the timing of her panic attacks and meals or snacks.

Nancy describes her mood as "a little down lately." Although her energy and motivation have been "consistently low" for at least a month, Nancy denies thoughts of dying, is not suicidal, and has never experienced suicidal impulses. She is about 30 pounds overweight and reports a longstanding history of sleep apnea, which she realizes is related to her weight. She uses a machine to assist her breathing while sleeping. Although she is dieting, she has been unable to lose weight. She has moderately elevated blood pressure, has regular menstrual periods, and does not experience hot flashes.

She does not have heart disease or other medical problems, and there is no history of head trauma, seizures, or loss of consciousness. Her only medications are mirtazepine and an antihypertensive to control her blood pressure. She also takes a multivitamin and a calcium supplement most days. There have been no recent changes in her medications or supplements. She does not have allergies to medications or food and has never experienced episodes of severe depressed mood, mania (or hypomania), generalized anxiety, social anxiety, agoraphobia, obsessions or compulsions, recurring nightmares, or flashbacks. She has never had psychotic symptoms, but she has noticed a seasonal pattern of depressed mood since her 30s and is generally more depressed in the fall months.

Nancy recalled her mother's "mental breakdown" when she (Nancy) was 14. Her mother was subsequently diagnosed with manic–depressive disorder (now known as bipolar disorder), and has been stable on mood stabilizers since then. Her father "gets moody sometimes," but no other relatives have serious mental health problems.

> *Note*: When working with a client who reports both depressed mood and anxiety, it is important to take a thorough history to obtain a clear understanding of the *symptom pattern* in order to discern whether the two symptoms are related or independent. Depressed mood often occurs together with anxiety, but Nancy denies symptoms that might be consistent with social anxiety, generalized anxiety, obsessive–compulsive disorder, or PTSD. The history suggests that the timing and intensity of panic attacks are unrelated to her depressed mood. When getting to know any new client who complains of recurring episodes of depressed mood, it is important to ask about symptoms that could be consistent with an evolving picture of bipolar disorder or a psychotic disorder. This is especially important when there is known family history of bipolar disorder. In this case the interview has established a seasonal pattern of depressed mood in the absence of apparent manic or psychotic episodes.

Nancy had a normal upbringing and family life, has three siblings, and recalls her mother as being a "devoted" parent. Nancy was a good student and did not have problems focusing in class or doing homework beginning in elementary school. Nancy denied alcohol or substance abuse currently or at any time in the past. She married her high school sweetheart at age 20, divorced at age 35, and has raised two "healthy children" who have both graduated from college, are pursuing careers, and are in stable, long-term relationships.

Nancy is a reliable historian and provides a coherent and believable story about her life and her medical, family, and psychiatric history. She is alert, oriented, and cooperative and maintains normal eye contact throughout the interview. Her thought process is logical. She is neatly dressed and appears well rested but yawns at several points in the interview. Dr. Reynolds notices that she sometimes "fidgets" when asked about work-related stresses, though she denies having problems at work. She doesn't think she has a heart problem even though she experiences "tightness" in her chest during panic attacks. To confirm that the panic attacks are not related to an undiagnosed heart problem, Dr. Reynolds decides to order an EKG.

> Panic attacks are frequently caused by abnormal heart rhythms that are often the result of benign heart problems such as sporadic skipped beats or mitral valve prolapse, but they may also be caused by an evolving and serious heart problem. For this reason it is always prudent to order an EKG in any client who has panic attacks.

Because of her weight problem Dr. Reynolds orders a thyroid panel and a fasting glucose level.

> Thyroid problems frequently manifest as depressed or anxious mood. *Hypo*thyroidism is an established cause of chronic depressed mood, but *hyper*thyroidism can also be an underlying medical cause of depressed mood. Panic attacks

and other forms of anxiety are frequently present with hyperthyroidism and generally resolve with successful treatment. Poor eating habits are often associated with rebound hypoglycemia and may be related to Nancy's dysphoric mood and the panic attacks. In this case an abnormal fasting blood glucose level may also be indirectly related to the appetite-boosting effects of mirtazepine.

Formulation

Nancy is a healthy adult woman with an unremarkable childhood who is approaching menopause, has a family history significant for her mother's probable diagnosis of bipolar disorder, and began to experience moderate depressed mood in her early 40s. At about the same time she had several panic attacks without apparent triggers. Her mother's history suggests a genetic predisposition to bipolar disorder, but at the age of 49 Nancy reports never experiencing a manic or hypomanic episode. From her history there is no evidence of any kind of severe or recurring psychiatric disorder, such as bipolar disorder, severe unipolar depression, generalized or social anxiety, a phobia, substance abuse, or a psychotic disorder. Panic attacks sometimes occur in the context of PTSD, but she has no history of trauma and denies experiencing recurring nightmares, flashbacks, or other symptoms that might be consistent with a diagnosis of PTSD. The timing of her panic episodes suggests that they may be triggered by anticipatory anxiety related to ambivalence about spending time with relatives, or perhaps by her current employment situation; however, other possible psychological explanations need to be explored in psychotherapy. There are no known cardiac problems or other medical problems that may underly her panic attacks. Nevertheless, an EKG is a prudent initial test to determine whether her panic attacks are being caused by an abnormal heart rhythm. Poor dietary habits resulting in episodes of hypoglycemia as well as disorders of the thyroid are established causes of both depressed mood and anxiety. Appropriate laboratory studies have been ordered to rule out these possibilities. Hormonal changes are frequent causes of depression and anxiety in middle-aged women, even when premenopausal.

However Nancy continues to have regular menstrual periods and is not experiencing hot flashes or other symptoms of menopause. Therefore, there is no indication to check her estrogen level at this time.

Depending on the results of the EKG, fasting glucose, and thyroid hormone levels, Nancy's history and current symptoms are probably consistent with two independent DSM-IV diagnoses: dysthymic disorder and panic disorder (without agoraphobia). However, the ongoing problems of sleep apnea, high blood pressure, and possible adverse effects of her blood pressure medication may be exacerbating her mental health problems or interfering with her response to treatment and should be addressed. Finally, and perhaps most signifantly, Nancy's symptom of moderate depressed mood has improved with conventional antidepressants, but she is strongly conflicted about taking any kind of medical treatment because of her religious beliefs as a Christian Scientist. This issue needs to be openly and actively addressed to ensure that Nancy will become invested in a relationship with her physician and her therapist.

Treatment Plan and Referrals

As the hour comes to an end, Dr. Reynolds hands Nancy slips for the EKG and blood work. He encourages her to engage in activities that will empower her to feel better about her life and have greater control over her weight, which may be contributing to her mental health problems. Specifically, she is encouraged to exercise more, join a support group for overeaters, and expand her yoga practice to include a regular class. Dr. Reynolds recommends that she take measures to change her eating habits and to avoid snacking on foods with high fat or sugar content. He also suggests that she take a high-potency B-complex vitamin in the morning for both her depression and anxiety symptoms and that she continue on the mirtazepine for the time being, until the the results of her medical workup are available and they identify an effective substitute treatment that is acceptable to Nancy's Christian Science perspective.

Noting that her depressed mood is not severe, Dr. Reynolds remarks that several nonconventional and integrative alternative therapies would probably help improve her mood. He emphasizes St. John's wort and SAMe as reasonable alternatives to conventional antidepressant medications that are supported by considerable research evidence. Nancy recalls that a friend once had problems with moderate depression and used St. John's wort with good results. She has read a popular book about St. John's wort and wishes to try this medicinal herb first. Dr. Reynolds briefly reviews research findings and safety information for St. John's wort, noting that a few recent studies show that the herbal may be as effective as conventional antidepressants, including sertraline (Zoloft) and paroxetine (Paxil) for moderate depressed mood.

Numerous research studies confirm that both St. John's wort and S-adenosyl-methionine (SAMe) are effective treatments of depressed mood. Some studies suggest that both natural products have antidepressant effects that are comparable to conventional antidepressants; however, findings to date are inconsistent. Compared to St. John's wort, the amino acid SAMe is probably more efficacious against severe depressed mood. These two natural products have different kinds of adverse effects, and both interact in ways that are synergistic or potentially unsafe with conventional medications and other natural products. For these reasons it is always prudent to defer to a qualified naturopathic physician or family physician when a client is interested in the science behind St. John's wort, SAMe, and other natural products.

Dr. Reynolds remarks that St. John's wort has also been evaluated as a naturopathic treatment for generalized anxiety, but not for panic attacks, and that the evidence for its antianxiety effects is uneven. Because Nancy is taking a relatively low dose of mirtazepine, and because only a few possible cases of serotonin syndrome have been reported when antidepressants are combined with St. John's wort, Dr. Reynolds is not worried about this adverse effect. Nevertheless, he tells that Nancy there is a small risk of developing this serious problem.

Serotonin syndrome is a serious, potentially life-threatening syndrome that begins with general feelings of anxiety and agitation and may progress to insomnia, increased blood pressure, stroke, coma, and even death. Rare cases of *possible mild* serotonin syndrome have been reported when St. John's wort is combined with SSRIs and other antidepressants that affect the brain's serotonin level. In this case the client, Nancy, is on a relatively low dose of an antidepressant that affects serotonin, though not as a reuptake inhibitor. Starting Nancy on a trial of St. John's wort and gradually increasing the dose while monitoring for symptoms that might indicate an incipient serotonin syndrome is a conservative and reasonable integrative strategy. If Nancy's symptoms improve with treatment (i.e., assuming the absence of serious adverse effects), her physician will have the option of further reducing, or possibly discontinuing, the conventional antidepressant.

After going over what Nancy might experience if she develops serotonin syndrome, Dr. Reynolds reviews the more common adverse effects of St. John's wort and recommends a reputable brand. They also talk about dosing and what to do if Nancy has adverse effects.

Dosing considerations raise many complex safety issues, including the relative risks of adverse effects and toxic interactions with conventional medications or natural products and when and how often, or by what amount, to increase or consider reducing the dose of a conventional medication or herbal. Conventionally trained physicians and naturopathic physicians have extensive training in this area, but psychologists do not. For these reasons, it is appropriate for you to suggest St. John's wort as a reasonable alternative in this case, but unless you are certified to practice psychopharmacology, *all questions about starting or discontinuing medications or changing doses should be discussed by the client and his or her physician)*

A follow-up appointment is scheduled in 1 month. Dr. Reynolds encourages Nancy to find a psychotherapist who can help her develop cognitive–behavioral strategies addressing her panic attacks and her eating while also working on achieving greater insight into longstanding issues that may be related to her depressed mood.

Follow-Up Sessions

A week later Nancy makes an appointment with Julie, a marriage and family therapist (MFT) recommended by a friend. She feels encouraged and optimistic after only one session, noting that "she really listens to me . . . every word!" Julie obtains Nancy's permission to request medical records from her family physician and affirms that Dr. Reynold's recommendation of St. John's wort is both reasonable and sensitive to Nancy's request to discontinue conventional medications.

> When working with any client who is also receiving advice from another clinician, it is important to let the client know that you understand and agree with that clinician's treatment recommendations. This will help diminish any hesitations or doubts your client may have when disclosing that he or she is being treated by someone else concurrently, while opening the door to communication and collaboration with the other clinician and broadening your referral network.

Sessions are divided between cognitive therapy aimed at Nancy's panic attacks and eating patterns, supportive-expressive therapy addressing work-related stress, appropriate concerns about her medical problems, and her ambivalence about spending time with her siblings. She has been taking the B-vitamin and has gradually increased her dose of St. John's wort, as directed. She hasn't noticed any adverse effects, has experienced a gradual lessening of daytime fatigue, but continues to have "too many down days." By the third weekly appointment her therapist has received a copy of Nancy's medical record, reviews the new treatment plan with Nancy, and makes a note in her chart about Dr. Reynold's recommendations, including dosing and potential safety issues with St. John's wort. At this point in the therapy, and with the support of others in an Overeaters Anonymous (OA) group who are struggling with destructive eating behaviors and weight problems, Nancy feels motivated to change her "dance with food."

One month after her initial appointment with Dr. Reynolds Nancy returns for a scheduled follow-up. He opens her chart and tells Nancy that her EKG and thyroid studies were normal but that her fasting glucose was somewhat elevated. "I don't think this is anything to worry about yet," he tells her. Nancy has already lost 8 pounds and her general outlook seems brighter. In the past month she has had only one panic attack which she describes as "mild" and "short." The panic attack occurred soon after eating lunch, "so I know it wasn't caused by not eating." She ascribes the reduction in panic attacks as largely due to cognitive strategies she has learned in therapy, her improved diet, and her recently renewed exercise routine. Nancy now takes 120 mg of St. John's wort twice daily (in the morning and evening) and is not experiencing adverse effects. Although she feels "a little more energized," there is no noticeable difference in her mood. With apparent frustration, she asks, "How long will it be until the herbs begin to work so I can finally get off the other drug . . . the mirtazepine?" Dr. Reynolds recommends staying on the mirtazepine until there is a clear, sustained response to the St. John's wort. He suggests continuing to gradually increase the herbal to the recommended therapeutic dose for moderate depressed mood and to take it with breakfast and dinner.

> The most appropriate dosing strategy and the best time to take a particular conventional medication, herbal, or other natural product is highly individualized and depends on many factors, including the age and weight of the client, medical problems, and potential interactions with other medications, natural substances being used medicinally, or diet. When your client asks you questions about the best time to take a medication or herbal, it is prudent to refer him or her back to their family physician or naturopathic physician. (If you are a psychologist who is certified to pre-

scribe psychotropic medications, you may of course elect to give specific medication advice in cases where you feel qualified to do so).

Dr. Reynolds praises Nancy's impressive progress managing her panic symptoms and losing weight and encourages her to continue in psychotherapy and attending OA.

One month later Nancy's appearance is noticeably different. She has lost 25 pounds in a little over 2 months and describes "a nice flow of energy" that helps keeps her motivated to exercise and "do my work in therapy." By this time she has been on St. John's wort at the recommended dose for about a month and about 3 weeks ago, she noticed "my mood starting to get level." She has not experienced adverse effects, such as nausea or sedation, or any symptoms that could point to a serotonin syndrome, such as severe agitation, increased blood pressure, or insomnia. In weekly psychotherapy she continues to work on cognitive–behavioral strategies aimed at preventing panic attacks and changing eating patterns. She has realized that she is conflicted about her job and her professional career path and is beginning to think about alternative careers. There are occasional "moments" of increased anxiety before meetings at work and important social events; however, Nancy has not had a panic attack for at least 6 weeks. Toward the end of her appointment Nancy remarked to Dr. Reynolds: "You may remember that I am a Christian Scientist, and I would still like to get off of everything—all medications, herbs, and supplements—if I can get away with it." They review her treatment plan and agree that it is reasonable to gradually reduce the mirtazepine over a few weeks, and if her mood does not worsen and panic attacks do not return, to discontinue that medication. Nancy feels enormous encouragement that she might not have to rely on medications to "function and feel OK." Over the next few weeks she reduces her bedtime dose of mirtazepine, as instructed. Although she has lost almost 30 pounds in 3 months and no longer needs her breathing machine when sleeping, she sometimes still has problems falling asleep.

One month after stopping the mirtazepine, her mood remains stable and there are no recurring panic attacks. She calls Dr.

Reynolds from time to time to ask for advice on managing occasional insomnia, "preferably without taking another pill," and is encouraged to use regular relaxation and guided imagery before bedtime. Her therapist helps her develop a routine that includes guided imagery and progressive muscle relaxation. Over the ensuing months Nancy is able to get adequate sleep most of the time by using simple relaxation techniques. She is encouraged to continue taking the St. John's wort for the time being and has routine follow-up appointments with her family physician about every 3 months.

Six months after going off the mirtazepine, Nancy's mood remains even and there have been no recurring episodes of panic. She has continued her weekly psychotherapy "to make sure that I stay with the plan," is actively considering a career move, and attends OA support groups on a regular basis. At her next appointment with Dr. Reynolds, Nancy asks when she can stop taking the St. John's wort. They review her progress over the previous 4 months and agree that it would be prudent to remain on the herbal at her current dose for another 2–3 months before discontinuing it, and at that time to taper the dose over several weeks with close follow-up to reduce the risk of relapse. Nancy is pleased and surprised that Dr. Reynolds is willing to work with her, even though she does not wish to continue on any kind of antidepressant therapy.

For reasons discussed above, considerations of tapering or discontinuing a conventional medication, herbal medicinal, amino acid therapy, or integrative treatment of depressed mood always fall in the domain of the client's family physician, psychiatrist, or naturopathic physician. Decisions to stop taking any antidepressant are important because the risk of relapse is generally higher when a treatment that has been effective is discontinued soon after the depressed mood begins to improve. This is especially true for more severe cases of depression.

Putting It All Together

Moderate depressed mood has many social, psychological, and biological causes and often responds dramatically and rapidly to simple changes in lifestyle, conventional antidepressants, select herbal therapies and supplements, and psychotherapy. The etiology of Nancy's panic attacks, which are unrelated to her depressed mood, never becomes clear as the narrative unfolds, but the panic attacks nevertheless resolve as her mood and overall psychological and physical health improve. Cognitive–behavioral strategies, guided imagery, yoga, and other mind–body practices and relaxation approaches are effective tools for lowering Nancy's level of anxiety and preventing panic attacks. Nancy has both sleep apnea and high blood pressure, which are frequently associated with depressed mood. However, her family physician's assessment rules out two other medical problems that frequently cause depression and anxiety: thyroid disease and a cardiac arrhythmia. Her weight problem, which is probably due primarily to poor eating habits and secondarily to the adverse effects of an antidepressant, is certainly the cause of her sleep apnea. As she exercises, works on stress management, and makes changes in her eating behavior using cognitive–behavioral strategies and a support group for overeaters, she successfully loses weight, and her sleep apnea and depressed mood begin to improve in tandem. The client's family physician is trained in integrative medicine and has thoroughly addressed Nancy's medical problems and appropriately referred her to a psychotherapist.

When working with moderately depressed clients who have medical problems that may be related to their mood symptoms, it is always prudent to refer them to their family physician, naturopathic physician, or psychiatrist for consultation and to exchange notes with their doctor to ensure that important aspects of their medical history and treatment plan are clearly understood and carefully documented *before discussing treatment alternatives or making referrals to alternative medical practitioners*. Because of Nancy's medical problems, her newly chosen family physician appropriately orders tests to check her thyroid, fasting glucose, and heart functioning at their first encounter, while also advising her to make proactive lifestyle changes such as changing her eating patterns and following a regular exercise program to lose weight.

When clients are motivated to do psychological work, psychotherapy can often help provide insight into stresses that may be contributing to a depressed mood or interfering with treatment response. Individualized cognitive–behavioral strategies can result in significant improvements in both depression and anxiety. When clients are motivated, lifestyle changes together with appropriate supplementation strategies—even in the absence of conventional antidepressants—are frequently effective when symptoms of depression are moderate. However, when depression is severe, and especially in cases where there is active suicidal ideation (see next section), lifestyle changes and natural supplements alone seldom constitute adequate treatment. Numerous research studies show that St. John's wort, high doses of B-vitamins, certain amino acids, and other natural products (see Table 4.1) ameliorate symptoms of moderate depressed mood. The most appropriate integrative treatment strategy will depend on conventional and non-conventional modalities that have already been tried, the relative evidence for treatments that would reasonably be expected to work, and your client's values and preferences. In this case both the physician and therapist honor Nancy's goal of finding effective ways to manage her mood and anxiety symptoms without needing to take conventional antidepressants or other biological therapies. The result is an open, trusting, and cooperative relationship between Nancy, her physician, and her therapist.

Severe Depressed Mood

Charles is a 33-year-old single male who is employed as a software engineer and has been struggling with depression for many years. He was started on an antidepressant by his family doctor about 3 years ago and continues to take it at the recommended dose. Although his mood has significantly improved, he experiences episodes of severe depressed mood two or three times every year, lasting 2 or 3 weeks, during which he is frequently suicidal and unable to work. In spite of his generally improved mood, Charles has been considering discontinuing the antidepressant because of these episodes, in addition to problems with weight gain and diminished libido. For over a month he has been severely depressed and has been fighting suicidal urges. His concentration and short-term memory have been severely impaired, and he has been on a leave of absence from his job but has not applied for disability. Charles eventually decided to go to an urgent care center and was seen by a physician assistant. After refusing emergency psychiatric hospitalization in response to intrusive suicidal thoughts, Charles agrees to call 911 if he becomes acutely suicidal, and he also agrees to an urgent appointment with a psychiatrist named Dr. Tomlinson the following day. The referral is for evaluation and management of recurrent severe depressive episodes with active suicidal ideation.

Intake

Charles has strongly ambivalent feelings about seeing a psychiatrist but at the last minute decides to go. As the first session with Dr. Tomlinson begins, Charles remarks, "I've been in one long depression since I was 28." He begins to cry as he describes years of "barely finding the resolve . . . to avoid suicide." He denies having had severe depressive mood episodes, suicidal thoughts, mood swings, or other serious mental health problems of any kind before the age of 28. He has been drinking moderately for a few years but denies a history of chronic alcohol abuse. He smokes marijuana occasionally "to take the edge off" but does not use or abuse other substances. Charles describes his life as "a comfortable middle class existence—you know, a nice car . . . good job . . . a few friends . . . the whole thing." His father struggled with severe depressive episodes much of his life "and I think he may have tried suicide once or twice. He never talked about it. My grandfather may have had depression genes also."

Charles's medical history is significant for a diagnosis of hypothyroidism "at about the time the depression started," and he has been a taking thyroid hormone supplement since that time. His thyroid levels have been consistently normal since starting treatment, although his most recent lab work was 2 years ago and he doesn't remember which hormones were checked. Although he claims to have "fought the urge to end my life" almost continuously for several years, Charles has never actually attempted suicide. Over the past 5 years he has considered hanging, carbon monoxide asphyxiation in his car, and—most recently—driving over a cliff on his way home from work on a winding mountain road. He has had difficulty sleeping through the night for several days and has been feeling "more agitated" during the same time. "I think the Paxil [paroxetine] helps with with the sleep." There is a history of generalized anxiety "but this hasn't been a problem for years, and it was never really too bad."

Charles has tried numerous conventional antidepressants as well as combinations of two or more antidepressants and mood stabilizers.

Conventional pharmacological treatments of severe depressed mood that fails to respond to single medications include "augmentation strategies" that may consist of combinations of medications from two different drug classes: for example, lithium carbonate in combination with an SSRI or other antidepressant; an atypical antipsychotic together with an antidepressant; and others.

Most conventional treatments "worked for a short time . . . maybe a few months" before Charles began to experience severe depressed mood again. Several medications—including paroxetine (Paxil), his current medication—have caused significant adverse effects, including loss of libido, agitation, weight gain, rash, heavy perspiration, and others, and were soon discontinued.

All of these are common adverse effects of selective serotonin reuptake inhibitors (SSRIs). Some are dose-related and become less severe over time. Others persist and eventually lead to discontinuation of the medication. All questions and concerns pertaining to adverse medication effects or possible safety problems should be referred to your client's prescribing physician.

Charles has remained on paroxetine because "I know it's helping, and I just have to learn how to *live* with the side effects." Charles repeatedly describes his brain as feeling "extremely unbalanced . . . the neurotransmitters just don't work the way they're supposed to . . . maybe they never have." He does not recall dealing with any serious stressors around the time he began to have severe depressive episodes.

He describes his work as "not very difficult . . . it's OK." His relationship with his current girlfriend is also "just OK . . . she's supportive."

In addition to trials on multiple single and combined conventional antidepressants, Charles has tried numerous nonconventional therapies alone or in combination with antidepressants. He has sought treatment from many alternative medical practitioners, including a naturopathic physician, a Chinese medical practitioner, a chiropractor, an Ayurvedic physician, and most recently, a Reiki master. Charles is very methodical and organized in his presentation. From a plastic file folder he takes out a typed report that list all conventional and alternative treatments he has tried together with start dates and discontinuation dates. Dr. Tomlinson goes over the list and asks questions about the nonconventional modalities that are unfamiliar to him, including certain Chinese and Ayurvedic herbal formulas. Among many others, Charles has tried large doses of B-vitamins, including folate, B-6, and B-12 in combination with conventional antidepressants, but he stopped taking these over a year ago because "I didn't think they were doing anything." He has tried St. John's wort alone and in combination with two SSRIs, as well as various Chinese medicinal herbal formulas alone and also in combination with fluoxetine; he has taken high doses of omega-3 essential fatty acids (up to 6 gm/day) in combination with sertraline, and most recently he tried DHEA (a prohormone that is a precursor of testosterone) together with sertraline. Each combined regimen was tried for at least 2 months. Charles describes all of them as "disappointing in general . . . equally ineffective."

A few years ago Charles tried chelation therapy to "cleanse the toxic metals and chemicals from my body," also without lasting beneficial effects on his mood. He has been taking paroxetine for about a year and receives semiweekly acupuncture treatments directed at restoring "diminished liver qi"—his Chinese medical diagnosis, and, he explains to Dr. Tomlinson, the apparent "energetic cause" of his depressed mood.

> According to Chinese medical theory chronic feelings of sadness or sorrow almost always originate from a deficiency

of vital qi energy in the liver. The general goal of treatment is to normalize the flow of qi using acupuncture, herbals, and *moxibustion* or energetic massage (*tui na*) so that symptoms of depressed mood resolve. The specific acupuncture points or herbal formula used will depend on the energetic assessment and pattern of emotional and somatic symptoms in which the depression occurs. For example, irritability or anger in conjunction with depressed mood imply a different kind of energetic imbalance than depressive symptoms associated with insomnia, mental slowing, or a specific somatic complaint.)

Charles takes a synthetic thyroid hormone (FT4) at the recommended dose, but he stopped taking all but a few supplements about 3 months ago because "they weren't working and they were expensive." He continues to take omega-3 essential fatty acids with high EPA content, phosphatidyl choline "for my memory," and a high-potency multivitamin. He takes all of these in the morning, does not have adverse effects, and notes "I think they give me a little more mental energy."

After summarizing the extensive list of vitamins, minerals, amino acids, and herbs he has tried over the years, Charles sighs deeply, becomes quiet, and stares at Dr. Tomlinson. "I don't even know what I hope to gain by coming here. I've tried everything there is to try and nothing works . . . nothing." Charles scores 27 out of 30 on the mini-mental status exam (MMSE) because of problems with concentration and short-term memory. His shirt is wrinkled, and he hasn't shaved for several days. He avoids eye contact when narrating his history, talking about supplements, and especially when describing events and feelings that are emotionally painful. His speech is deliberate, punctuated with frequent pauses, and reflects a logical but slowed thought process. Charles denies psychotic symptoms, including auditory hallucinations and paranoid ideation, and any history of mania or hypomania. He admits to frequently thinking about suicide and is finding it increasingly difficult "to resist giving into it. Staying alive is getting to be more painful than dying."

Many severely depressed individuals become hopeless and demoralized out of the belief that they have tried every possible treatment and have found nothing that works. An important part of your job when beginning to work with clients who are profoundly depressed is to instill hope that they will feel better and to offer resources and referrals for assessment and treatment that will help clarify why their symptoms are unresponsive and identify promising therapies that haven't been tried.

Assessment

Dr. Tomlinson orders a thyroid panel, including FT3, FT4, and TSH to confirm that Charles's thyroid levels are in the normal range.

Thyroid panels ordered by physicians typically check for FT4 and TSH (thyroid stimulating hormone) but not FT3. In some cases FT3 can be low even when FT4 and TSH levels are normal. Abnormal findings in any of these thyroid hormones can point to a thyroid problem that can cause depressed mood or interfere with optimal response to antidepressants. Evaluating thyroid function, including FT3, is an important part of the routine laboratory evaluation of severe depressed mood.

He also suggests specialized studies of the urine to determine whether there may be deficiencies in the neurotransmitters serotonin, dopamine, and norepinephrine.

Although research findings about the relationships between urine levels of neurotransmitter metabolites and brain neurotransmitter levels are inconclusive, emerging evidence suggests that analysis of urinary neurotransmitter metabolites may provide useful indirect indicators of relative deficiencies or imbalances of certain brain neurotransmitters associated with some cases of depressed mood. Many laboratories perform the analysis using a 24-hour urine sample to measure concentrations of byproducts of serotonin, dopamine, and norepinephrine, and on this basis, infer relative brain neurotransmitter levels. In cases where functional testing may provide useful clinical information, it is important to refer your client to a conventionally trained or naturopathic physician who knows how to use these tests.

Formulation

Charles has a long history of severe depressed mood with suicidal ideation that is poorly responsive to both conventional and nonconventional treatments. He has a family history of depressed mood but not mania or psychosis. He also has a history of generalized anxiety, which is not a cause of his current distress. His mood symptoms do not appear to be related to severe stressors at work or in his social life. However, these issues need to be explored in psychotherapy. It is possible that his hypothyroidism has resulted in a chronic worsening of his mood and interfered with his response to both conventional and nonconventional treatments. Although he is taking hormonal replacement therapy it is possible that the nature of his thyroid problem has not been correctly diagnosed or adequately treated. A repeat thyroid panel including FT3, and possibly an endocrinology consult, is an important part of his assessment. Although the onset of severe depressive episodes occurred about the time his hypothyroidism was diagnosed, Charles's lifelong struggle with depression cannot be completely ascribed to this relatively recent medical problem. Moderate alcohol consumption and recreational marijuana use do not account for his mood symptoms, and he may be using both substances to self-treat depressive episodes.

Treatment

After recommending thyroid studies and urinary analysis of neurotransmitter metabolites, Dr. Tomlinson briefly summarizes his clinical impressions and confirms a diagnosis of severe depressed mood that has been only partially responsive to a broad range of conventional medications, alternative biological therapies, and integrative treatment strategies. He asks Charles about the intensity and urgency of his suicidal thoughts and gently encourages him to accept voluntary psychiatric hospitalization for his own safety. Charles has strong negative feelings about being hospitalized "in a nut house" and, as before, agrees to call 911 or go to the emergency room of the local hospital if his suicidal urges become "too hard to resist." "I brought myself here—I think I can do this again without going to a hospital." In his chart Dr. Tomlinson notes that Charles refused a recommendation of voluntary hospitalization for suicidal ideation and is competent to enter into a no self-harm contract.

> When working with any suicidal client who refuses hospitalization, a maxim among all mental health professionals is to clearly document that they strongly advised the client to accept hospitalization but that he or she refused.

As they begin to review previous treatments Dr. Tomlinson remarks that Charles has not yet been on therapeutic trials of several conventional antidepressants as well as augmentation strategies that include combinations of specific atypical antipsychotics, mood stabilizers, and antidepressants. Charles stares at the floor "I think the Paxil is working OK . . . not very much . . . but nothing has worked better."

Dr. Tomlinson goes over the list of alternative therapies Charles has tried and notices that one of the few nonconventional treatments Charles has not tried that might be effective for severe depressed mood is the amino acid SAMe. Charles nods. "OK, so tell me about the downside of my different options." Dr. Tomlinson reviews the advantages and possible adverse effects of the various conventional drug regimens Charles has not yet tried as well as SAMe. Charles remarks, "You know, the reason I've stopped taking most antidepressants before I might get a steady benefit is the bad side effects." He recounts weight gain on fluoxetine (Prozac) "and then the effect wore off," loss of libido on sertraline (Zoloft), increased blood pressure and anxiety on venlafaxine (Effexor), and currently weight gain and libido problems with paroxetine (Paxil).

He remarks that he has had to become his own advocate in seeking a safe and effective treatment for depression. He has read about the risks of developing a "metabolic syndrome," associated weight gain, and diabetes with the newer atypical antipsychotics, which can sometimes be helpful augmentation strategies in the management of severe depressed mood. On this basis he declines Dr. Tomlinson's suggestion of taking one of these medications in combination with paroxetine.

After several more minutes of comparing the conventional and nonconventional treatment choices, Charles decides to try SAMe "mainly to avoid all the downside of the usual treatments." Dr. Tomlinson explains that most studies done on SAMe have evaluated this amino acid therapy in individuals who are moderately depressed, and only a few studies suggest that the amino acid is effective for severe symptoms of depression. Dr. Tomlinson reviews possible adverse effects of SAMe, including the risk of serotonin syndrome when combining SAMe with paroxetine, and he describes the symptoms Charles might experience if he developed serotonin syndrome.

> Serotonin syndrome is uncommonly associated with SAMe alone. However, many cases have been reported when SAMe is combined with antidepressants that affect brain serotonin levels, including paroxetine, sertraline, and the other SSRIs. Serotonin syndrome can manifest as symptoms of acute agitation, anxiety, and insomnia. As noted previously, if these symptoms, persist your client should be referred immediately to an urgent care center or emergency room for evaluation and treatment. More common and less severe adverse effects of SAMe include upset stomach and mild anxiety.

Charles has already read about these risks and still wishes to try SAMe. "I just have a feeling that adding this might make a difference," he comments. Dr. Tomlinson suggests that he start SAMe at 200 mg in the morning before breakfast and gradually increase the dose by increments of 200 mg to 400 mg twice daily before breakfast and lunch. A gradual titration schedule generally reduces the risk of adverse effects with conventional medications as well as amino acid therapies and other natural products. Dr. Tomlinson recommends a reputable brand of SAMe that is available at a local health food store. In addition to SAMe, Dr. Tomlinson recommends a high-potency B-complex vitamin to be taken in the morning "to boost the effect of the SAMe."

> Certain B-vitamins are necessary for the synthesis of the amino acid SAMe into the neurotransmitters dopamine, nor-epinephrine, and serotonin. Although a healthy diet includes these vitamins, taking a B-complex supplement probably increases the rate of synthesis of SAMe into neurotransmitters, thereby boosting its antidepressant efficacy).

He writes down the brand name of SAMe and his recommendations for gradually increasing the dose and jots down a note about taking a B-complex in the morning.

Next Dr. Tomlinson writes down the title of a self-help book on cognitive therapy for depression. He recommends the book to Charles, saying "Depression is not only about brain chemistry. Sometimes working on changing your thoughts can help lift your mood. This book has strategies that will show how you how to do that." Charles discloses his intention to apply for disability, and Dr. Tomlinson offers to provide a supporting letter. In the final minutes of the first session Dr. Tomlinson suggests a follow-up appointment in 1 week. He writes down the number of the suicide hotline and askes Charles to call that service if it becomes too difficult to resist suicidal urges. Charles nods his head slowly, and for the first time in the session makes eye contact with Dr. Tomlinson. "Sure. I can do this. I think this approach makes sense, but I also think we've used up all our time. Thank you." He rises slowly, turns stiffly, and walks out to the waiting room where he writes a check in payment for the session as the minute hand on the wall clock behind him moves to exactly 3:50 P.M.

Follow-Up Sessions

One week later Charles reports continuing suicidal thoughts but adds that he does not have a plan and there is less urgency. He has contacted the human resources manager at his place of employment and has started the process of applying for disability. He is relieved at being "officially" on long-term disability leave at his company and is asking for retroactive coverage, starting with the first week taken off work. Charles is taking the recommended dose of SAMe (400 mg) twice daily, before breakfast and lunch. He is experiencing mild nausea after breakfast, "but it's not too bad" and "there might have been some lifting in my mood in the past few days . . . it's hard to tell." He has continued to take paroxetine. There are no symptoms suggestive of a possible serotonin syndrome. "My thinking is still impaired. I just can't make my brain work." He expresses concern over being away from his job for so long: "My boss is a good guy, but he knows I have a big problem with this."

Charles hands Dr. Tomlinson a long list of all the vitamins, herbs, and other supplements that have been recommended over the years by naturopaths, herbalists, Chinese medical practitioners, a homeopathic doctor, and a few family physicians. The list is two pages long and includes precise doses, times and durations of the various natural products Charles has taken for depression "and getting my brain to work." "I know some of this stuff probably works, but I'm not sure what. Different people tell you different things," He asks Dr. Tomlinson to advise him about "what is more important and what doesn't work."

> Many individuals who have struggled with chronic severe depressed mood have been evaluated and treated by multiple practitioners: family physicians, psychiatrists, psychologists, naturopaths, Chinese medical practitioners, herbalists, energy healers, and others. Out of frustration or desperation, many severely depressed individuals see two, three, or more clinicians who have completely different perspectives and different ways of understanding and treating depressed mood. Being seen by many clinicians often results in confusion and a very long list of medications and supplements, many of which are unnecessary or potentially unsafe. An important initial task of an M.D. or naturopathic physician is therefore to carefully review this list, evaluate which conventional medications and supplements are safe and appropriate,

and make recommendations about tapering or discontinuing certain treatments. Although many physicians have some familiarity with integrative medicine, no one has mastery over all systems of medicine. The work of reviewing a long list of medications and supplements often takes several sessions and involves consultation with Web-based resources or authoritative textbooks on alternative medicine.

Dr. Tomlinson looks over the list and quickly realizes that many of the supplements and herbs Charles has tried are unfamiliar to him. Fortunately, Dr. Tomlinson subscribes to several expert Web-based resources on alternative medicine that provide comprehensive and up-to-date reviews of efficacy and safety data for the range of nonconventional therapies. (See Appendix A for useful books on the range of nonconventional and integrative therapies, and Appendix B for Web resources.)

Dr. Tomlinson relies on Web-based resources because they are updated on a regular basis and, for the most part, report research findings in the absence of advertising. After going over the 15 or so supplements that he knows about, Dr. Tomlinson opens his laptop, which has a wireless connection, and searches for current reviews of the remaining 10 supplements about which he has limited knowledge. As he scrolls through summaries of the various natural products Charles is using, he jots down notes on the list and makes comments to Charles about their efficacy for depressed mood or their safety. By the end of this process, which takes about 15 minutes, Dr. Tomlinson remarks that several natural products Charles has tried over the years are supported by some research evidence, but the majority, including certain Chinese herbal formulas and Western herbs, have never been formally evaluated as treatments of severe depression.

This is a relatively common scenario. Although many conventional, nonconventional, and integrative modalities are used to treat severe depressed mood, relatively few are supported by compelling evidence. Many severely depressed individuals end up using modalities that have never been evaluated as treatments for the severe symptoms they are experiencing.

This results in prolonged suffering, hopelessness, social and occupational impairment, and possibly also an increased risk of suicide. It is incumbent on the ethically responsible physician or alternative medical practitioner to always carefully review the evidence before recommending or endorsing a particular conventional, nonconventional, or integrative treatment for severe depressed mood (or other severe mental or emotional symptoms).

Several herbals have safety warnings that Charles was not told about when they were recommended. Dr. Tomlinson recommends discontinuing those herbals and notifying the clinician who initially recommended taking them. He recommends resuming omega-3 essential fatty acids with high EPA content because of their beneficial effects on depressed mood.

Emerging research findings suggest that taking the omega-3 essential fatty acid EPA together with a conventional antidepressant is an effective and safe augmentation strategy for depressed mood.

Charles notices that he feels optimistic about this new "more scientific approach to my treatment" and remarks, "I got to a place where I didn't know what to try, so I guess I tried everything." He continues to receive acupuncture treatments, "and I think they really help my mood and my nervousness." Dr. Tomlinson supports Charles's choice to continue with acupuncture and remarks "acupuncture is another matter. It helps many people feel better, and there's no potential risk of interactions when taking medications and supplements."

The evidence for acupuncture as a treatment of severe depression is uneven. Several sham-controlled studies show mood-enhancing effects of certain acupuncture protocols, including regular manual acupuncture, electro-acupuncture, and laser acupuncture. However, systematic reviews point out problems with research designs and inconsistent findings. The effectiveness of acupuncture in severe depression probably depends on the skill of the acupuncturist and the specificity of the treatment protocol with respect to each client's unique energetic pattern obtained through history and pulse diagnosis.

Charles has not gone to a laboratory for the thyroid and urine tests and has not purchased the self-help book Dr. Tomlinson recommended. "I just don't see how changing my thinking could get me out of this slump. . ." Dr. Tomlinson gently encourages Charles to get the lab work done and to buy the book. As the session ends, Dr. Tomlinson recommends further increasing SAMe to 1600 mg (dividing the total dose between breakfast, lunch, and later afternoon) over the next few weeks so long as significant adverse effects do not emerge. A follow-up appointment is scheduled in 2 weeks.

At their third session Charles appears more energetic, and Dr. Tomlinson notices that his speech is not as slow. Charles makes direct eye contact much of the time, and his eyes are brighter. He reports feeling "energized by the SAMe. When I got to about 1200 mg a day I started to really notice it." He has experienced increasing nausea with the morning dose of SAMe and has started taking it after breakfast, which has helped. He now takes a B-complex and omega-3s every day and feels more "in control of how I'm handling this. I'm not just taking pills and concoctions day and night, and the main ones I'm taking seem to be making a difference." He still has not gone to a local laboratory for the tests Dr. Tomlinson ordered, stating, "I don't think that is really necessary." It is clear that Charles has chosen not to follow through with the recommended lab work, and Dr. Tomlinson does not force the issue. Suicidal thoughts have lessened in severity and frequency and his "mental faculties appear to be returning." He is on disability now but is "thinking about" returning to work: "I think it would do me good, but I don't yet trust my brain."

Charles purchased the self-help book on depression and has started to read. "I think I recognize some of my self-defeating tendencies in the stories, and this cognitive therapy approach sounds interesting." Dr. Tomlinson encourages Charles to continue with the book and suggests that he consider starting regular psychotherapy sessions. Charles has never tried psychotherapy: "I didn't think that *talking* helped depression. I thought it was all about correcting a chemical imbalance or the energetic imbalance, as the Chinese do." Dr. Tomlinson comments on the evidence that cognitive therapy is often as effective as conventional medications for depression, "and besides, it will give you a deeper understanding of patterns of thinking and behavior that may be keeping you stuck." Dr. Tomlinson writes down the names of three marriage and family therapists (MFTs) whose skill he highly respects, and encourages Charles to contact one of them for ongoing work, including cognitive therapy. "Bring that book with you and tell whomever you choose what we've been talking about here."

Charles is clearly relieved to have more energy and improved mental functioning. Dr. Tomlinson takes this as an opportunity to recommend regular exercise. "You know, there's a lot of evidence supporting the benefits of exercise for depression. It really works. It might even work as well as antidepressants." Charles appears brighter and tells Dr. Tomlinson that he used to be a distance runner "before this all started. Maybe this is a good time to go back to my running." Dr. Tomlinson nods and tells Charles that he was a runner also. "I've read a lot about exercise and depression and really think there's something to it."

> Many studies show that regular aerobic or strengthening exercise has significant mood-enhancing effects in depressed individuals. Some studies have found that exercise has antidepressant efficacy that is equivalent to SSRIs. Advising a severely depressed client who is profoundly lethargic to exercise will likely result in further frustration, as he or she will probably be unable to follow through with your advice. When a client begins to experience increased energy, however, it is reasonable to recommend regular exercise, which generally adds to the beneficial effects of the antidepressant regimen.

As the session closes Charles asks if it would be "OK" to wait a few weeks before his next session. "I think I'd like to do this on my own for a while."

By their next session Charles has found a psychotherapist and has continued to read the self-help book. His mood has been "solid" for 3 weeks on the same dose of SAMe, and the nausea has "gotten a little better," though he needs to take an antacid before meals "to get through it." He casually announced, "Hey, I finally had those labs done . . . the ones you ordered a few months ago." Dr. Tomlinson had received the faxed results that morning and tells Charles that analysis of his urine indicates relatively low brain levels of two neurotransmitters—dopamine and norepinephrine—possibly related to his chronic depressed mood and disappointing responses to both conventional antidepressants and alternative therapies. Dr. Tomlinson confirms that SAMe is a logical choice in view of these findings because this amino acid therapy results in increased brain levels of serotonin, norepinephrine, and dopamine, directly addressing the findings of Charles's urine study. Charles purchased a new pair of running shoes after the last session with Dr. Tomlinson and has been jogging. "I can't tell you how good it feels to get out there and move again." He returned to work about a week ago and is comfortable doing his job. "The brain fog seems to have lifted most of the time." He has occasional suicidal thoughts but no specific plan and no feeling of urgency.

Charles appears to be genuinely interested in continuing the work of cognitive therapy with his therapist—"I'm realizing that my way of thinking is just negative and maybe I'm too rigid. I think these traits get me into these spirals of depression." Therapy sessions have already given Charles important insights into how his personality "has been getting in the way" of his efforts to stay healthy. "Now I realize that I have choices." As the session ends, Charles asks Dr. Tomlinson if it is "OK for my therapist to call you to get an update on what we've been doing here." Charles plans to continue in weekly therapy sessions and schedules a routine follow-up appointment with Dr. Tomlinson in 1 month.

As noted previously, it is always helpful to be in contact with other clinicians who are working with your client in parallel to ensure that all clinicians have a clear and up-to-date understanding of the treatment plan. However, your client must first consent to the exchange of information between his or her physician or other health care provider and you.

Ongoing Treatment

Charles's mood remains stable 3 months after his first appointment with Dr. Tomlinson, and he continues to take SAMe at a dose of 400 mg three times daily. He is exercising on a regular basis and is actively engaged in psychotherapy, where he is beginning to explore dynamic issues that "may be keeping me depressed most of the time" and learning cognitive strategies for "getting myself out of the next slump." He has started dating and asks Dr. Tomlinson if it would be safe to stop the paroxetine because of sexual side effects. They discuss the risk of a recurring severe depression if the paroxetine is stopped, and Dr. Tomlinson suggest gradually reducing the dose from 30 to 20 mg (to reduce sexual side effects) while remaining on his current dose of SAMe, omega-3 fatty acids, and a high-potency B-complex and continuing to exercise. He also suggests that taking ginkgo biloba might help reduce the diminished libido caused by paroxetine.

There is evidence that taking the Chinese herbal ginkgo biloba can counteract the sexual side effects of paroxetine and other conventional antidepressants. Ginkgo is generally well tolerated and when used at recommended doses is associated with infrequent mild adverse effects including upset stomach, skin allergies, dizziness, and headache. Ginkgo interferes with normal blood clotting and therefore should not be used soon before or following surgery. For the same reason, Ginkgo should not be used by pregnant women who are going into labor. Ginkgo has been reported to cause seizures in individuals who are taking medications for a seizure disorder and should be avoided in this population. For these reasons ginkgo should be recommended only by a physician after determining that it is safe to take for a particular patient).

Charles is optimistic as the session ends, and they agree to a routine 1-month follow-up appointment.

Three months later Charles returns for a routine follow-up appointment. He never started the ginkgo. *His new relationship recently ended* and he is talking about "fighting suicide." He is staring at the floor, and Dr. Tomlinson notices dark circles under his eyes. "I was feeling so good I decided to go ahead and get off the Paxil [paroxetine] and the SAMe all together and see how things would go. I felt fine at first. Then I just caved in after about a month." Charles does not have a specific suicide plan, does not own a gun, and has told a close friend about his struggle with suicidal thoughts. As they begin to discuss treatment options a tear begins to move slowly down Charles's left cheek, and he emits a barely audible sigh.

Putting It All Together

This case illustrates the complex psychological, social, familial, and medical issues often found in severe depression. When working with a severely depressed client it is vitally important to accurately assess suicide risk and to provide resources, including psychiatric crisis services, for rapid triage if your client is actively suicidal. Psychiatric hospitalization should be discussed up front, and if your client refuses, your note should document that you know about the client's suicide risk, suggested hospitalization, and that the client refused. In such cases it is always appropriate to refer a severely depressed client to a psychiatrist on an urgent basis (and, if possible, to confirm that the initial appointment takes place) while also providing the phone number of a suicide hotline or psychiatric crisis service in the community.

Anxiety, insomnia, and mental slowing often accompany severe depression and often resolve when a client responds to therapy. When working with any severely depressed client, it is important to address medical problems that may cause the depression or interfere with treatment. Hypothyroidism is commonly associated with depressed mood. If you suspect hypothyroidism or another untreated medical problem, it is important to refer your client to his or her family physician or naturopathic physician for evaluation and treatment. Thyroid hormone replacement therapy can result in dramatic and rapid improvement in mood.

At least two-thirds of severely depressed individuals self-treat with a variety of nonconventional therapies or see alternative medical practitioners while taking conventional antidepressants concurrently, yet relatively few nonconventional treatments of severe depressed mood are supported by strong evidence. Because most individuals who use nonconventional therapies do not disclose this information to their family physician or psychiatrist, there is often a great deal of confusion about "what works and what doesn't," and there is also a very real risk of adverse effects and toxic interactions when herbals and other natural substances and medications are used concurrently.

You can provide a valuable service to your client by familiarizing yourself with expert information resources on nonconventional therapies, such as those mentioned in the vignette and listed in Appendix B Using these tools, you will be able to point your client in useful directions, safely away from nonconventional modalities that are probably ineffective, unsafe, or both. "Paring down" a long list is a valuable service to a client who is taking 15 supplements and has little understanding of what is beneficial and safe or unnecessary and unsafe. In complicated cases (such as this vignette), where a client is taking many natural products together with conventional medications, an important first step is to thoroughly document what is being taken. With your client's permission you can forward this information, together with your clinical impressions, to the family physician, naturopathic physician, or psychiatrist for evaluation of possible medical risks associated with different natural products, and for advice about supplements or medications that your client should continue or stop taking. Developing a good working relationship with your client's physician is in everyone's interest. Clearly documenting communication with your client's physician or psychiatrist will also reduce your own liability in the event your client attempts suicide.

When symptoms of fatigue and mental slowing begin to improve, it is appropriate to encourage your client to exercise, work on stress management, and—if your client has insight and is motivated—consider regular psychotherapy, including cognitive therapy. When clients who have been severely depressed respond to treatment and wish to discontinue a medication because of adverse effects—in this case, reduced libido—it is appropriate to send them to the psychiatrist, family physician, or naturopathic physician who is managing their care to discuss the risk of relapse and review alternatives. In such cases, a reasonable integrative treatment plan might entail reducing the dose of the medication that is causing the adverse effects while continuing and possibly increasing a nonconventional therapy that has proven effective (in this case, SAMe), adding an herbal therapy that helps to improve libido, or continuing and increasing doses of augmentation therapies such as B-vitamins and omega-3 fatty acids.

The way in which this vignette ends is unfortunately typical of many severely depressed individuals who choose to discontinue all treatment—often against the advice and encouragement of their psychiatrist, family physician, and therapist—soon after their mood symptoms improve. Stopping an effective conventional or integrative treatment too early is associated with a high risk of relapse. For unclear reasons, resuming a conventional antidepressant that was previously effective may result in little or no improvement, and the work of finding an effective conventional or integrative treatment plan must begin all over again.

CHAPTER 5

~

Cyclic Mood Changes and Mania

W HEN evaluating a client who describes cyclic mood changes that shift between depression and euphoria (or irritability), it is often difficult to distinguish symptoms of mania, hypomania, or depression from those of agitation, anxiety, and psychosis. Furthermore, endocrinological and neurological disorders sometimes manifest as cyclic mood changes. An underlying medical problem or the adverse effects of a prescription medication can also cause *apparent* mania. For example, hyperthyroidism, seizure disorders, multiple sclerosis, and other medical or neurological problems can mimic the cyclic mood changes seen in bipolar disorder, and certain prescription medications have stimulating effects that can "look like" mania or acute anxiety. Stimulant abuse, including cocaine or methamphetamine (speed) and certain prescription medications (e.g., methylphenidate [Ritalin] and amphetamine [Adderall]) can also result in cyclic mood changes that are actually the "highs" and "lows" of substance abuse. Clients who report mood changes sometimes experience psychotic symptoms when "up" or "down." Depending on the timing and severity of psychotic symptoms, the most likely diagnosis—suggesting the most appropriate treatment—may be bipolar disorder, schizoaffective disorder, schizophrenia, a severe personality disorder, or a complicated picture involving more than one primary psychiatric disorder. Failure to correctly diagnose bipolar disorder has important implications for clinical management, because using inappropriate medications (e.g., antidepressants) can worsen your client's condition or result in hypomania or mania. Emerging findings suggest that individuals diagnosed with bipolar disorder may have abnormally low blood levels of folic acid (Hasanah, 1997). As mentioned previously, a specialized kind of brain-wave analysis, quantitative electroencephalography (QEEG), is currently used as a research tool in this population and may eventually provide useful diagnostic information that will help guide treatment planning (Hughes, 1999).

TREATMENT

Conventional Treatments

Bipolar patients often experience a broad range of mood symptoms in addition to anxiety and psychosis during severe episodes. The result of this variability is that treatment is individualized in relation to the most prominent symptoms at different times in the course of the illness. For example, antidepressants are used during the acute depressive phase of the illness, mood stabilizers and possibly atypical antipsychotics are used as maintainence therapy and during acute manic episodes, and antidepressants and mood stabilizers are used in combination when an individual is experiencing a "mixed episode" involving symptoms of both depressed mood and mania. Specialized medication regimens are used to treat the so-called "rapid cycling" variant. Along these lines, a bipolar patient who reports symptoms of anxiety or cognitive impairment in the context of a broader pattern of cyclic mood changes should also be treated for those symptoms.

It has been estimated that roughly half of all conventional medications used to treat bipolar mood symptoms are used in the absence of compelling evidence of efficacy (Boschert, 2004), so it is not surprising that conventional pharmacological treatments have a mixed record of success. A systematic review of randomized controlled trials of mood stabilizers as maintenance therapy for bipolar disorder reveal markedly differing profiles of efficacy and tolerability for different medications. Lithium and and the atypical antipsychotic olanzapine were found to be most effective for reducing manic relapses, whereas lamotrigine (Lamictal) and valproate significantly reduced the risk of depressive relapses. Discontinuation because of adverse effects was twice as likely with lithium compared with valproate and lamotrigine (Smith et al., 2007). Mood stabilizers including lithium carbonate, valproic acid (Depakote), carbamazepine (Tegretol), as well as lamotrigine and other more recently introduced medications are associated with significant adverse effects, such as weight gain (which can lead to diabetes), hypothyroidism, hair loss, tremor, loss of libido, and others. It has been estimated that as many as 50% of individuals treated with conventional mood stabilizers discontinue treatment against medical advice because of concerns over adverse effects.

Augmentation strategies that combine antidepressants and mood stabilizers are frequently used to treat cases of bipolar disorder that do not improve with single medications; however, combining two or more medications is probably no more effective in bipolar disorder than using single mood stabilizers (Ghaemi, 2001). Transcranial magnetic stimulation (TMS) is an emerging treatment that stimulates specific brain regions using a high-intensity pulsing magnetic field. Findings on the use of TMS for bipolar disorder remain inconclusive at the time of writing (Nahas et al., 2003; Kaptsan et al., 2003). The limitations of conventional treatments of bipolar disorder have resulted in a growing interest in nonconventional therapies that are being used alone or in combination with prescription medications.

Nonconventional Treatments

Relatively few nonpharmacological treatments of bipolar disorder have been rigorously evaluated in Western-style research studies, compared to unipolar depressed mood, and findings are more preliminary. Emerging findings suggest that taking daily supplements of omega-3 essential fatty acids reduces the severity of mood swings in bipolar disorder and possibly also in some personality disorders (Freeman et al., 2006). There is limited research evidence that taking omega-3s alone is beneficial, whereas some outcome studies support an adjunctive role of omega-3s in combination with conventional mood stabilizers (Lin & Su, 2007; Parker et al., 2006). Preliminary findings suggest that an amino acid drink that excludes tyrosine and phenylalanine may reduce the severity of mania and improve cognitive functioning in acutely manic individuals (Gijsman et al., 2002; McTavish et al., 2001). A proprietary multi-ingredient nutrient formula is being widely used to self-treat the mood swings of bipolar disorder (Kaplan et al., 2001). This formula aims to improve brain functioning in general, and consists of high-potency vitamins, minerals, certain amino acids, and proprietary herbs. Case studies and open trials are very encouraging. The first randomized placebo-controlled trials on the formula for individuals diagnosed with bipolar disorder are starting, and no data are available at the time of writing (Simmons et al., 2003; Simmons, 2002). Case reports and the findings of a small pilot study suggest that daily exercise may lessen the severity of mania and reduce the frequency of hospitalizations in individuals diagnosed with bipolar disorder (Ng et al., 2007). Regular early morning bright light exposure probably lessens the severity of symptoms in some cases of bipolar disorder, especially in individuals who report a seasonal pattern of mood changes. However, cases of mania induction have been reported with bright light therapy, and individuals who use this approach should be closely monitored (Golden et al., 2005).

By learning about nonconventional treatments that work and are safe, you can help guide clients who experience cyclic mood changes to appropriate nonconventional therapies that may help stabilize their mood symptoms while directing them away from therapies that will probably be of little benefit or potentially worsen their symptoms. Table 5.1 summarizes promising nonconventional therapies for bipolar disorder.

TABLE 5.1 Nonconventional and Integrative Treatments of Mania and Cyclic Mood Changes

More substantiated:

• There are no strongly substantiated nonconventional treatments of bipolar disorder at the time of writing.

Less substantiated:

• Omega-3 essential fatty acids alone or with mood stabilizers
• Amino acid drink that excludes tyrosine and phenylalanine
• Proprietary multi-ingredient nutrient formula
• Regular exercise
• Bright light exposure (*caution*: can induce mania)

CASE VIGNETTES*

Moderate mood swings

Intake

Jack is 35 years old, works as a financial advisor, and was recently divorced. His family physician referred him to a psychotherapist in the community when he complained of "feeling down lately. I guess the divorce thing has really gotten to me." He makes an appointment with Angela Wilson, a highly respected marriage and family therapist, for the following week. As the session begins, Angela notices that Jack's shirt is stained and badly wrinkled and he seems to be fatigued. Jack falls into the leather chair and slouches forward. He appears distracted and begins to tap his left foot on the carpeted floor while staring at a Monet print over Angela's left shoulder.

"Nice painting. What is it supposed to be about?"

---

* Individuals who have cyclic mood changes caused by bipolar disorder or other mental health problems frequently experience anxiety, depressed mood, insomnia, and other symptoms in addition to mania. Some nonconventional therapies used in the vignettes are directed at symptoms other than cyclic mood changes and are addressed in other chapters.

"It's about summer in France. It's a French impressionist paint-ing. What about it interests you, Jack?"

"Nothing . . . I don't know . . . I used to enjoy painting land-scapes, never tried the French approach. I know how hard it is to capture nature—*understand* it—the way it really is."

Jack pauses, again staring at the floor. "I really don't know why I'm here. What good can words do for my problem?"

"Why don't you begin by telling me how you got to where you are now . . . how life became so hard?"

Jack replies, "It's a long story. Sure you want to hear it?"

He begins by describing recent financial problems caused by a slow-down in the housing market. In the past few months his income has plummeted to about half his usual earnings, and he has experi-enced considerable anxiety over "this financial hit. I'm not sure where the market will end up, and it's starting to worry me. I have to bring in the money. I have to pay the bills . . . alimony. . . . don't know where it's going to end."

Until about 3 months ago, when the divorce became final, Jack had been an avid hiker and runner. "I was always proud of doing the work to stay in shape. I guess exercising kept me calm." Since letting go of his exercise routine he has gained about 15 pounds. "I don't really care how I look anymore. From my ex I know the only thing I'm good for is rescuing her, paying bills, and keeping everyone in the green."

Angela listens, nodding empathically as Jack tells his story: a stormy 10-year marriage; two affairs on his side; possible infidelities on her side; always struggling to stay even; and—finally—the intense disappointment of realizing that his wife could not become pregnant. "I guess that was the final straw for us. After that there was really no reason to continue on."

Angela asks Jack to talk about his marital conflicts. "I get into angry bouts. I don't know . . . I get very *irritable*. It's just there—it comes from out of *nowhere*—and I feel myself getting wound up, and I say nasty things to people. I think my wife just got tired of my temper."

As Angela listens, Jack goes on to describe a long history of erratic mood changes that cycle from "feeling great" to "my Mr. Hyde persona—dark, irritable, *angry*." He has been experiencing mood changes like this about three to four times a year since his early 20s and is not aware of particular stressors, thoughts, or events that trigger them. "My father also had a reputation for his temper, but everyone *respected* him, and people loved him when he was having a good day. I never had enough people skills to make up for my temper, like my Dad could."

Jack continues, describing "mental problems" managing financial details in his real estate business when feeling down. "The brain isn't as sharp when I'm in a downward cycle. When I get really bad, I cry . . . especially in the morning . . . and I can go into this *rage* thing. I feel like it's getting worse lately."

Jack has never assaulted anyone when experiencing rage, nor has he contemplated or attempted suicide. He denies experiencing symptoms that are consistent with severe mania, including racing thoughts, pressured speech, diminished sleep lasting days at a time, spending beyond his means, grandiosity, or psychotic symptoms. Jack enjoys a beer after work but has never had a "real problem" with alcohol or drug abuse. There are no major medical problems in his history, and he has never been hospitalized. Jack takes a multivitamin "when I remember it" but does not take prescription medications. He has never sought treatment for his mood symptoms or any other mental health problem. "I guess I thought I could take care of this on my own, like my Dad. Anyway, I'm not *crazy*."

When Angela asks him about his childhood, Jack remarks, "You know, the usual. Dad was always working. I was just there . . . trying to stay out of the way." There is no history of abuse or neglect. "I was an average student and got along with everyone pretty well until my temper started to cause problems in my 20s." Jack notes that his father began to experience similar "temper problems" at about the same age.

In the final minutes of the session Angela tells Jack: "You may have the milder kind of bipolar disorder, but I don't know yet. Anyway, it's more important to understand what's driving your mood swings and treat them than to give you a label." Jack appears startled. "But I've never had a problem sleeping. I thought people with manic–depression stayed up all night for days and got into trouble for doing all kinds of crazy stuff." Angela explains the difference between bipolar I, characterized by episodes of severe mania, and bipolar II, in which milder symptoms of mania alternate with periods of depression.

> *Note:* The DSM-IV-TR diagnosis of bipolar I disorder requires a history of *at least* one severe manic episode lasting several days, in which the individual experiences a reduced need for sleep, euphoric or irritable mood, racing thoughts, pressured speech, and in some cases psychotic symptoms, including delusions of grandeur, auditory hallucinations, or others. Together, these symptoms often result in seriously impaired social or occupational functioning. In contrast, bipolar II, the milder form of this disorder, is characterized by less severe mood symptoms that do not result in severe impairments in functioning. Bipolar II symptoms may include elevated or irritable mood, reduced need for sleep, but *never* psychotic symptoms. Other variants of bipolar disorder include *mixed states*, in which symptoms of depression and mania occur at the same time, and *rapid cycling*, in which an individual experiences at least three complete cycles of mania (or hypomania) alternating with depressed mood during a 1 year period.

Angela invites Jack to continue in psychotherapy with her to learn how to use cognitive and behavioral strategies for managing his mood swings and to develop insight into his "temper problem," and she encourages him to see a psychiatrist to discuss other treatment options. "There are many ways to approach your problems. Since we're at the beginning of your journey, I think it would be useful to explore a range of treatment options." Jack is upset. "I have no *intention* of seeing a shrink . . . crazy people see shrinks." After letting Jack emote for a few minutes, Angela tells Jack about a psychiatrist in the community who prescribes medications but also treats patients using EEG biofeedback and has expertise in Western herbal medicine and nutritional approaches to mental health care. "Dr. Streeter doesn't just prescribe medications and check in with you for 15 minutes every 3 months. He's different. You owe it to yourself to find out what he has to offer. I think there are some supplements that might help you feel better. And in the meantime, I'd like you to practice relaxing every day. There are some CDs I'd like you to get." Angela tells Jack about a guided imagery program used for deep relaxation. "It's nice music, and if you take time to listen every morning and every evening, I think it will help your brain feel calmer. You might sleep better also." As the session ends Jack remarks, "I guess I should be relieved to know that what I have can be treated and that I have many choices." They agree to a follow-up appointment in 2 weeks. "I'd really like you to see Dr. Streeter before then."

Assessment and Formulation

The initial interview by the therapist is quite thorough and provides a great deal of useful clinical information. In view of the absence of significant medical or psychiatric history and no ongoing medical problems, there is no indication for more formal psychological or medical assessment at this time. The emotional and financial stresses from his recent change in income and his contentious divorce together with his erratic diet and sedentary lifestyle may help account for some of the symptoms of anger and emotional lability he is experiencing at present. Jack has never had a severe depressive episode or periods or elevated or irritable mood that suggest a full-blown manic episode. Longstanding issues of anger and emotional lability in the context of his father's history of "having a bad temper" are consistent with a milder form of bipolar disorder. However, according to the DSM-IV-TR, Jack's symptoms may be consistent with an impulse control problem associated with anger or an adjustment disorder. Making a formal DSM-IV-type diagnosis in this case may not be necessary and, in fact, may add an unnecessary psychological burden to the client's already overwhelming situation. Such a burden would interfere with achieving the important goals of establishing a good working relationship and focusing on basic treatment outcomes.

Intake with Psychiatrist

One week later Jack finds himself outside Dr. Streeter's office, which is located on the second floor of an old Victorian house on a quiet, tree-lined street. A sign above the entrance reads "Integrative Mental Health Care." Jack recognizes the medium-size tree in a planter on the landing as a ginkgo. Inside the waiting room there are books on herbal medicine, energy medicine, yoga, biofeedback, hypnosis, and psychotherapy as well as conventional pharmacological treatments. Classical guitar music plays softly in the background, and there is a slight scent of lavender in the air. Jack picks out an illustrated book on herbal medicine and sits down to browse. In a few minutes Dr. Streeter opens the door to his office. He invites Jack inside. "Nice to meet you. I'm Dr. Streeter. I'm happy we were able to meet this soon." Dr. Streeter gestures to a suede-upholstered chair next to an end table on which a small fountain bubbles quietly. Jack realizes he is feeling calmer just being in Dr. Streeter's office. "It's peaceful here. The music and the lavender make me feel quiet inside."

"Thank you. I've tried to create a healing environment," Dr. Streeter replies. "I know Angela suggested that you see me, but maybe you're tired of telling your story to different people."

"It's not a problem," Jack replies. Anyway, I think talking is probably good for whatever's ailing me." During the next 10 minutes Jack emphasizes aspects of his story that seemed interesting to Angela. Summing up, he remarks: "Angela thinks I have bipolar disorder but not the serious type. She said you won't just throw medications at me right off, and you might have other ideas, more natural approaches that could help."

Dr. Streeter nods his head. "I see. Well, first let's talk a bit about what it is that *you do have*, and then go over some approaches that might help you feel better, perhaps give you more control over the anger and the mood swings." Dr. Streeter says that he agrees, in general, with Angela's diagnosis of bipolar disorder II but notes, "One could also describe your issue as an anger problem or a kind of self-defeating behavior pattern. Sometimes symptoms fit into a formal diagnosis such as bipolar disorder, and sometimes they don't clearly fit. In any event, I treat symptoms. In my experience, codes designating a particular diagnosis are mainly for the insurance people, so let's focus on the symptoms that are causing you the most distress." Dr. Streeter adds: "I think psychotherapy would be very helpful for what you have, but I also think that medications, certain supplements, or other kinds of treatment might add to the benefits of psychotherapy. Psychotherapy is about engaging in a dialogue with the goal of figuring out what is bothering you and learning skills that will help you change self-destructive habits. My understanding is that you're planning to continue in psychotherapy with Angela, so in our work together I'll focus on the rest."

> In this case a psychotherapist and a psychiatrist who know and respect one another's perspectives have chosen to work together. Splitting care is generally a reasonable approach assuming that two mental health professionals have similar values and communicate with one another effectively to avoid working at cross-purposes. In this instance the client is seen initially by a marriage and family therapist, who subsequently refers him to a respected psychiatrist. Their shared integrative perspective will ensure that the client is approached in ways that are consistent and mutually reinforcing. Referring a client to a psychiatrist who understands and agrees with your clinical orientation and shares your treatment philosophy is always preferable to making a blind referral, and will probably result in a more satisfying collaborative experience for everyone involved.

It soon becomes clear from their conversation that Jack does not want to take a conventional medication. However, to do his work with integrity and to ensure that Jack is fully informed about the range of conventional and nonconventional treatment choices, Dr. Streeter briefly describes conventional medications in addition to alternative modalities for which there is good evidence of both efficacy and safety. "I want to make sure that you know about all your options before eliminating any of them. There are many viable approaches to managing your symptoms, and each one has its own pros and cons."

> The majority of nonpharmacological treatments used in mental health care are not formally endorsed by the American Psychiatric Association or other professional medical associations. For this reason, when a psychotherapist, psychiatrist, family physician, or alternative medical practitioner is considering recommending any nonconventional modality to a client, it is always expedient to clearly and completely inform

him or her about both conventional and nonconventional modalities that represent reasonable treatment choices. Fully informed consent includes a discussion of the potential therapeutic benefits and established or predictable adverse effects of all modalities that are being considered, and limiting your own liability requires that you clearly document in your client's chart that you have done so.

In his review of medication options and nonconventional modalities, Dr. Streeter makes it a point to distinguish between treatments that are reasonable to consider for the more severe form of bipolar disorder versus the milder form of this disorder, which is probably consistent with Jack's symptom profile. Dr. Streeter starts by listing several conventional mood stabilizers and antidepressants as well as sedative/hypnotics that are frequently prescribed for bipolar II disorder, and mentions some of their more common adverse effects. He then remarks that the skillful, consistent practice of mind–body approaches, certain kinds of biofeedback, exercise, and certain nonpharmacological approaches may be as effective as prescription medications for the management of moderately severe symptoms of anger, agitation, and cyclic mood changes, while avoiding risks of potentially serious adverse effects associated with mood stabilizers.

When planning treatment for symptoms of moderate severity, it is important to emphasize that many nonpharmacological modalities, including stress reduction, dietary changes, exercise and certain supplements, can result in significant clinical improvement. Providing a range of treatment choices to clients early in the course of therapy will help them stay hopeful and actively engaged in treatment.

Jack appears uneasy at the mention of conventional medications. "I really don't want to start with the big guns, Doc. I have to say, I'm scared to try those medications because of what I've been reading about people gaining weight, or feeling drugged, or developing a tremor or something."

Dr. Streeter nods. "Many people have understandable concerns like yours, but sometimes the conventional medications are the best choices in the long run—sometimes they're the treatments that work best."

"Yeah, I know, Doc, but can we try the other stuff first, you know, the natural remedies?"

"In your case that is reasonable because your symptoms aren't too serious, but if your symptoms were serious, I would have to advise you to try conventional medications first . . . and if your symptoms get worse at some point, I'll will probably feel better about recommending the Depakotes and Lamictals of the world rather than the alternative approaches."

"I understand, and that sounds reasonable," replies Jack. "In other words, we'll find out what works best—whatever that may be—and stick with that."

"Exactly, that's integrative medicine." Dr. Streeter then mentions the amino acids 5-hydroxytryptophan and L-theanine, which can have a significant calming effect in individuals who experience anger and mood swings. He also describes a proprietary nutrient formula that has helped many individuals diagnosed with bipolar disorder regain control over the intensity of their mood swings while permitting some to significantly reduce doses of mood stabilizers, and in some cases, to completely stop taking conventional medications. After talking about amino acid therapy Dr. Streeter mentions that he also uses a machine that "trains the brain to be calmer. EEG biofeedback, or neurofeedback, achieves a kind of retuning of the brain."

> EEG biofeedback, or "neurotherapy," is widely used mainly by psychologists to treat anxiety and improve attention. The goal of EEG biofeedback is to change the dynamic characteristics of brain electrical activity, thereby ameliorating emotional or cognitive symptoms. Protocols addressing particular brain regions or specific frequency ranges are most efficacious depending on the target symptom(s) being treated.

After some back and forth with Dr. Streeter, Jack says he would like to try amino acids. "I'd like to keep this simple, if possible." Dr. Streeter explains that taking specific amino acids can help compensate for a deficiency or imbalance in certain neurotransmitters that may underlie Jack's mood swings. Dr. Streeter explains: "Taking amino acids will also improve your nutrition in general, and I think an important part of the plan should be to think about changing the way you eat. Your mood might be going up and down because your brain's on empty too much of the time."

5-hydroxytryptophan (5-HTP) is the immediate precursor of serotonin, as noted previously. This amino acid is prepared from a natural source, is taken orally, and goes into the brain more readily than a related amino acid, L-tryptophan. L-theanine is derived from green tea and other natural substances and affects the activity of brain receptors that result in a calm or mildly sedated feeling. Because naturally occurring amino acids are not very potent and are metabolized in the body fairly rapidly, they are generally taken several times daily. When treating depression, mood swings, anger, or anxiety, 5-HTP and L-theanine can be safely combined. However, questions about advice on dosing should always be deferred to a family physician, naturopathic physician, or psychiatrist who can inform your client about possible adverse effects or toxic interactions when amino acids are combined with conventional drugs or other naturally occurring substances.

Dr. Streeter takes this opportunity to shift the conversation from a discussion about the evidence for amino acid therapy to a more general discussion about the importance of good nutrition, starting with regular meals balanced in protein, fats, and complex carbohydrates. "It's basically about getting the nutrients your body and brain need and avoiding too much sugar and caffeine." Jack realizes that his eating habits have been poor or erratic since childhood. "I know I need to clean up my act, Doc." In the closing minutes of the session Dr. Streeter goes over a conservative plan for starting 5-HTP at an initial dose of 25 mg twice daily, and gradually increasing the dose to 50 mg three times daily, assuming there are no or moderate adverse effects. They agree that if Jack experiences significant relief from his anger and improved mood using 5-HTP alone, he will continue to take only this amino acid. They agree to revisit the idea of adding L-theanine to his regimen at their next appointment. Dr. Streeter invites Jack to call or e-mail with questions or problems, and they agree to a 3-week follow-up.

Second Session with Angela

A week after his intake with Dr. Streeter, Jack returns to see Angela. He talks enthusiastically about the appointment with Dr. Streeter. "I can't tell you how nice it was to be able to talk about treatments that aren't limited to the usual medications," he comments. Jack goes over the new treatment plan, explaining that he has been taking 5-HTP since seeing Dr. Streeter and is now up to 100 mg twice daily. So far he hasn't experienced any side effects. There have been fewer crying episodes and no anger outbursts for several days. "I think the 5-HTP may be helping me feel more even lately, but there hasn't really been anything to get upset about since starting it."

"Dr. Streeter also told me about his EEG biofeedback machine. We might try that in the future if the 5-HTP doesn't do the job," Angela comments. Jack reports also working on improving his diet, including less sugar, more vegetables, and fewer late-night snacks. "I think the new approach to eating might also be helping me feel smoother." Since changing his eating habits Jack has noticed fewer "lows and highs" during the day.

> Brief episodes of hyperglycemia, followed by relative hypo-glycemia, often affect people who eat high-sugar snacks or have poor or erratic eating habits. Alternating cycles of hyperglycemia and hypoglycemia are often associated with transient feelings of increased energy or improved mood and diminished energy or worsening mood, respectively, which can mimic the cyclic mood changes experienced in the mild form of bipolar disorder. Dietary changes resulting in stabler blood glucose levels can be a strategic intervention in individuals complaining of cyclic mood changes.

Angela and Jack use the balance of the session to discuss the overall plan and to go over mind–body practices. "Following a simple routine a few times a day can really bring down your stress level," Angela notes. She then describes the calming benefits of regular deep breathing and introduces Jack to the principles of guided imagery. Jack is obviously interested in learning more about mind–body methods and realizes that practicing a few simple skills may give him significantly more control over his stress level, his "moods," and his temper problem. "I think the deep breathing and guided imagery will be very helpful before the next mediation session," Jack remarks. Angela suggests a follow-up appointment in 2 weeks, but Jack is using his savings to finance therapy sessions, so they agree to a follow-up appointment in 1 month. "I think I'm doing a lot better, and I'd like to take some time to see how the new plan works. Anyway, I have an appointment with Dr. Streeter in 2 weeks."

Second Appointment with Dr. Streeter

As Jack sits down 1 month after their initial session, Dr. Streeter notices dramatic differences in both his demeanor and apparent level of distress. "You seem much calmer than before, Jack." Jack replies that he has been taking the 5-HTP for about 6 weeks now at a dose of 100 mg in the morning and late afternoon and another 200 mg at bedtime. "I think it makes me more relaxed in general, but I'm doing a lot of other things at the same time, so it's difficult to know what is really helping." Jack continues to follow a healthy, consistent diet and has avoided high-sugar snacks. "I really think that cleaning up my eating routine has made a big difference in my temper." He describes feeling "much more in control of my moods" in general and when interacting with his estranged wife during mediation. "I think being able to stay calm makes a big difference in the mediation sessions. The anger isn't getting in the way as much." He has been following Angela's advice on deep breathing for relaxation, especially in the mornings. "I think it helps to tune me to a calmer level, Doc." Jack has also been using a guided imagery CD in the evenings before going to bed. "I think I sleep more deeply when I'm more relaxed."

Dr. Streeter nods his head. "I think you're doing a great job with everything, Jack. I'm wondering if it would be helpful for you to try some biofeedback to consolidate your gains." Dr. Streeter describes the basic theory of EEG biofeedback. "It's a technique that helps *retune* the brain."

EEG biofeedback is a treatment approach that uses information from the brain's electrical activity as feedback in the form of a pleasing image or progress in a computer game. Specific settings of "reward" or "inhibit" frequencies essentially *train* the brain to hold on to patterns of electrical activity that translate into sustained clinical improvement in one or more target symptoms. In a case like this one, involving anger and emotional reactivity, training the brain using feedback from electrodes positioned at specific locations over the right temporal and parietal regions can help achieve calmness and greater emotional stability.

Jack is clearly interested in the idea of EEG biofeedback, and they schedule an initial session for the following week. Dr. Streeter suggests using a simple biofeedback program at home between EEG biofeedback training sessions in his office. The program, Journey to the Wild Divine™, is affordable and can be downloaded to a home computer. "It's a simple biofeedback program, not as powerful as what I can offer you in my office, but it will start you in the right direction," Dr. Streeter explains. Jack writes down the name of the program. "I think this is really going to make a difference, Doc."

In the final minutes of the session Dr. Streeter talks about using the various approaches Jack has learned to "get the best outcome." "For example, you can practice deep breathing during guided imagery or when doing the computer game. It's important to keep taking the 5-HTP also. It's what your brain needs to stay calm and even." In closing, Dr. Streeter suggests that they meet about every 2 or 3 months, assuming Jack's mood remains "level." He also encourages Jack to continue seeing Angela. "You know, Jack, the 5-HTP, the breathing, the guided imagery, and the brain training don't replace psychological work. I think it would be of tremendous value for you to continue in psychotherapy for a while." Jack nods and agrees to continue seeing Angela when it isn't too much of a financial strain.

Putting It All Together

This case illustrates that it is not always necessary to regard clients' symptoms and problems from the perspective of the DSM in order to understand the causes or meanings of their distress and provide effective conventional or integrative treatment. Because of his "temper problem," Jack's father would probably qualify for a diagnosis of bipolar II if he were evaluated by a conventionally trained psychiatrist. One could argue that Jack's symptoms are probably also consistent with a diagnosis of bipolar II. However, giving him this formal diagnostic label for insurance billing purposes would be tantamount to telling him that he has a permanent serious mental disorder. There are several problems with this approach. First of all, diagnosing a client with a serious psychiatric disorder is a powerful act, in and of itself, which may cause more personal harm than good. A formal psychiatric diagnosis can be received as a pejorative label implying that the person is *defined* by his or her symptoms. Diagnostic labels often result in intense feelings of personal shame and social stigma. In my view diagnostic labels are often unnecessary and may, in fact, interfere with the goals of compassionate treatment.

Second, the validity of many psychiatric disorders—including bipolar II and other so-called variants of bipolar disorder—continue to be debated in the academic journal literature in working groups that are currently reevaluating the methodology and criteria sets used to diagnose these psychiatric *disorders*. This process will conclude with the publication of the DSM-V in 2012. There is considerable disagreement and debate in academic circles over whether the same symptom pattern of emotional reactivity and lability is more consistent with a particular personality disorder, mood disorder, or a disorder of impulse control.

Third, practical treatment considerations in the day-to-day management of clients are more often based on particular symptoms that cause the greatest amount of distress or impaired functioning at any given period in an individual's life, and only secondarily on a formal psychiatric diagnosis that is presumed to adequately characterize the nature, causes, and extent of a complex pattern of mental illness averaged over the lifetime.

Finally, assigning a client a fixed diagnostic label often precludes consideration of significant new information or emerging symptoms that may be more consistent with other disorders. In other words, giving a client a formal diagnosis can take away the therapist's motivation to remain open to new ways of understanding the client's distress and finding new—perhaps more effective—therapeutic interventions.

In this case, the absence of a formal diagnosis does not limit or interfere with thorough, multilevel assessment and treatment planning while ensuring that the client's therapist and psychiatrist remain focused on symptoms that are causing Jack the greatest amount of distress and impairment. Open, collaborative relationships between the client and both clinicians ensure that the client's symptoms are clearly identified—and agreed on—before any treatment recommendations are made. In this collaborative context a multimodal treatment plan emerges that addresses the psychological, neurobiological, and energetic causes and meanings of the client's distress.

The treatment plan starts with general considerations of dietary change, exercise, deep breathing, and guided imagery, then progresses to more specific interventions including amino acid supplementation addressing the client's mood symptoms and EEG biofeedback to assist the client in brain retraining for sustained emotional stability. In a case like this one, where moderately severe symptoms do not warrant urgent, dramatic treatment, a client can experience significant improvement through simple lifestyle changes such as diet and regular exercise. After the client's general physical and emotional well-being has improved—in this case through improved diet and regular exercise—more specific interventions are added targeting specific symptoms that continue to cause distress or interfere with functioning. Perhaps most important of all, the psychotherapist and the psychiatrist carefully listen to Jack, acknowledge his distress, and take into consideration his hesitations and preferences when discussing a range of treatment choices. Respectful, collaborative relationships between a client and his or her therapist(s) ensure that the client is actively engaged with the treatment process, is motivated to stay in treatment, and will convey any problems that arise in a timely way. As this story ends, the client is feeling more confident and self-empowered to take care of his general well-being and mental health needs, he is actively engaged in treatment, and he is looking forward to continuing the work of staying healthy with both his therapist and psychiatrist.

Severe Mood Swings

Intake

Marsha found Dr. Alvarez through a Yellow Pages ad describing her integrative psychiatric practice. As she sits down at her first session, she says, "I'm extremely sensitive to medications, and I knew you would be the one who could help me find the right alternative therapies." Marsha is 42 years old, works as a medical illustrator and is devoted to her yoga practice. "I think the glue that holds my life together is yoga." Marsha describes feeling "empty and unfulfilled" in her technical career and notes that she began to practice yoga "to feel more integrated." She has read widely about the world's great spiritual traditions and soon realized that "I never really fit what I've been trying to do with my life . . . you know, the whole career thing. I needed something more spiritual, but my career was necessary to pay the rent."

A year of psychotherapy helped Marsha clarify alternative career choices, and she finally decided to pursue Chinese medicine "because it challenges me technically and also honors my need to evolve as a spiritual person." She recently ended a 3-year relationship because "he said he couldn't deal with my mood cycles any more. It's always been that way. I don't know how to stay in a relationship." Marsha is distraught and tearful as she describes years of "swinging from lows to highs and back again and all the chaos in my life from this craziness." During the past 6 months she has been consistently "down, crying much of the time—even at work." Recently she has had fantasies of committing suicide by veering into oncoming traffic on the drive to work. She adds that these suicidal impulses "aren't too bad most of the time." She reports having a "breakdown" 3 days ago when she realized, "I just can't work . . . the mental fog." She discloses feeling overwhelmed and lonely since breaking up with her boyfriend.

As she narrates her history, Marsha describes herself as a "truth seeker." Last year she traveled to China for 3 months with her boyfriend after completing advanced training in traditional Chinese medicine. She has found the study of Chinese medicine fascinating, but adds, "It was just too difficult to keep up with the demands of studying because of the mental fog I've been in." Marsha describes being unable to focus enough to study for months at a time. She did well enough in her courses to pass, but "I think I barely did the minimum." She had been looking forward to beginning a private practice in Chinese medicine with her boyfriend, who also finished his degree work last summer. "But there's no possibility of that now."

Marsha describes a happy childhood without abuse. She has two older sisters, both in good health. Her father was diagnosed with bipolar disorder and took mood stabilizers most of his adult life. He had a brilliant career as a professor of history before succumbing to Alzheimer's disease in his early 70s. There is no other known family history. Marsha reports having a drinking problem in her early 20s but denies current alcohol or drug abuse. She experienced her first major depressive episode at age 20 during finals of her junior year. Her symptoms eventually resolved without treatment, and she graduated with a B.S. in computer science. Over the following 12 years she designed software programs for a large computer game company in the San Francisco Bay Area. During that time she began to notice mood cycles that felt like she was "crashing against rocks and then being lifted up to the warm sun." She has not been hospitalized, though she recalls "barely avoiding going to the hospital" several times when manic. She has never experienced psychotic symptoms, including paranoia or auditory hallucinations, when manic or depressed, but sometimes "I begin to think about suicide." She has not attempted suicide.

After 3 years of constant struggle with her mood symptoms, a friend encouraged her to see a psychiatrist. She was diagnosed with bipolar disorder at age 35 and since then has tried multiple mood stabilizers, antidepressants, and antipsychotics alone and in combination. A combination of lithium carbonate and quetiapine (Seroquel) resulted in improved functioning and "fewer sharp jags." She continued to take quetiapine for several more months but eventually chose to discontinue that medication because "I was just too spacy all the time." Soon afterward she discontinued lithium because of weight gain, tremors, and lithium-induced hypothyroidism. "I just couldn't accept that I had to be 30 pounds overweight and have a tremor . . . and then the thyroid problem happened." She was started on thyroid hormone therapy, and her most recent thyroid panel, done

3 months ago, showed normal FT3, FT4, and TSH levels. Because of poor control of her manic symptoms, her psychiatrist recently added lamotrigine (Lamictal) to her regimen, which she discontinued in 2 weeks because of severe nausea. "I don't know if anything might have worked because I felt sick all the time and I couldn't stay on any of them long enough to find out."

Discontinuation of conventional mood stabilizers early in treatment because of serious adverse effects is very common. Although many individuals diagnosed with bipolar disorder experience improved functioning with conventional mood stabilizers, as many as 50% stop taking them after only a few months because of weight gain, the so-called "metabolic syndrome," tremor, kidney problems, elevated liver enzymes, and other serious adverse effects.

At various times Marsha has also tried several SSRI antidepressants, including paroxetine (Paxil), fluoxetine (Prozac), and sertraline (Zoloft). Sertraline "seemed to do the job most of the time" and was especially helpful in "smoothing out my mood just before my [menstrual] period." Yet she discontinued sertraline after only 1 month because "it made me feel too flat."

Many bipolar patients who do not tolerate mood stabilizers are able to achieve greater control of cyclic mood changes with SSRIs or other antidepressants but are uncomfortable with the "flat feelings" that can sometimes result. Although antidepressants can help control the depressive phase of the illness, taking them carries a risk of inducing mania. Therefore, anyone diagnosed with bipolar disorder who takes an antidepressant should be closely monitored by a psychiatrist.

About a year ago her psychiatrist referred Marsha to a gynecologist when it became clear that her cyclic mood changes became worse just before menstrual periods. She had been diagnosed with premenstrual dysphoric disorder, "but I also had bipolar disorder, so I didn't know which one it really was." She was treated with estrogen for her premenstrual symptoms, "but it just made my spacy." Last week she was started on progesterone by her gynecologist and has been feeling "a little steadier" since then.

During the past 2 years Marsha has been treated for her mood symptoms by a naturopathic physician, an acupuncturist, a gynecologist, a Reiki master, and an endocrinologist. She currently takes over 20 vitamins and supplements in addition to thyroid replacement therapy. She briefly tried several amino acids, high-potency vitamins, and Chinese herbals, but soon discontinued all of them because of adverse effects. "I think there is a great deal of validity to Chinese medicine and nutrient therapy for my mental problems. I'm just very sensitive to side effects and haven't found the right formula yet. But energy healing may make the greatest difference in my mood."

Marsha sleeps well most of the time, meditates, and does daily yoga stretches. She eats fish but not meat and has excellent nutrition. While continuing with several alternative therapies, Marsha remains open to trying conventional medications "to smooth me out." Her psychiatrist recently started her on a very low dose of escitalopram (Lexapro) solution, and in the past 2 weeks she has gone up from 1 to 3 mg/day. "I don't know whether this is making a difference, but I want to believe it works and at least I can tolerate it."

At the time of the initial consultation Marsha is taking only Lexapro solution, a very low dose of levothyroxine (Synthroid), and some "fish oil." She expresses intense frustration at her lack of progress with both conventional and nonconventional treatments and states that she wishes to simplify her regimen of medications as well as natural remedies as much as possible. "I guess from this point on my goal is to take *only what I need*—whether it's synthetic or natural. I just want to be healthy."

Assessment

Dr. Alvarez decides to check Marsha's thyroid hormones even though she reportedly had normal laboratory results as recently as 1 year ago. It is possible, though unlikely, that a primary thyroid problem is causing Marsha's cyclic mood changes or interfering with response to treatment.

It is important to evaluate thyroid function in this case even though Marsha's thyroid studies have been within the normal range. Subclinical hypothyroidism and associated mood problems can occur when thyroid stimulating hormone (TSH) is in the lower end of normal. In such cases, mood symptoms often improve when the dose of FT4 or FT3 is slightly increased. If you suspect that your client may have a subclinical hypothyroid picture, it is appropriate to refer him or her to an endocrinologist for a specialized evaluation.

Because of her history of premenstrual dysphoric disorder Dr. Alvarez suggests a follow-up appointment with her gynecologist, for a hormone panel to check serum estrogen and progesterone levels. Marsha's positive experience using mind–body practices and Reiki— as well as her spiritual values and intellectual fascination with these approaches—suggests that a formal energetic assessment by an experienced Chinese medical practitioner might yield valuable diagnostic information about "energetic imbalances" possibly associated with her cyclic mood symptoms and possibly explain her sensitivity to conventional and alternative therapies in energetic terms.

According to Chinese and Ayurvedic systems of medicine, "energetic imbalances" can manifest as both physical and emotional symptoms. Formal energetic assessment by a skilled Chinese medical practitioner or Ayurvedic physician can help characterize the nature of an underlying energetic imbalance and point to appropriate conventional or nonconventional treatments that will correct them.

Because of her strong interest in Chinese medicine, Dr. Alvarez encourages Marsha to obtain a thorough assessment by a highly respected professor at the college of Chinese medicine where she was trained.

Formulation
Marsha describes cyclic mood changes starting at age 20. Although she was drinking heavily when her symptoms started, her cyclic mood changes have persisted in the absence of ongoing alcohol or substance abuse. There is a family history of bipolar disorder on her father's side. There is no history of childhood abuse or trauma. How-

ever, a longstanding pattern of failed relationships, emotional lability, and erratic, unrealistic—and possibly self-destructive—life choices may be consistent with a severe personality disorder. Several therapy sessions will be needed to determine whether Marsha's relationship history and symptoms are more consistent with rapid-cycling bipolar disorder or a personality disorder, possibly borderline personality disorder. The absence of psychotic symptoms eliminates schizoaffective disorder from consideration. She has at least two documented medical problems that probably contribute to her cyclic mood symptoms or interfere with her treatment response: hypothyroidism (caused by chronic lithium use) and a dysregulation of her reproductive hormones, of unknown etiology. Marsha is taking a synthetic thyroid hormone for her thyroid problem, but it is not clear from her history if her current treatment regimen is adequately addressing the underlying causes of this problem.

At present, Marsha is not receiving conventional or nonconventional therapy for her reproductive hormone problem. Like many individuals treated for bipolar disorder, Marsha is unable to tolerate therapeutic doses of many conventional medications as well as alternative biological treatments. Reasons for her "sensitivity" to adverse effects are not clear but may include both psychological and genetic, physiological, or postulated "energetic" factors. Because of her strong spiritual orientation, meditation and yoga help "balance" Marsha energetically. Regular Reiki treatments may also be beneficial at a subtle, energetic level of mind–body functioning.

> Sensitivity to adverse effects of biological therapies can be related to psychological factors, such as negative expectations and anticipatory anxiety, as well as biological factors at multiple physiological or genetic levels, including problems of liver metabolism, regulation of neurotransmitter receptors in the brain, genetic predisposition, and others. According to Chinese medical theory and Ayurveda, the inability to tolerate biologically active substances may also be related to specific kinds of energetic imbalances.

Treatment

After interviewing Marsha, Dr. Alvarez summarizes her clinical impressions: a probable bipolar disorder complicated by a thyroid problem that may be partially treated, gynecological issues that may also related to hormonal problems, and a possible energetic imbalance. Dr. Alvarez has attended lectures on Chinese medicine and tells Marsha that she is open to both conventional Western and non-Western ways of understanding and treating mental and emotional problems. Marsha is visably relieved to find a psychiatrist who is open-minded about Chinese medicine, and on Dr. Alvarez's recommendation, she agrees to schedule an appointment with one of her former professors for a thorough Chinese medical energetic assessment. Marsha also agrees with a recommendation to see her gynecologist to check her estrogen and progesterone levels. However, she doesn't think that her thyroid is the cause of her mood problems and does not wish to repeat thyroid function tests. Marsha makes a visable shudder when Dr. Alvarez asks her if she is open to increasing the escitalopran. "I just can't go there now, Doctor. I need to keep the Lexapro where it is for a while until I've tried everything else." Dr. Alvarez sees that the Lexapro is a very sensitive matter and does not force the issue. She comments on the importance of essential fatty acids for mental health.

Emerging research findings suggest that the omega-3 essential fatty acid EPA (ecosapentanoic acid) is beneficial in bipolar disorder, as well as depression and possibly schizophrenia. To date, an optimum source (i.e., fish vs. flax seed oil) and dose have not been determined. However, many studies suggest that 1–2 gm daily of a purified form of EPA result in consistent improvements in mood.

Dr. Alvarez explains that the omega-3 essential fatty acid EPA is probably the most important component of fish oil for cyclic mood changes and asks Marsha to check her omega-3 supplement to find out how much EPA she takes daily. She also encourages Marsha to find a quality brand of fish oil that contains both omega-6s and omega-3s. She recommends taking a quality fish oil preparation with meals for a total daily dose of 2 gm of EPA. Dr. Alvarez also suggests that Marsha start on an herbal called golden root (*Rhodiola rosea*) in the morning, explaining that this medicinal herbal is beneficial for depressed mood in general and is widely used to treat mood changes related to imbalances of the reproductive hormones, such as occur in premenstrual dysphoric disorder.

> Golden root has been used in Russia for decades for its stimulant and immune-boosting properties and is becoming increasingly used in Western Europe and North America to treat depression and fatigue and especially mood disorders in women. Golden root has no known serious adverse effects, and no cases of mania have been reported in bipolar patients. However, the herbal is highly energizing and should be taken in the morning to reduce the risk of excess stimulation.

Before the session ends, Dr. Alvarez suggests that Marsha consider psychotherapy and recommends a self-help book on cognitive–behavioral therapy for depression. Marsha smiles. "My other psychiatrist didn't think therapy would make a difference, so I guess I've never considered trying it." Dr. Alvarez writes down the names of two family therapists.

First Follow-Up Session

At her 2-week follow-up session, Marsha appears anxious and distracted. "I'm really having high anxiety today. I think I may have taken the wrong dose of something this morning." She continues to feel "overwhelmed and unfocused" much of the time. "I think I'm a little more level with the golden root," which she has been taking at the recommended dose since the last session. She has also seen her endocrinologist, who increased her T3 dose slightly on the basis of a TSH level in the low-normal range. She has been evaluated by her former professor of Chinese medicine, who diagnosed her with liver qi stagnation. Marsha is optimistic as she describes Dr. Lee's findings. "He concluded that I am energetically *stuck*, that my liver qi was congested. I told him I didn't want herbals at this point, so we scheduled two acupuncture treatments to address the energy problem." She has a new boyfriend and mentions that they are "already thinking of moving in together. I know this is going too fast, but. . . ."

She has started another brand of omega-3s with the recommended balance of omega-6 to omega-3 fatty acids and daily amount of EPA, and has not experienced adverse effects such as upset stomach.

Marsha is visibly agitated and tearful as she describes an upcoming European family vacation. "I get tight inside. I know it's going to be the same pathological family dance." She is considering inviting her "very new boyfriend . . . as a buffer" but also realizes that this choice may result in greater awkwardness with her family during the vacation. She has tried to meditate in the mornings but is seldom able to remain focused long enough "to clear out." Marsha shows Dr. Alvarez a bottle of a proprietary nutrient formula she learned about when researching alternative treatments for bipolar disorder. She has already purchased a month's supply. "It looks promising . . . and it also looks safe."

> The proprietary nutrient formula contains minerals, vitamins, and trace elements developed for use by individuals diagnosed with bipolar disorder. The ingredients of the nutrient formula are believed to reduce the severity of cyclic mood changes by compensating for metabolic problems that cause neurotransmitter imbalances that manifest as the symptoms of bipolar disorder. To date, all of the evidence for this nutrient formula comes from reports of individuals who use it to self-treat symptoms of bipolar disorder. According to the manufacturers, a significant percentage of users have experienced dramatic improvements in the severity of bipolar symptoms and are able to reduce their doses of conventional mood stabilizers. Two large randomized, placebo-controlled studies are now in progress, with the goal of rigorously evaluating the therapeutic claims of this promising nutrient formula.

Marsha is not worried about reacting to the nutrient formula "because I know it is entirely natural." The supplier recommends starting out with several capsules daily. However, Dr. Alvarez advises Marsha to begin with only one capsule of nutrient formula and gradually increase the dose to four capsules twice daily over the next 3 weeks, explaining that gradually titrating the dose will reduce the risk of adverse effects. As the session ends, Dr. Alvarez asks Marsha if she is reading the self-help book on cognitive therapy for depression. "I guess I don't really see the relevance of a psychological approach for my problem. It's clearly biologically driven." Dr. Alvarez remarks, "You know, the causes of symptoms are probably *always* biological and *always* psychological. I think you might get some useful ideas from browsing through the book." Marsha pauses for a few seconds, quietly stares at the floor, and agrees to bring the book with her on the family vacation. A follow-up appointment is scheduled for about 1 month later, a few days after Marsha returns from her vacation.

Second Follow-Up Session

Four weeks later Marsha is relaxed and appears to have gained some weight. There were no "catastrophes" during her family vacation. She decided not to invite her new boyfriend: "It would have made things too unsteady for me." Marsha has been taking the proprietary nutrient formula for about 3 weeks and gradually increasing her daily dose according to plan. There have been no adverse effects except for mild upset stomach soon after the morning dose. Taking the nutrient formula with food helps lessen that problem. She is taking the omega-3s and her thyroid medication and appears motivated to continue taking these. She received two acupuncture treatments before her vacation. "The first session was powerful . . . I felt so much calmer and clearer." Marsha had a second acupuncture treatment 1 week later, which "helped me to center but wasn't as powerful as the first one." She intends to continue with acupuncture therapy and is optimistic that her "energetic imbalance is being addressed as well as my brain chemistry."

Dr. Alvarez encourages Marsha to continue receiving acupuncture treatments from Dr. Lee and wants her to know that she believes acupuncture therapy is a legitimate treatment. "I think there's a great deal of validity to acupuncture, and Dr. Lee's treatments certainly seem to be making a difference." Marsha discloses that she had several important conversations with her mother, "the matriarch of our clan," during her family vacation. She relates feeling "clearer about the big picture, and calmer" following those conversations. Marsha also describes feeling more confident about recent life choices, including her decision to pursue a career in Chinese medicine.

"Mom has never been that supportive before. I can't tell you how good it feels!" Dr. Alvarez uses Marsha's newfound confidence to encourage further exploration through psychotherapy. This time Marsha is receptive. "I know you're right about therapy. I just wanted to level out the neurotransmitters before doing hard psychological work." Dr. Alvarez writes down the names of two psychotherapists in the community, suggesting that Marsha call both and "feel out who is the best match for you." Marsha asks Dr. Alvarez if she thinks it is "safe" to stop taking the Lexapro now that her "neurotransmitters have leveled out." Dr. Alvarez recommends remaining on the escitalopram for 1 month, at her current dose, then gradually discontinuing the SSRI over another month. "I think this is the safest approach to take at this point. We don't want to change things too fast and get back to where we were . . . and it's only been 2 months." Marsha finds this "middle ground" approach acceptable. "Could we meet in about 2 months? We can see how I'm feeling off the Lexapro and maybe I'll get something out of psychotherapy in the meantime." As the session closes, Dr. Alvarez reminds Marsha to continue taking the nutrient formula at her current dose and writes down the week-by-week plan for tapering and discontinuing the escitalopram.

Putting It All Together

Complex psychological, familial, medical, and possibly energetic issues frequently contribute to the causes of cyclic mood changes and are often present when there is a diagnosis of bipolar disorder or a personality disorder. When there is a history of hypothyroidism, it is important to determine whether a hormonal deficiency or imbalance is driving mood symptoms or interfering with response to treatment. As in Marsha's case, many individuals who are taking thyroid replacement hormone therapy remain symptomatic because of subclinical hypothyroidism. Therefore, it is prudent to refer anyone who is taking a thyroid supplement to see an endocrinologist in order to ensure that subtle physiological and emotional symptoms related to thyroid function are being adequately addressed. Specialized laboratory panels sometimes reveal a deficiency or imbalance of specific thyroid hormones when standard laboratory findings are within normal range.

As noted above, a significant percentage of individuals who experience cyclic mood changes choose to discontinue conventional mood stabilizing medications early in the course of treatment because of adverse effects. Finding an alternative or integrative treatment strategy for a medication-sensitive individual that is both effective and safe poses many challenges. Recommendations about medications or medicinal herbs are the domain of Western medical specialists or alternative medical practitioners, and treatment recommendations should always be based on the research evidence in the context of your client's preferences and financial constraints. In this case the client is open to the range of nonconventional modalities and has already tried numerous conventional medications, naturopathic remedies, and energy therapies before seeing a psychiatrist. Perhaps the greatest contribution the psychiatrist makes to Marsha's mental health care is providing an open-minded and rigorous dialogue about possible underlying causes of her symptoms in terms of both conventional medical theory and energetic imbalances, and the range of conventional and nonconventional treatment choices that may effectively address those causes. In this case, as in many cases where the chief complaint is cyclic mood changes, the client does not receive a definitive diagnosis of a particular disorder corresponding to her symptoms, which probably match DSM criteria for a personality disorder or a variant of bipolar disorder. Even in the absence of a diagnostic label, the open-minded approach taken by her psychiatrist leads to useful new insights about likely causes of Marsha's symptoms at many psychological, biological, and possibly energetic levels. Acupuncture addressing energetic imbalances takes place in parallel with appropriate biological therapies, and Marsha gradually achieves sufficient resilience to engage in the hard work of psychotherapy. Through a collaborative process the integrative strategy that ultimately proves to be effective involves an herbal (golden root), omega-3 essential fatty acids, acupuncture treatments, a nutrient formula, a small adjustment in the dose of thyroid hormone therapy, a small (tolerable) dose of an SSRI (escitalopram), and ongoing psychotherapy.

CHAPTER 6

Generalized Anxiety, Panic Attacks, and Obsessions and Compulsions

A SKILLFUL interview will generally provide enough information to determine whether a significant anxiety problem exists. When a client discloses a medical problem, further assessment may be warranted. For example, many heart problems are associated with anxiety symptoms. Disorders of the thyroid and other endocrinological disorders sometimes cause anxiety. When there is reason to suspect an underlying medical problem, it is always appropriate to refer clients to their family physician or naturopathic physician for further evaluation and medical treatment.

Nonconventional Approaches

In addition to established approaches used to assess the causes of anxiety, nonconventional approaches are coming into broader use. Different kinds of changes in brain electrical activity are associated with different anxiety symptoms. For example, decreased alpha activity often accompanies generalized anxiety, whereas increased theta activity is associated with obsessions and compulsions, and panic attacks are often accompanied by paroxysmal activity in the EEG (Hughes & Roy, 1999). Studies suggest that quantitative electroencephalography (QEEG) may predict the response of a person with obsessive–compulsive disorder (OCD) to conventional medications or biofeedback (Princhep et al., 1993). Preliminary research findings suggest that analysis of heart rate variability (HRV) may help clinicians decide which treatment will most likely be effective (McCraty et al., 2001). In contrast to depressed patients, who are more likely to have abnormally low serum cholesterol levels, individuals who experience generalized anxiety, panic attacks, or obsessions and compulsions tend to have elevated cholesterol levels (Peter et al., 2000). Emerging findings suggest that dietary deficiencies in vitamins B-6, niacin, C, and E and the minerals magnesium, selenium, and phosphorous may be associated with anxiety, and correcting these through supplementation may be beneficial in some cases (Heseker et al., 1992; McCleane & Watters, 1990).

EDST (electrodermal skin testing) is an assessment approach based on Chinese medical theory, which is used to measure qi energy in the body's meridians. EDST is also used by healing touch practitioners and other energy healers to help determine which conventional pharmacological or energetic treatments of anxiety will be most efficacious for a particular client's anxiety problems (Forbes et al., 2004). Research findings suggest that postulated energetic changes measured by EDST may reflect changes in the body's "bioenergy" field when pharmacological and energetic treatments of anxiety are successful (Stouffer et al., 2003).

TREATMENT

Conventional Treatments

Established conventional treatments of anxiety include cognitive–behavioral therapy and medications. However, many individuals do not improve significantly with these therapies. A meta-analysis of placebo-controlled studies found inconsistent evidence for many conventional pharmacological treatments of anxiety disorders (Westen & Morrison, 2001). Furthermore, many individuals with chronic anxiety or panic disorder are at risk of becoming dependent on potent sedative hypnotic drugs required to manage their symptoms. Generally anxious individuals may require lower doses of conventional medications to control symptoms of anxiety (Chaudhary et al., 1988). A significant percentage of anxious individuals are also depressed and have problems sleeping.

Nonconventional Treatments

A great deal of research has been done on a few natural substances used to treat anxiety, including kava-kava (*Piper methysticum*) and the amino acids L-theanine and 5-HTP. A systematic review of placebo-controlled double-blind studies concluded that kava is superior to placebo for the short-term management of generalized anxiety (Pittler et al., 2004). The antianxiety effects of standardized kava preparations compare favorably to conventionally used antianxiety medications (Boerner et al., 2003). Rare cases of liver failure following kava use have been attributed to manufacturing processing errors (Dragull et al., 2003). L-theanine is a natural constituent of green tea. This amino acid reduces generalized anxiety by increasing alpha activity and stimulating increased synthesis of GABA (the brain's principle inhibitory neurotransmitter) (Mason, 2001). Numerous research studies show that 5-HTP has consistent antianxiety effects (Soderpalm & Engel, 1990; Kahn et al., 1987) and may also help prevent panic attacks in some cases (Schruers et al., 2000).

Aromatherapy, using the essential oils of lavender, passion flower, and lemon balm, may help lessen anxiety in some cases (Diego et al., 1998; Akhondzadeh et al., 2001). Exercising 20–30 minutes daily can significantly lower anxiety levels in individuals who have generalized anxiety (Paluska & Schwenk, 2000), and regular massages have been found to reduce symptoms of generalized anxiety (Kim et al., 2002). Mind–body therapies, including yoga and mindfulness-based stress reduction, have been evaluated in research studies and found to be beneficial for many individuals who experience generalized anxiety (Keefer & Blanchard, 2001; Lau et al., 2006). Preliminary findings suggest that a specialized kind of yogic breathing may reduce symptom severity in individuals diagnosed with obsessive-compulsive disorder (Shannahoff-Khalsa et al., 1999), and combining daily yoga and mindfulness training has been shown to significantly reduce symptoms of generalized anxiety (Miller et al., 1995).

Frequent listening to soothing music reduces the overall level of autonomic arousal and generalized anxiety (Kerr et al., 2001), and exposure to certain frequency patterns of binaural sound can result in a calm, relaxed state (Atwater, 1999). Virtual reality graded exposure therapy (VRGET) is a recently introduced form of therapy that uses computers to create high-quality images that stimulate an anxiety response, which the client then works to extinguish through relaxation training. Numerous studies have confirmed that VRGET is an effective treatment of specific phobias, generalized anxiety, panic disorder with agoraphobia (Wiederhold et al., 2002; Vincelli, 2003), and PTSD (Riva et al., 2001). In fact, VRGET may ultimately prove to be more effective than conventional exposure therapy or medications for the treatment of phobias and PTSD.

Different kinds of biofeedback are widely used to treat generalized anxiety. Studies show that the anxiety-reducing effects of regular EEG or EMG biofeedback are comparable to conventional antianxiety medications (Rice et al., 1993; Sarkar et al., 1999). EEG biofeedback is now widely used to treat a range of anxiety disorders, reportedly with consistently good outcomes and few or no adverse effects. Heart rate variability (HRV) biofeedback training reduces stress and improves feelings of general well-being (McCraty et al., 2001).

Cranioelectrotherapy stimulation (CES) uses very small electrical currents to stimulate the muscles of the neck or head. This approach, which was pioneered in the former Soviet Union, is growing in popularity in the United States and other Western countries as a self-treatment for anxiety, insomnia, and chronic pain disorders. A systematic review of sham-controlled trials concluded that regular CES treatments effectively reduced symptoms of generalized anxiety (DeFelice, 1997). Sham-controlled studies on manual and electroacupuncture support its use for the treatment of generalized anxiety, although the anxiety-reducing benefits of acupuncture probably depend on the specific form and needling protocol used (British Acupuncture Council, 2002). Preliminary findings suggest that acupuncture may be an effective treatment of PTSD. In a small 12-week randomized controlled pilot trial, individuals with a DSM-IV diagnosis of PTSD were assigned weekly acupuncture sessions using a specific protocol vs. weekly group cognitive-behavioral therapy or a wait-list which received no treatment (Hollifield, Sinclair-Lian and Hammerschlag 2007). Individuals treated with acupuncture or CBT experienced comparable improvements in PTSD symptoms, and outcomes of both interventions were superior to improvements reported by the wait-list group. Furthermore, beneficial effects of acupuncture (and CBT) were maintained three months after the end of treatment. Limited evidence suggests that energy healing approaches including Reiki (Shore, 2004; Dressen, 1998), healing touch (Wardell, 2000; Guevara et al., 2002), and qigong (Lake, 2001) have anxiety-reducing effects. Table 6.1 summarizes the nonconventional treatments of anxiety.

TABLE 6.1 Nonconventional and Integrative Treatments of Anxiety

More substantiated:

- Kava-kava
- 5-hydroxytryptophan
- L-theanine
- Essential oils of lavender, passion flower, and lemon balm
- Mindfulness training and meditation
- Yoga

Less substantiated:

- Virtual reality graded exposure therapy
- EEG biofeedback
- HRV biofeedback
- Cranioelectrotherapy stimulation
- Acupuncture
- Qigong
- Healing touch

CASE VIGNETTES

Moderate Anxiety

Intake

Tom is 24 years old, married, and employed as an accountant in a high-tech startup company. He experienced his first panic attack 2 months ago when he was trapped in an elevator during a power outage. "I thought I was having a heart attack. I couldn't breathe, I started to have chest pain, and I thought I was going to pass out." Two weeks later he had another panic attack while sitting in traffic during rush hour. "I couldn't get out and I couldn't go anywhere . . . then things caved in!" Tom was so worried about his heart that he went to an emergency room the following day. His EEG was normal and after confirming that Tom was in excellent health, exercised regularly, and had never previously experienced chest pain or shortness of breath, the emergency room physician reassured him that his electrolytes were in the normal range and his heart was in excellent condition.

> Note: It is prudent to refer any patient complaining of new-onset panic attacks associated with chest pain and shortness of breath to the nearest hospital emergency room or urgent care center for immediate medical evaluation, including laboratory studies to check blood electrolyte levels and an electrocardiogram (EKG) to rule out a myocardial infarction or potentially serious cardiac arrhythmias. Mitral valve prolapse is a relatively common condition associated with a benign cardiac arrhythmia that may cause untriggered panic attacks; however, other cardiac arrhythmias associated with panic attacks are potentially life-threatening.

Tom was enormously relieved to learn that his heart was strong. He returned home and resumed his normal work and social routine. One month later, when standing in line at a market, Tom again experienced shortness of breath, tightness in his chest, and feelings of dread. This time he understood that he was having a panic attack, but there were no apparent reasons for it. It was a quiet Saturday afternoon, he felt rested, he hadn't been worrying about work, and— unlike his first two episodes—he was not confined in a small space. After sitting quietly in his car for several minutes, breathing deeply and "just trying to relax," Tom drove home slowly. He told his wife what had happened, and she hugged him as he began to cry. Over the next few weeks, he had more panic attacks; once in a supermarket and twice in a mall.

Like other symptom patterns, panic disorder can transform over time. Symptoms that were initially triggered by identifiable stressors or circumstances now occur spontaneously, without apparent precipitating factors. Panic attacks appear to take on a life of their own.

With the encouragement of his wife, who had been receiving acupuncture treatments for a chronic pain condition, Tom found an integrative psychiatrist who combined acupuncture with psychotherapy and medication management. Two weeks later he found himself at his initial appointment with Dr. Jeffers, a psychologist. "My understanding is that I've been having panic attacks." During the intake interview Tom discloses ongoing feelings of generalized anxiety dating back many years, but no history of panic attacks prior to being trapped in the elevator approximately 1 month ago. "I think I get too stressed out at work sometimes, and I carry it around with me." There is no history of depression or other mental health problems, including substance abuse, and no one in Tom's family had ever had a serious mental health problem. His medical history is significant for a head injury with loss of consciousness sustained in a motor vehicle accident at the age of 18. He was not drinking at the time of the accident, when he was rear-ended on the highway. Tom felt fortunate to be alive and ever since the accident has experienced a vague "queasy" feeling when driving on the highway. He had two concussions while playing high school football at about the same age. "I still have headaches sometimes but no more neck pain." About 1 year ago his family physician diagnosed him with hypertension and prescribed a medication. Tom's blood pressure has been normal since then, and he does not have medication side effects. After reviewing his own history in detail Tom remarks, "I guess I've had reasons for feeling anxious for some time, but you know, Doc, I really don't want to take pills for the rest of my life. I understand you do acupuncture. Can that help my problem?"

In reply to Tom's question Dr. Jeffers suggests that they first clarify the specific nature and possible underlying causes of Tom's symptoms in order to determine the most appropriate treatment plan. "There are many approaches, but let's take a moment to think through our options and talk about ones that best fit your situation." Dr. Jeffers starts with questions about diet and lifestyle. It is soon apparent that Tom's diet has been erratic for some time. In recent months he has often worked through lunch and delayed dinner until 8 p.m. On the day of his first panic attack he could not recall whether he had eaten lunch. "It's all a blur, Doc. All I can remember is being inside the elevator." Dr. Jeffers explained that hypoglycemia, caused by prolonged fasting, can precipitate feelings of acute anxiety, which are often accompanied by clammy skin and dizziness. Tom recalled that his symptoms had resolved soon after getting out of the elevator, *before* he had eaten again, and he did not remember feeling dizzy or perspiring while inside the elevator or during the subsequent panic attack. Dr. Jeffers asks Tom if he has noticed an irregular heart beat, feels cold much of the time, or has experienced anxiety, agitation, or intolerance of heat or cold in recent months.

These are common symptoms of hyperthyroidism which can sometimes manifest as panic attacks.

Tom has not experienced any of these symptoms but on Dr. Jeffers's advice agrees to have his thyroid hormone levels checked. By the end of their initial session it seems likely that Tom's symptoms were not caused by physiological factors, such as hypoglycemia, an electrolyte disturbance, or hyperthyroidism, and medical conditions commonly associated with panic have been reduced to a low probability. Furthermore, since Tom has not experienced neurological symptoms (e.g., changes in the level of consciousness, headaches) since his 18th birthday, there is no reason to suspect that the new-onset panic attacks are somehow related to his head injury or concussions. Finally, his first two panic attacks followed the same pattern, in that they were apparently triggered by feelings of loss of control when Tom was confined in a closed space. His third attack seemed to reflect a somewhat different theme: being in line and having to wait to get out of the store. His subsequent attacks continue to generalize this theme. On this basis, by the end of the first session, Dr. Jeffers concludes that Tom's panic attacks are most likely related to psychological factors. As the session ends Dr. Jeffers suggests that Tom purchase a self-help book on panic attacks, explaining: "This book will walk you through cognitive and behavioral strategies that will give you a better handle on this situation." He also asks Tom to make notes on any habits, situations, or circumstances that might function as triggers of future panic episodes, including eating habits, stressors, and the amount and timing of caffeine he consumes in the form of coffee, tea, or soft drinks. Dr. Jeffers concludes, "We'll use this information to put together a treatment plan next time I see you. Remember to get the thyroid studies done for good measure." They schedule a follow-up appointment in 2 weeks.

Assessment

Although Tom had a serious head injury at age 18, he denies experiencing headaches, vision changes, impaired concentration or other neurological or psychiatric symptoms in the intervening years since then. The emergency room physician who evaluated Tom following his first panic attack went a long way toward ruling out the most likely medical causes of his symptoms—a cardiac arrhythmia and abnormal electrolytes. However, many kinds of abnormal heart rhythms are difficult to detect with a resting EKG, and an extensive cardiology workup may be required before they are accurately diagnosed. For this reason Dr. Jeffers asks Tom about subjective perceptions that may suggest an underlying cardiac arrhythmia. Dr. Jeffer's history has already eliminated hypoglycemia as a likely cause of Tom's symptoms. Hyperthyroidism stands out as the only other common medical cause of panic attacks that has not yet been checked, but in view of the absence of typical symptoms of hyperthyroidism and the circumstances of his first two panic attacks, it is more likely that Tom's panic symptoms were triggered by intense feelings of loss of control when confined. Although a myriad of less common medical problems can cause panic-like symptoms, there are no other *apparent* or *highly probable* medical reasons for new-onset panic attacks that are appropriate to evaluate in this case. At the end of the initial session Dr. Jeffers makes a provisional diagnosis of panic disorder, commenting that thyroid studies are being done to rule out hyperthyroidism.

Formulation

This young adult male had no serious medical or psychiatric problems prior to experiencing a panic attack when trapped in an elevator 2 months ago. Medical evaluation following the initial panic attack confirms the absence of serious underlying medical causes. Factors identified during psychotherapy include fatigue, chronic work stress, and erratic eating habits. Because severe anxiety symptoms sometimes result from disorders of the thyroid, it is reasonable to order laboratory studies to rule out this possibility. However, hyperthyroidism is an unlikely cause of panic symptoms in this case because of the initial circumstances of onset and the patient's young age, excellent health, and the absence of physical symptoms that would suggest hyperthyroidism. Tom's panic attacks have evolved into non-cued episodes of intense anxiety when in supermarkets and shopping malls. In view of his benign medical and psychiatric history and the nature and progression of his symptoms, panic disorder with agoraphobia is the most appropriate diagnosis at this time, pending normal thyroid studies.

Treatment

Two weeks later Tom arrives at Dr. Jeffers's office carrying a notebook. "I've taken notes on the anxiety symptoms. There may be a pattern." As Tom reviews what he has written, it becomes apparent that, on an average workday, he drinks five or six cups of caffeinated coffee. There are also many days when he skips lunch because of work. "I think my lifestyle has been going in the wrong direction for some time." Dr. Jeffers remarks that excessive caffeine can result in both chronic anxiety and fatigue, may increase chances of uncued panic attacks in predisposed individuals, and may also cause irregular heart beats. "Your thyroid is normal, as we thought it would be. I think your symptoms are probably a result of chronic work stress, too much caffeine, and possibly also hypoglycemia in the afternoons when you skip lunch." Tom listens attentively and then begins to speak slowly. He describes his work environment as a "pressure cooker that just keeps getting worse—there's never a letup in the pace." It is clear that Tom has not felt in control of his time for many years. "I'm like that rat running in the maze, but I never seem to stop running."

Dr. Jeffers explains how lowering his baseline stress level through regular exercise, improved diet, and a mind–body practice such as yoga will not only reduce Tom's day-to-day anxiety level but also help control the frequency and intensity of panic attacks. "It's about retuning your central nervous system so you'll feel calmer in general and will have fewer episodes of extreme anxiety. The goal is to do whatever it takes to interrupt your panic attacks before they become a more established pattern." Dr. Jeffers goes on to describe various conventional and alternative therapies that are known to be effective for anxiety reduction and preventing panic attacks. He first mentions sedative hypnotic drugs such as clonazepam and lorazepam as the conventional pharmacological treatments used to lower generalized anxiety and to interrupt panic attacks when they occur. "These are the most established mainstream treatments for panic and they are often quite effective."

> Clonazepam, lorazepam, and other drugs in the benzodi-azepines class are frequently prescribed for management of panic attacks. These conventionally used medications are often effective at reducing both the frequency and intensity of panic attacks. However, many individuals who take them experience significant adverse effects, including excessive daytime sedation and impaired attention and short-term memory. Chronic benzodiazepine use is also associated with a high risk of dependence, which is especially problematic in the elderly, who are at increased risk of falling with cata-strophic consequences.

Dr. Jeffers then describes various natural treatment options used to lower the general level of anxiety, including the herb kava-kava and the amino acids 5-HTP and L-theanine, remarking that there is solid evidence for kava but less evidence for 5-HTP and L-theanine as treatments for generalized anxiety but not panic attacks or other severe anxiety symptoms.

> As noted previously, extensive research supports the use of kava for the treatment of generalized anxiety, but there is lit-tle evidence that the herbal is effective against panic attacks.

Research evidence suggests that L-theanine ameliorates moderate but not severe anxiety symptoms. The amino acid 5-HTP is also beneficial for symptoms of moderate generalized anxiety. It is absorbed orally, crosses into the brain, and is synthesized into the neurotransmitter serotonin; 5-HTP can be taken in the daytime for anxiety, but doses greater than 100 mg should be taken at bedtime to avoid sedation.

Dr. Jeffers then briefly talks about the evidence that a regular yoga practice can reduce generalized anxiety.

Many studies suggest that the regular practice of yoga reduces the severity of generalized anxiety. However, no studies to date have evaluated the effectiveness of yoga as a preventive "therapy" for panic attacks.

Dr. Jeffers continues: "I offer a specialized form of biofeedback, called EEG biofeedback, which can also help reduce general anxiety levels, but I don't think this kind of therapy will reduce the frequency or severity of your panic episodes. Acupuncture is also sometimes helpful for reducing generalized anxiety, but again, it doesn't directly treat panic attacks."

Tom is hesitant about taking a strong antianxiety medication. "I've heard it's difficult to get off those once you begin. Anyway, I think the larger problem is my overall anxiety level. I've thought about trying yoga for a long time. Maybe it's finally time. The natural treatments also appeal to me—even though they might not be as strong as the drugs. I would prefer treatments that are not potentially addictive. Getting hooked on an anxiety pill would essentially be replacing one problem with another."

Dr. Jeffers replies: "Many people feel the same way. However, the bottom line is finding a treatment that works. I understand that you want to try the alternatives first. We'll work together on this; perhaps yoga will help, but if one of these alternative approaches doesn't alleviate your symptoms, we may have to resort to conventional medications. I also want to encourage you to reduce the amount of coffee you drink to no more than two cups a day. I think the caffeine is keeping you revved up. You also need to start taking breaks a few times every day, including time to eat lunch, and learn how to relax. Here is a great guided imagery CD you may borrow. We're not talking about medications yet. Are you OK with this approach?" Tom nods his head in agreement. "What you're saying sounds reasonable, and I appreciate your guidance with the alternative approaches before prescribing a drug."

> Integrative mental health care can begin with alternative therapies and progress to more mainstream treatments, or vice versa, depending on the relative strength of evidence for different approaches, your client's preferences, and the affordability and availability of conventionally trained or alternative practitioners who can provide the desired treatment or expert consultation. In this case, although the evidence for alternative modalities is not strong, the client prefers an initial treatment plan that emphasizes specific natural products, dietary changes, a regular mind–body practice, and guided imagery for stress reduction. The integrative clinician is flexible in his or her approach to clients, and is open to considering more conventional treatment options if the initial treatment strategy is not successful.

Dr. Jeffers recommends a quality brand of kava, goes over safety issues associated with this herbal, and suggests starting with 60 mg for the first few days. He instructs Tom to gradually increase the dose to 300 mg/day, divided into three doses, and to remain at the lowest dose that consistently reduces feelings of generalized anxiety. Tom agrees to enroll in a yoga class and use the guided imagery CD twice daily: in the morning before work and after work. He also agrees to cut down his consumption of coffee and other caffeinated beverages. "I know this is about making healthier choices. I can do this." They agree to a follow-up appointment in 4 weeks.

Follow-Up Session

Tom appears relaxed and his speech is evenly paced. He explains that he has just listened to the guided imagery exercise while sitting in his car before the appointment. "That stuff really works." He has been taking kava three times daily for a total dose of 180 mg. He has not experienced adverse effects and describes his anxiety level as "much better . . . I feel smoother throughout the day." Tom now has two cups of coffee most days, one at breakfast and one in the early afternoon. "I can see that the coffee was really winding me up." He has been enjoying yoga for almost a month, attends classes three times a week, and practices yoga stretches for 10 minutes each morning before going to work. His wife has started to practice yoga with him. "I think this is helping our relationship get to a calmer place. My life is no longer just about working all the time and rushing in and out of the house." Tom has not had panic attacks since his appointment with Dr. Jeffers. "I'm hoping that this panic stuff is behind me, Doc." Dr. Jeffers praises Tom for the proactive lifestyle changes he has made and for his commitment to yoga: "I think the yoga is the strongest medicine you are taking. The kava is probably also helping to reduce your overall anxiety." Tom wants to continue taking kava and enjoys doing yoga. Dr. Jeffers does not recommend other treatments. "I think you've gotten this under control, Tom." Tom smiles, "What if I check in with you in about 3 months, Doc?"

Putting It All Together
Panic attacks can rapidly evolve into a debilitating disorder if not treated soon after they begin. Individuals who experience panic attacks often have a history of chronic stress and generalized anxiety. A thorough medical evaluation is prudent when a client reports new-onset panic attacks. History frequently points to diet and other lifestyle issues that may increase the risk of panic attacks. This case illustrates the integrative management of new-onset panic attacks uncomplicated by other significant medical or psychiatric problems. After underlying medical causes of panic have been ruled out, engaging in a regular mind–body practice such as yoga, guided imagery, or other stress reduction strategies, reducing caffeine and other stimulants, and taking kava or other natural products known to have calming effects on the central nervous system can significantly reduce generalized anxiety, thereby increasing the threshold needed to trigger future panic attacks, and effectively interrupting a recurring pattern of panic attacks before it evolves into a chronic debilitating disorder.

Severe Anxiety

Intake

Sandy is 68, retired, and recently separated from her spouse of 22 years. "The marriage never worked—there were always conflicts." During the past year she has experienced steadily increasing anxiety. In recent weeks she has been "unhappy, maybe even depressed," which she ascribes to a contentious divorce settlement that is now in mediation. Sandy has not been able to sleep through the night for at least 6 months. "I stay awake worrying and just can't seem to quiet my mind." A friend suggested psychotherapy and today she finds herself in the waiting room of Karen Bateson, a licensed clinical social worker. A barely perceptible fragrance of lemon and soft guitar music give her a relaxed feeling. "I'm a spiritual person. I think I should be more resilient," Sandy comments, noting her disappointment over "caving into negative emotions" around her marital troubles. Although she has been an avid meditator and yoga practitioner for decades, her anxiety has worsened in the past few years. She has been taking the SSRI paroxetine (Paxil) for 2 years. At first her anxiety level was somewhat less, but soon the beneficial effects of the drug seemed to "just fade." Her family physician increased the dose, but there was no further improvement in her mood and Sandy noticed adverse effects, including excessive perspiration and a rash. At that point, about 6 months ago, she was started on clonazenam at bedtime and twice during the daytime. She also continued on paroxetine and there were no significant adverse effects. "My sleep was better, and I felt free of anxiety for the first time in years, but I also felt spacy most of the time, and there were days when it was difficult to focus and stay awake. Then I found that I needed to take more pills to keep the anxiety away."

> The benzodiazepines clonazepam, lorazepam, and valium are widely prescribed for insomnia and anxiety disorders. However, their long-term use may result in increased tolerance, manifesting as a need to steadily increase the dose to achieve the same sedating or anxiety-reducing effects that were initially achieved using a much lower dose. Higher doses of benzodiazepines are often associated with daytime fatigue.

Sandy recalls being depressed for several months following the birth of her second son, but her symptoms eventually resolved without treatment, and she has had no subsequent episodes of depression. She has never experienced panic attacks or chronic generalized anxiety, and denies a history of alcohol abuse. There are no serious medical problems, including heart disease or hypertension, and Sandy has never had seizures, experienced loss of consciousness, or had a serious head injury. She denies a history of childhood trauma or abuse, and her parents and grandparents did not have mental health problems. Sandy had an uneventful menopause starting in her mid-50s and has not experienced mood changes or health problems related to menopause. She does not take estrogen or other hormonal replacement therapy.

Sandy has three adult children, two of whom have recently been diagnosed with depression. For the past 6 months she has been drinking two or three glasses of wine before bedtime "to help relax myself," but still wakes up in the middle of the night. Her appetite has been diminished for some time, and she often has to force herself to eat regular meals. Sandy has lost 15 pounds in the past 6 months and discloses that she feels generally weak much of the time. Her most recent annual physical exam was about 3 months ago. Routine laboratory findings, including complete blood count and electrolytes, were normal except for low total serum cholesterol. Her resting EKG was also normal. A thyroid panel was ordered, but Sandy "forgot" to bring the slip to the lab. During the past several months, Sandy has experienced a gradual "dulling" in her mood, diminished energy and interest in life, and has become increasingly withdrawn. She denies thoughts of suicide but reports that "sometimes I don't think I can go on." Her family physician recently recommended switching to another SSRI. Sandy remarks: "I don't think I'm getting anywhere with this approach. The medications seem to work for a short time or just make me feel numb, but I don't think I'm really getting better. I want to try something different."

Assessment

Psychological issues that need to be evaluated in this complex case include those underlying Sandy's generalized feelings of anxiety, insomnia, and depressed mood—all probably related to the stress of her divorce. Recent changes in cognitive functioning and mood may be related to chronic fatigue due to insomnia, poor dietary habits, or adverse effects of medications. The seriousness of Sandy's alcohol abuse needs to be evaluated. Possible underlying medical causes of her psychiatric symptoms are being evaluated by appropriate conventional laboratory tests, including thyroid studies and serum cholesterol. Elevated serum cholesterol may be associated with increased risk of many anxiety problems, including generalized anxiety and panic attacks. Deficiencies in vitamins B-6, C, E, and thiamin, and the trace minerals magnesium and selenium—in some cases due to chronic poor nutrition—may increase the risk of developing generalized anxiety.

Formulation

Sandy is a healthy 68-year-old woman with a history of postpartum depression that resolved without treatment. She has not experienced recurring depressive episodes and has not had other major mental health problems. Insomnia, generalized anxiety, and moderate depressed mood have continued for 6 months coinciding with a stressful divorce and uncertainty over the future. Her family history and medical history are unremarkable. Assessing prescription benzodiazepine abuse and dependence and associated changes in mood, energy, and cognitive functioning should be a priority in this case. There is a question of general malnourishment and hypoglycemia related to low vitality, anxiety, fatigue, and depressed mood. A pattern of alcohol use at bedtime is probably disrupting sleep, interfering with the therapeutic effects of her antidepressant, and potentiating the sedating effects of the clonazepam.

Treatment

As the initial session ends, Ms. Bateson asks Sandy whether she told her family physician about her pattern of drinking before bedtime. "I didn't think that was a problem. After all, it's not so much and I don't have hangovers in the morning." Ms. Bateson briefly comments on the risks of drinking when taking any sedative.

Consuming alcohol together with benzodiazepines or other sedative hypnotics amplifies the sedating effects of these potent drugs; increases the risk of overdose, disorientation, and falling; and can result in significant memory problems and impairment in cognitive functioning. Chronic alcohol use also interferes with the therapeutic benefits of SSRIs by activating liver enzymes that subsequently reduce blood levels available to the brain.

"It sounds like you're waking up at about the same time a few hours after going to sleep, then having trouble getting back to sleep." Ms. Bateson attributes Sandy's sleep issues to a combination of rebound insomnia caused by alcohol and chronic stress due to preoccupation with her divorce. "One of the first issues we should address is getting a good night's sleep. If we can find ways to help you sleep through the night, I think things will get better overall."

Chronic insomnia can exacerbate anxiety and depression while interfering with cognitive functioning and causing debilitating daytime fatigue. Paradoxically, many conventional treatments of insomnia rapidly lead to tolerance and dependence, and there is a significant risk of withdrawal if they are abruptly discontinued. It has been established that prolonged use of potent sedative hypnotic drugs impairs short-term memory and general cognitive performance and exacerbates depressed mood, thus interfering with the beneficial effects of antidepressants.

Ms. Bateson is a certified neurotherapist and has considerable experience treating anxiety with this approach. She briefly describes the concepts of EEG biofeedback to Sandy, who appears intrigued by this approach. "It's about retuning the brain to reduce the overall level of anxiety. It's like playing a computer game with your brain." Ms. Bateson gives Sandy a DVD that introduces the basic concepts of neurotherapy, and they agree to start EEG biofeedback training at the next appointment. Ms. Bateson recently attended a lecture on targeted amino acid therapy (TAAT) and recalls that certain amino acids can be used to ameliorate both anxiety and depression. Although Sandy has not tried alternative therapies, her disappointment with conventional medications, due to her poor response and concerns over adverse effects, suggests that she is open to trying

TAAT. Ms. Bateson briefly reviews the evidence for 5-HTP and L-theanine and suggests that Sandy try a combination of these two amino acids, known to have general calming effects on the central nervous systsm. Before starting the amino acid regimen, however, Ms. Bateson wants to find out whether Sandy's neurotransmitter levels are low or out of balance. She gives Sandy a form she can use to order a kit for collecting urine and sending it to a laboratory for testing. Ms. Bateson suggests that Sandy have the results sent to herself as well as her physician so that they will both know about any abnormal findings. In closing, Ms. Bateson encourages Sandy to improve her general nutrition, to take a high-potency B-complex and multivitamin, and to try to be "more aware" of her eating habits. She also encourages Sandy to cut out wine around bedtime and to try meditating or sitting with relaxing music in the final hour before sleep.

First Follow-Up Session

Two weeks later Sandy appears more rested. She remarks that not drinking wine and instead meditating with calming music about 30 minutes before bedtime have resulted in more restful sleep and fewer awakenings. She ordered the self-test kit and returned a urine sample to the lab about a week ago. She has been more attentive to her dietary preferences and has managed to eat three balanced meals almost every day, though her appetite continues poor. "The anxiety is still there, but I think that it is generally less when I sleep well and take in enough nutrients." She has been taking the vitamins recommended by Ms. Bateson and believes they give her more energy and improve her mental focus. Sandy left a message with her family doctor to let him know about the work she is doing with Ms. Bateson, including the urine testing to check for neurotransmitter deficiencies. "I don't know if my doctor believes in this approach, but I think it's important to let him know what I'm doing." The previous she learned that her thyroid levels are all in the normal range. Fifteen minutes into the session Ms. Bateson brings Sandy to an adjoining room where she does neurofeedback training. After walking her through the routine and selecting a game that involves "walking" in a meadow and finding wildflowers, she attaches two electrodes over Sandy's ears and adjusts the settings with the goal of normalizing the electrical brain activity underlying Sandy's anxiety symptoms.

An appropriate neurofeedback protocol in this case might involve placing electrodes over the temporal lobes on both sides of the head to address the client's high arousal level. Training at prefrontal areas is also helpful for calming what neurotherapists refer to as "mental overactivity" associated with generalized anxiety states. After her anxiety symptoms resolve, a different neurofeedback protocol, possibly involving training over the right temporal and occipital regions, might be used to modulate regional brain activity associated with her depressed mood.)

Thirty minutes later Sandy has completed her first session of neurofeedback training. She reports a pleasant, calm feeling and is more focused. "This is really interesting!" Ms. Bateson explains that the goal of training is to learn how to maintain the more balanced brain states achieved during neurofeedback sessions on a day-to-day basis. As the session ends, Ms. Bateson tells Sandy about a hand-held biofeedback device that she can use on her own to regulate her pulse and respiration, thereby lowering her general arousal and anxiety levels. She explains that by using the device for several minutes two to three times daily, Sandy will reinforce the benefits of neuro-feedback and make more rapid and sustained progress in lowering her general level of anxiety. "This is a loaner. If it works, you can get one for yourself."

Inexpensive and portable feedback devices are now available for monitoring heart rate and temperature, providing feedback in the form of light or vibration cues to help clients (1) become more aware of the connection between their heart and body temperature and their anxiety and (2) eventually learn how to change their heart rate and temperature while reducing their arousal level and improving their capacity to focus.

Because of her financial situation, the earliest time Sandy can schedule a return appointment is in 2 weeks.

Second Follow-Up

Sandy has been using the portable biofeedback device almost daily, including just before bedtime. She feels calmer for the hour or so afterward, sleeps better, but continues to experience significant anxiety much of the day. She ascribes her generally improved mood and energy level to better sleep and the vitamins she is taking. She continues to take her medications as before. Since her last appointment, findings of the specialized urine test have returned, showing that a metabolite of serotonin in her urine is lower than usual. "I think I'd like to try one of those amino acids and get off the Paxil." Ms. Bateson checks a textbook on amino acid therapy and remarks that daily doses of 5-HTP could help increase Sandy's brain serotonin level. She advises Sandy to consult with her physician before stopping the SSRI or starting amino acids or other biologically active natural products. "Amino acid therapy is generally very safe, but since you are already taking a medication, you should discuss this option with your family physician before trying it. "Stopping an SSRI too fast can also send you into a tailspin."

> Abrupt discontinuation of all SSRIs (with the exception of fluoxetine [Prozac]) can result in an unpleasant constellation of symptoms including insomnia, acute anxiety, and agitation. The chances of this taking place are generally increased with higher doses and longer duration of treatment. It is prudent to advise clients who wish to discontinue an SSRI, or any other conventional medication, to consult with their family physician or psychiatrist first.

Third Follow-Up

Sandy has been taking 5-HTP at doses of 100 mg at breakfast and lunch and 200 mg just before bedtime. She brought the lab findings suggesting reduced brain serotonin levels to her family physician and has gradually reduced her Paxil to 20 mg over the past 2 weeks. "My head feels better; I think the anxiety is less, I sleep better, and I think my mood is better also." There has been progress in her mediation sessions with her estranged husband, and she is hopeful of an amicable settlement in the near future. Sandy tells Ms. Bateson about how her family physicians instructed her to gradually increase the 5-HTP from 50 mg twice daily to a dosing regimen that "works for me." So far, other current regimen, there are no adverse effects. She uses the hand-held biofeedback device three times daily, including 10 minutes right before sleeping. "I think it's really helping with my anxiety and my sleep. Now that I'm rested most of the time and my anxiety is lower, my brain seems to be working better." She has continued to follow a healthy diet and has regained 8 pounds since seeing Ms. Bateson the first time. "At this point I would really like to get off the clonazepam. I don't think I need it any more." Ms. Bateson suggests that this is probably a reasonable choice, given that Sandy is now generally less anxious and depressed and taking a natural therapy that is helping with sleep. "But it is always safer to change medications after speaking with your doctor. We've come a long way and don't want to get tripped up at this stage," Ms. Bateson cautions her.

When going off any sedative hypnotic drug, it is always prudent to follow a gradual taper with the advice and supervision of a physician. Abrupt discontinuation of benzodiazepines and other sedatives can result in a serious withdrawal syndrome that includes feelings of intense agitation or anxiety, increased heart rate, and insomnia.

They enter the neurotherapy suite, and Ms. Bateson attaches the electrodes. "I think I'll try a new game today," Sandy comments. After 30 minutes Sandy is relaxed and focused. She remarks, "You know, my personal gadget gives me the same kind of quiet, centered feeling that I get from your machine. Maybe this and my meditation practice are all I need at this point." Ms. Bateson acknowledges Sandy's progress and encourages her to continue meditating and using the hand-held biofeedback device. A follow-up is scheduled in 1 month.

Putting It All Together

This case illustrates the integrative management of anxiety complicated by depressed mood, insomnia, chronic fatigue, and moderately impaired cognitive functioning. A conventional treatment regimen typically includes an SSRI (or other antianxiety medication) in combination with a sedative hypnotic at bedtime for insomnia and at a lower dose during the day for anxiety. Although SSRIs often provide symptomatic relief of both anxiety and depressed mood, for reasons that are not well understood, many experience a "wearing off" effect after taking an SSRI for several months. Trials on other conventional medications, including augmentation strategies, are often effective. However, clients who are frustrated by the lack of a consistent response or by significant adverse effects may wish to try alternative therapies at this point.

Meditation, improved nutrition, and a simple biofeedback approach comprise a first-line integrative strategy for improving sleep, reducing the general level of stress and anxiety, and finding out to what degree the client's cognitive problems are related to adverse medication effects versus poor nutrition. Neurotherapy (i.e., EEG biofeedback) is primarily directed at reducing the general level of arousal and anxiety but often results in improvement in overall cognitive functioning. Amino acid therapy is introduced when the client's baseline symptoms have already started to improve. Progress made through ongoing neurofeedback sessions in the therapist's office is reinforced by use of a simple hand-held biofeedback device between sessions. Symptoms of moderate depressed mood often improve when anxiety is reduced via multimodal treatment, and neurotherapy sessions address residual depressed mood symptoms after the client's baseline arousal level has responded to treatment. When the client is stable and motivated to continue following an integrative regimen, it is reasonable to consider tapering conventional medications, but only under the supervision of a family physician, naturopathic physician, or psychiatrist. Abrupt discontinuation of most SSRIs, benzodiazepines, and other medications carries the risk of an uncomfortable, potentially destabilizing withdrawal syndrome. This case illustrates how a highly motivated client who is experiencing chronic anxiety, insomnia, and moderate depressed mood can benefit from an integrative strategy that includes improved nutrition, amino acid therapy, neurofeedback, and a mind–body practice.

CHAPTER 7

Hyperactivity and Distractibility

A PATTERN of hyperactivity, distractibility, or both that is not caused by another psychiatric or medical problem, and that begins in childhood and persists into adolescence and adulthood, is typically diagnosed as attention-deficit/hyperactivity disorder (ADHD). It has been estimated that up to one-third of the world population experiences persisting symptoms of inattention, distractibility, impulsivity, or hyperactivity consistent with the Western psychiatric diagnosis of ADHD (Barkley, 1998). Three subtypes of the syndrome can be diagnosed depending on which symptoms cause the greatest degree of social or occupational impairment. Some individuals are primarily affected by inattention and distractibility, whereas others are impulsive and always moving. A third group of individuals diagnosed with ADHD experiences both kinds of symptoms. Most children and adults who have this syndrome have not been correctly diagnosed and treated, resulting in enormous productivity losses in the workplace as well as relationship problems. Many individuals with ADHD also have learning disorders, depressed mood, anxiety, and substance abuse problems (Newcorn et al., 2007). The syndrome is believed to be caused by genetic factors, birth trauma, exposure to environmental toxins before or after birth, or early childhood abuse and neglect (Swanson et al., 2007). Certain food colorings and preservatives probably exacerbate the syndrome. Standardized symptom rating scales are used by therapists, parents, and teachers to assess the type and severity of ADHD in children and self-rating scales are used for adults.

Nonconventional Approaches

There may be a causal relationship between low zinc levels and dysfunction of brain regions important for maintaining attention and processing auditory information (Arnold, et al., 2005). Large prospective studies are needed to verify that zinc supplementation in deficient children results in consistent improvements in ADHD symptoms and to determine the optimal dosing strategy. Low serum iron levels in children with ADHD who are not anemic may also be associated with an increased risk of hyperactivity (Oner et al., 2008). Neuroimaging studies have shown that the symptoms of ADHD correlate with abnormal patterns of regional brain metabolic and electrical activity. A specialized, quantitative kind of electroencephalography, QEEG, is used to "map" electrical brain activity. A persisting pattern of relative underarousal in the frontal cortex—the part of the brain that is necessary for sustained attention—is present in 90% of individuals diagnosed with ADHD (Butnik, 2005). Using QEEG analysis to determine the specific pattern of abnormal brain electrical activity associated with ADHD may help guide the selection of the optimal EEG biofeedback protocol.

TREATING HYPERACTIVITY AND DISTRACTIBILITY

Conventional Treatments

Conventional treatments of ADHD include stimulant medications, a nonstimulant medication (atomoxetine), SSRIs, clonidine, and others. The choice of medication depends on the type and severity of ADHD symptoms. Research findings suggest that extended release stimulants are associated with fewer adverse effects. Behavioral modification is a widely used technique aimed at rewarding desirable behaviors and extinguishing disruptive or inappropriate behavior.

Supportive psychotherapy can help children and adults reduce anxiety and cope with feelings of loss of control. Many children and adults diagnosed with ADHD use nonconventional modalities together with stimulants or other conventional pharmacological treatments, but fewer than 10% disclose this information to their physician (Chan et al., 2003). Frequent adverse effects associated with stimulants include insomnia, decreased appetite, and abdominal discomfort (Schachter et al., 2001). It has been established that chronic stimulant use during childhood interferes with normal growth rate, and long-term stimulant use is associated with increased risk of substance abuse in adults but not children (Faraone & Wilens, 2003). In addition to these safety issues, there are growing concerns about potential neurotoxic consequences of long-term stimulant use on the brain.

Nonconventional Treatments

Emerging nonconventional treatments of ADHD include elimination diets, omega-3 essential fatty acids, EEG biofeedback, zinc and iron supplementation, certain herbals, yoga, massage, and "green" play environments. Specialized diets that eliminate food colorings, additives, and specific foods (e.g., eggs, dairy products, wheat, corn, nuts) may substantially reduce the severity of ADHD symptoms—symptoms that recur when those foods are reintroduced. Research findings on elimination diets are inconsistent and large, and well-designed studies are needed to confirm their findings (Rojas & Chan, 2005). The amount of sugar in the diet may be related to the severity of ADHD symptoms. However, there may be a closer correlation between the glycemic index—the relative rate at which foods are converted into glucose in the blood—and ADHD symptoms (Weber & Newmark, 2007). Although omega-3 fatty acids are widely used to treat or self-treat ADHD, research findings to date are mixed. A recent pilot study found that very high doses of omega-3s—up to 16 gm/day of mixed dehydroascorbic acid (DHA) and EPA—may be significantly more efficacious than lower doses (Sorgi et al., 2007). Electroencephalographic (EEG) biofeedback training is a rapidly evolving therapy in which brain electrical activity is normalized, with associated reductions in symptoms of inattention, impulsivity, and hyperactivity (Monastra et al., 2005). Studies on the use of certain herbals and plant-derived products in the treatment of ADHD have yielded promising results. A standardized extract of the bark of the French maritime pine tree, called Pycnogenol, is probably a safe and effective treatment of ADHD, but larger studies are needed to confirm its efficacy and determine optimal dosing strategies (Trebaticka et al., 2006). *Bacopa monnieri* ("Brahmi") is an important medicinal herbal in Ayurveda, the traditional medicine of India. The herbal is traditionally used to increase energy and enhance memory and mental performance and is now being used in the United States and other Western countries to treat children with ADHD and learning disorders. Only one study has been published on the use of this herbal for ADHD, to date, and it reported positive results.

Findings of a large controlled trial suggest that supplementation with zinc in individuals who are deficient in this trace element may reduce hyperactivity, but it has little effect on inattention and distractibility (Bilici et al., 2004). A daily iron pill may also be beneficial in children with ADHD who are iron deficient, but more studies are needed to confirm therapeutic benefits of iron before supplementation can be generally recommended (Konofal et al., 2008). Taking an iron supplement with a stimulant medication may be more effective than taking a stimulant alone. There is some evidence that the amino acid acetyl-L-carnitine, in doses ranging from 1 to 3 gm/day, is beneficial for symptoms of inattention (Torrioli et al., 2008). Certain homeopathic remedies may reduce symptoms of inattention and impulsivity; however, better-designed studies are needed before homeopathy can be generally recommended for the treatment of ADHD (Frei et al., 2007). Results of an 8-week study suggest that adolescents and adults who engage in a regular mindfulness practice experience improvements in symptoms of ADHD as well as anxiety and depressed mood (Zylowska et al., 2008). Finally, yoga and massage therapy have been investigated for their beneficial effects in children diagnosed with ADHD, with positive results (Jensen & Kenny, 2004; Khilnani et al., 2003). Table 7.1 summarizes the nonconventional treatments of ADHD.

TABLE 7.1 Nonconventional and Integrative Treatments of ADHD

More substantiated:

- EEG biofeedback training
- Zinc supplementation (primarily for hyperactivity; may be beneficial alone or in combination with stimulants)
- A standardized extract of the bark of the French maritime pine tree (Pycnogenol)

Less substantiated:

- Elimination diets
- Reducing dietary sugar intake
- Daily iron in individuals who are iron-deficient
- Acetyl-L-carnitine (primarily for inattention)
- High-dose essential fatty acids (DHA/EPA)
- Bacopa monnieri ("Brahmi")
- Mindfulness training
- Yoga
- Massage therapy
- Homeopathy

CASE VIGNETTES

Moderate Symptoms

Intake

Billy's parents had always experienced their son as "a very active little soul." They recalled how fussy he had been as a baby and all the accidents requiring frequent visits to the pediatrician "to take care of scrapes and bruises." Fortunately there had been no broken bones or other serious injuries. "Sometimes he just moves too fast for us to keep an eye on him," his mother explained. Billy was delivered on a sunny July morning after a full-term pregnancy without complications. Throughout her first pregnancy Nancy had been meticulous about her diet, avoiding alcohol and all medications and eating healthily. Billy has achieved all of his developmental milestones on schedule, has not had any serious illnesses, and is strong for his age.

Nancy noticed that Billy had a "sweet tooth" and seemed to "rev up" after dessert. She and her husband Tony have been conscientious about limiting the amount of sugar in Billy's diet, and they have recently become concerned about possible food allergies. As he squirms in his mother's lap in the office of Karen Pearson, MA, Nancy recalls how much Billy loved to play chase and climb on the "monkey bars" in preschool. "He just couldn't stop moving," she comments. At age 6 Billy had grown into a vital, energetic, and self-confident boy. By all accounts he is bright and socially appropriate for his age. Billy's first-grade teacher recently told Nancy and Tony about her concerns that their son "just can't sit still and isn't able to pay attention long enough" to benefit from school. "I don't know if Billy has ADHD, but his first-grade teacher told me he does! I don't want to label my son, but if there's a problem I want to be proactive." A friend suggested Karen Pearson because of her reputation for being an "open-minded" therapist specializing in the integrative management of children who have been labeled with ADHD.

Nancy has always been "mellow" but her husband Tony was "a holy terror" as a child, and although he no longer struggles with symptoms of hyperactivity, he continues to have problems focusing at work. Ms. Pearson briefly talks about the evidence for genetic contributions to ADHD.

> Evidence from twin studies has confirmed that ADHD is a highly heritable disorder. Genes involved in the regulation of attention and behavior are believed to affect brain activity of dopamine and serotonin, the neurotransmitters targeted by conventional treatments of the syndrome. Exposure to toxins soon before or following birth probably increases the risk of developing ADHD. There is evidence that food colorings and additives as well as certain foods may exacerbate the symptoms of ADHD.

Nancy appears worried. "I don't want to start Billy on stimulants. I've read too many bad things about them. I want to try other approaches first." Karen reassures Nancy and Tony, "If your son does have ADHD, there are many useful approaches other than stimulants. Let's get a sense of where the problem is first and discuss this next time."

Assessment

Ms. Pearson gives Nancy two copies of the Conners' Rating Scales—one for parents and one for teachers—and asks her to fill one out and give the other one to Billy's teacher. "This will give us a sense of Billy's behavior and whether the problem is ADHD or something else." She explains to Nancy that anxiety problems and some learning disorders can sometimes "look like" symptoms of ADHD. Ms. Pearson encourages Nancy and Tony to take notes on Billy's diet and behavior and to bring them to the next appointment to help determine whether there are relationships between certain foods and periods of relatively greater hyperactivity or distractibility.

Formulation

Billy is a healthy 6-year-old who was delivered after an uncomplicated full-term pregnancy. His mother has no medical or psychiatric disorders and does not smoke or drink. There is no evidence of possible exposure to toxins during fetal development, infancy, or currently, nor have there been serious medical illnesses or injuries. Billy's father probably had childhood ADHD, although he has never been formally diagnosed or treated. His parents are caring and conscientious, and there is certainly no evidence of neglect or abuse. Although there is no apparent evidence of a primary learning disorder or an anxiety disorder, these possibilities are being considered by the pediatrician. Billy's behavior does not suggest oppositional defiant disorder. Food additives, colorings, or specific food items may be causing Billy's symptoms. Good record keeping by his parents will help determine whether dietary factors are contributing to Billy's hyperactivity or distractibility. There is no indication for formal laboratory tests or a referral for specialized diagnostic evaluation.

Treatment Plan

Nancy and Billy return to Ms. Pearson's office 3 weeks later. Ms. Pearson hears the receptionist "negotiating" with Billy in the waiting room, with little success. His parents' impressions and the teacher's score on the Conners' scale confirm that Billy has moderate to severe symptoms of hyperactivity and distractibility consistent with a diagnosis of ADHD, combined type. There is no evidence of a primary anxiety disorder or other psychiatric problem. In class Billy is keeping up with his peers but is unable to focus for more than a few minutes, his behavior is disruptive, and he frequently blurts out answers or comments. Nancy has been carefully monitoring Billy's eating habits and believes he is "more hyper" in the morning hours, after breakfast. His usual breakfast consists of a hot wheat cereal with walnuts, a dab of honey, and soy milk. "I think his breakfast might be starting young Billy out at a disadvantage," Ms. Pearson remarks, adding that the carbohydrate-laden foods in Billy's breakfast might be contributing to his symptoms. Nancy asks about the Feingold diet, and Ms. Pearson tells her that this particular approach hasn't been supported by research.

Developed in the 1970s, the Feingold diet was the first highly restrictive diet used as a therapeutic intervention for children diagnosed with ADHD. The diet essentially eliminated all processed foods. Early findings reported by Dr. Feingold (1975) claimed dramatic improvements in ADHD symptoms with this diet. Unfortunately, these findings have not been borne out by controlled trials, and other so-called "elimination diets" have been developed (Wender, 1986).

Ms. Pearson then describes a more recently developed restrictive diet called the oligoantigenic diet. "The idea is that certain foods result in a kind of allergic response that can affect the brain and behavior."

Several restrictive diets have been explored as treatments of ADHD, starting with the Feingold Diet in the 1970s. The most scientifically validated restrictive diet investigated as a treatment of ADHD is the oligoantigenic diet, which eliminates food colorings and additives, diary products, sugar, wheat, corn, citrus, eggs, soy, yeast, nuts, and chocolate. Several controlled studies on this highly restrictive regimen have reported significant reductions in the severity of hyperactivity, which returns to baseline when children are subsequently "challenged" with a particular food item. Although this diet brings relief to many children, the research studies on which it is based have been criticized because of methodological flaws, including the absence of standardized outcome measures, high dropout rates, and, in some studies, nonblinded raters (Rojas & Chan, 2005).

Nancy listens intently and nods her head. "I wonder if this would be a good thing to try with Tony also." Ms. Pearson smiles, "It probably wouldn't hurt."

Nancy asks Ms. Pearson about sugar. "I've read that sugar is really the culprit in ADHD, and I know that Billy goes after sugar whenever he can find it." Ms. Pearson explains that the "verdict on sugar isn't in yet." Removing sugar might help with some of Billy's symptoms, but the research evidence on this is inconsistent."

Sugar is widely believed to play a causal role in ADHD, but research findings do not support this view. In a placebo-controlled study there were no behavioral differences between children randomized to diets high in sugar, aspartame, or saccharin (Wolraich et al., 1994). It has been suggested that symptoms of hyperactivity or distractibility may be more related to the glycemic index of foods rather than sugar content per se. High-glycemic-index foods contain simple sugars that result in rapid increases in blood sugar levels and associated insulin secretion followed by relative hypoglycemia, which may manifest as the symptoms of hyperactivity, distractibility, irritability, or "moodiness" that often accompany ADHD. Examples of high-glycemic-index foods are fruit juices, citrus fruits, candy, and honey (Weber & Newmark, 2007).

As they wrap up the session, Ms. Pearson suggests specific changes in Billy's breakfast routine and advises Nancy to eliminate sugar and high-glycemic index foods from his diet. In the last few minutes of the session, Ms. Pearson introduces Nancy to the concepts of behavioral modification therapy, recommending a popular book to help her get started. She also suggests Nancy use a chart with gold stars to reinforce Billy's desirable behaviors. Lastly, Ms. Pearson tells Nancy about an inexpensive computer game that includes a simple kind of biofeedback that helps children learn how to focus and is reportedly beneficial in some cases of ADHD.

> Several commercially available computer games incorporate biofeedback based on changes in heart rate or respiration. Although not yet formally evaluated in sham-controlled studies, consistent anecdotal reports suggest that regular use of these biofeedback "games" can ameliorate symptoms of inattention and distractibility.

As Nancy and Billy leave, Nancy becomes tearful. "His teacher told me that if things don't change very soon, I may have to find a special school for my son. She asked me why Billy isn't taking Ritalin . . . I feel like I'm being forced to put him on stimulants." Ms. Pearson reassures her, "We'll cross that bridge when we get to it. First let's try what we've talked about and see how things work."

Follow-Up Session

Four weeks later Billy and his mother return for a routine follow-up. Ms. Pearson is pleased to see Billy sitting in the waiting room turning the pages of a picture book. "Hello, Ms. Pearson," Billy smiles. "I eat different and I feel quiet." Nancy tells Karen about the dramatic shift in Billy's behavior that occurred when she changed his diet and eliminated high-glycemic index foods and sugar. "After this I think I've become a believer in 'You are what you eat!'" In addition to being able to pay attention in class, Billy is less irritable after school and "it seems like he's a happier little person overall." Nancy and Tony have been giving Billy gold stars on charts for good days at school and good weekend days at home. He is enjoying playing the computer game with the finger pulse sensor in the mornings before going to school and in the evenings before bedtime. "It feels like he's in a different space when he's playing, and then he's calm afterward." Nancy tells Ms. Pearson that Billy's teacher is no longer "pushing Ritalin at my son," and is praising Billy for good behavior. Billy is clearly engaged with the efforts of his parents and teacher and smiles with satisfaction, "I'm a good boy and now I don't have to be too busy." Nancy hugs her son and tears come to her eyes.

Putting It All Together

This vignette illustrates the integrative management of childhood ADHD that is not complicated by other medical or mental health problems. Billy's parents and first-grade teacher work in tandem to clarify the type and severity of his symptoms. His parents provide valuable information that helps the therapist and pediatrician make inferences about possible causal relationships between specific dietary factors and Billy's symptoms, which are addressed in a proactive manner using an elimination diet. A behavioral modification program is aimed at rewarding appropriate behaviors at school and home and empowering Billy to take control over symptoms that interfere with his ability to function at school and home. A simple biofeedback "game" is strategically used at the beginning and end of each day to further develop Billy's improving capacity to stay calm and maintain his focus. If Billy remains on a closely monitored restrictive diet and continues to benefit from regular behavioral modification therapy and biofeedback training, the use of stimulants, other conventional or biological therapies (including omega-3 fatty acids, herbals, etc.), may not be needed.

Severe Symptoms

Intake

Margaret is 48, divorced, and works as a landscape architect. "A friend told me I have attention deficit syndrome. For as long as I can remember, I get distracted easily and have problems being on time and staying organized. I'm sure it's also affected my personal life. Guys can't handle my 'disorganized mind' after a short time." Margaret has been taking 30 mg of methylphenidate (Ritalin) twice daily for several years, and it has moderately increased her ability to concentrate at work, but her last two performance reviews were poor and she was recently overlooked for a promotion. "My manager knows that I'm bright, but I just can't stay on task and get things done. My work is suffering!" Margaret had two previous architecture jobs but eventually lost both because "I just can't seem to control the monkey mind, and I end up spinning and getting nothing done much of the time." Recently she has felt anxious and is anticipating being placed on probation because of her poor performance. She has also felt very tired for years. "Maybe it's the stress . . . I don't know." Her diet has been erratic for as long as she can remember. She sometimes works for days without eating a healthy meal and often eats fast food on the way to or from work. "I just forget to eat sometimes, and I haven't had much of an appetite for years." Margaret tells Dr. Janson that she has thought about stopping the methylphenidate because of frequent upset stomachs, headaches, and problems sleeping, but "I know I would be even worse without it." She has been depressed for about a year, which she ascribes to relationship problems with her boyfriend and work stress. She found Dr. Janson's ad in the Yellow Pages and was intrigued by the mention of "integrative medicine." She made an appointment for the following week.

"I understand you do integrative medicine but I'm not sure what that means." Dr. Janson explains that he prescribes medications, does psychotherapy, and also teaches patients "about nutrition, healthy lifestyle changes, supplements, and a range of treatment choices based on solid medical evidence."

A complete history clarifies that Margaret has had difficulty focusing since childhood but has never had problems with hyperactivity or impulsive behavior. She has never had a head injury or seizures and has no known medical problems currently. She does not smoke cigarettes and occasionally drinks a few glasses of wine with dinner. She sometimes smokes marijuana "to take the edge off" after long days but has never abused marijuana or other drugs. Margaret denies a history of mania or hypomania and has never experienced severe depressed mood; however, she has struggled with moderate depressed mood since her early 20s. "I eventually went in for treatment, and I've been on several medications for ADHD and depression over the years," including three different SSRIs and buproprion. Margaret discontinued all of these medications after days or weeks either because of adverse effects, such as reduced libido, rash, and excessive perspiration, or because "they just didn't make a difference. I feel better for a short time, but then they wear off and I feel the same old way . . . or the side effects get to me, and I just can't deal with the meds anymore."

Margaret describes her parents as "healthy, average" people but notes that her father might struggle with depression "some of the time." She denies allergies to medications or foods and admits frequently eating sugary snacks. She once practiced yoga but had to "let that go" a long time ago "because I just didn't have the energy." Margaret does not take vitamins or other supplements, only methylphenidate. Dr. Janson encourages Margaret to work on changing her eating habits by avoiding fast food and high-sugar snacks whenever possible. In the final minutes of the session he introduces the concept of EEG biofeedback to Margaret. "It's a machine that you use to retrain your brain so that it is easier to stay focused." Margaret is interested but remarks in an exasperated tone, "At this point I'm open to anything that might work."

Assessment

A thorough history has established that Margaret's severe symptoms of distractibility have resulted in chronic occupational impairment. Formal assessment using the Conners' adult ADHD rating scale is unnecessary in this case. In view of Margaret's erratic diet, laboratory studies to check baseline nutritional status are warranted, including a complete blood count and a blood glucose level.

In view of her chronically poor nutrition, Margaret's fatigue might be caused by an iron-deficiency anemia. Chronic depressed mood can also result from anemia.

It is prudent to check thyroid hormone levels because of the relationship between hypothyroidism, depressed mood, and fatigue. Finally, Dr. Janson orders a special laboratory study to check Margaret's serum zinc level. Recent research findings suggest that many individuals diagnosed with ADHD have abnormally low plasma zinc levels, which may interfere with optimal brain functioning and manifest as symptoms of distractibility and inattention (Yorbik et al., 2008; Arnold et al., 2005).

Formulation

Margaret has a history of severe distractibility and inattentiveness starting in childhood and continuing to the present, as evidenced by negative professional and relationship consequences of her "disorganized mind," and an inability to stay focused at work and complete assignments in a timely manner. There is no known history of anoxic brain injury at birth, early childhood abuse or neglect, or toxic exposure. There is no history of a learning disorder, medical disorders, or substance abuse that might underlie symptoms of distractibility. Margaret's parents and other first-degree relatives do not have attention-deficit disorder. She has tried numerous conventional medications, including SSRIs and stimulants, but discontinued these conventional therapies (except for methylphenidate) because of lack of efficacy or adverse effects. She is currently taking methylphenidate, a stimulant medication, at a therapeutic dose but is experiencing little or no benefit.

Margaret's history and symptoms are a sufficient basis for a diagnosis of attention-deficit disorder, inattentive type, but transient worsening of her baseline symptoms of distractibility might be related to hypoglycemia caused by her erratic and high-sugar diet. Chronic work stress, poor nutritional habits, and the absence of exercise or a plan for managing stress may be contributing significantly to Margaret's depressed mood, anxiety, and fatigue. Symptoms of chronic moderate depressed mood, in the absence of episodes of mania or severe depressed mood, may be consistent with a primary diagnosis of dysthymic disorder but do not qualify for a diagnosis of major depressive disorder. More recent symptoms of generalized anxiety, absent a history of previous anxiety problems, do not justify a diagnosis of a specific anxiety disorder at this time. Furthermore, symptoms of anxiety could be related to episodes of hypoglycemia following periods of fasting, or to reactive hypoglycemia following high-sugar snacks. Chronic fatigue often goes together with depressed mood, but Margaret's fatigue could also be related to nutritional factors, chronic work stress, or both. Reduced appetite, anxiety, and fatigue are commonly described adverse effects of chronic stimulant use—an issue that should be explored in subsequent sessions. Although there is no evidence of an underlying medical problem, it is prudent to do laboratory studies to rule out a thyroid disorder that could manifest as depressed mood, anxiety, and fatigue. Other laboratory studies, including a blood glucose level and a complete blood count, are appropriate in this case to evaluate the role of nutritional factors in possibly causing chronic fatigue and depressed mood or exacerbating Margaret's baseline symptoms of distractibility.

Treatment Plan

Three weeks later Margaret returns after having done all the recommended laboratory studies. Her serum zinc level is borderline low. A random glucose level is also in the low-normal range, but results of her thyroid test are normal. She has been working conscientiously on improving her nutrition. "I've been trying to be more mindful about my eating habits, and I think my energy level is better. My anxiety is quite a bit better, but my concentration is still all over the map . . . and the depression hasn't changed." Margaret usually has a healthy breakfast with balanced protein and complex carbohydrates. She has been eating high-protein bars when she misses a meal and has managed to avoid high-sugar snacks. Dr. Janson tells Margaret about her laboratory findings, reassuring her that her thyroid is healthy, "and everything else can be corrected through improving your nutrition." He suggests that she take a zinc supplement, and he briefly summarizes the research evidence for this trace element.

> Most evidence for the use of zinc in ADHD is anecdotal. However, studies suggest that a daily zinc supplement of 150 mg is a safe and effective adjunctive treatment, when combined with stimulant medications, that significantly reduces the severity of ADHD symptoms (Bilici et al., 2004; Akhondzadeh et al., 2004). Although zinc supplementation is a widely used alternative therapy for ADHD, the only randomized controlled trials were done with children and resulted in improvements in hyperactivity, not distractibility. The evidence for zinc in adult ADHD is largely anecdotal, and large placebo-controlled trials are needed to establish whether this trace element has therapeutic benefits in adults diagnosed with ADHD.

Dr. Janson also recommends that Margaret take omega-3 essential fatty acids. "The omega-3s might help both your depression and your ADHD."

Omega-3s essential fatty acids are deficient in the average American diet (Simopoulos, 1991). It has been established that omega-3s decrease the risk of arrhythmias and atherosclerosis, lower serum triglyceride levels, and improve hypertension (Kris-Etherton et al., 2003). Studies on omega-3s in depressed mood show consistent beneficial effects when used together with antidepressants (Lin & Su, 2007; Keshavarz et al., 2008). It has been hypothesized that fatty acid deficiencies during fetal development, infancy, and early childhood are associated with an increased risk of ADHD (Richardson & Puri, 2000). Research findings on omega-3 essential fatty acids as a therapeutic intervention in ADHD are inconsistent, with some studies reporting benefits and others reporting no difference between omega-3s and placebo (Voigt et al., 2001; Stevens et al., 1995; Sinn & Bryan, 2007). Findings of a pilot study suggest that higher doses and longer treatment periods than examined in studies done to date may be needed to achieve lasting therapeutic effects. A small pilot study on omega-3s in nine children with ADHD found significant improvements in both hyperactivity and distractibility with high doses of omega-3s up to 16 gm/day (Sorgi et al., 2007). These results are interesting but should be viewed as preliminary pending confirmation by large controlled trials on high-dose omega-3s in adults diagnosed with ADHD.

Finally, Dr. Janson suggests a daily folate supplement for Margaret's depressed mood.

Several studies confirm that a highly absorbable form of folate called methylfolate, used adjunctively with conventional antidepressants, increases their efficacy (Glória et al., 1997; Passeri et al., 1993). Folate used alone may also reduce the severity of depressed mood.

Dr. Janson suggests continuing on the Ritalin for now. Margaret frowns, "I had hoped that I could stop taking it once I started these natural treatments." Dr. Janson remarks, "When you begin to feel more even, we'll talk about reducing your dose on the Ritalin, perhaps even going off of it." Margaret smiles, clearly encouraged by this prospect, and agrees to begin all three supplements at the recommended doses.

The balance of the session is taken up with a conversation about EEG biofeedback. Margaret has watched the DVD: "I think this is very interesting, and I'd like to try it." Dr. Janson describes the procedure involved in EEG biofeedback from start to finish. "There's a specific approach that has been found to be effective for reducing symptoms of distractibility. It may take several weeks of training, but I think it could really make a difference."

> Inattention and distractibility may be caused by "under-arousal" of the frontal cortex. EEG biofeedback works by normalizing brain electrical activity and improving the cognitive and behavioral symptoms of ADHD (Monastra et al., 2002). Two principle EEG biofeedback protocols that have been validated as effective treatments of ADHD are verified sensory motor rhythm (SMR) training and "theta suppression." SMR training is often beneficial for reducing impulsivity and hyperactivity, whereas theta suppression is used primarily to treat inattention and distractibility (Monestra et al., 2005).

Dr. Janson hands Margaret a handwritten note with the supplements and doses they discussed. They schedule the six EEG biofeedback sessions at weekly intervals with Dr. Janson's half-time neurotherapist and a follow-up appointment with Dr. Janson in 6 weeks.

First Follow-Up

Margaret appears more rested 6 weeks later. "I don't remember ever feeling this relaxed," she reports. She smiles as she tells Dr. Janson how she has "discovered" tai chi chuan since seeing him. "I know tai chi will be an important part of my plan from now on. It's amazing how calm and clear I feel after doing tai chi chuan."

> Tai chi and other mind–body practices, including qigong and yoga, are beneficial for reducing symptoms of anxiety as well

as symptoms of distractibility in individuals with ADHD. These practices also empower clients to feel in greater control over their symptoms without relying exclusively on medications or supplements.

Margaret has been enjoying the EEG biofeedback sessions in which she uses a protocol aimed at theta suppression. "I see it as a kind of high-tech yoga for ADHD." At the neurotherapist's advice Margaret is using a small, portable biofeedback device between EEG biofeedback sessions "to keep my nervous system tuned in the right way." Since starting evening yoga classes, Margaret has put limits on her work schedule and now leaves work promptly at 5:00 P.M. "It's amazing. I'm spending less time at work but getting more done, so no one is complaining."

Margaret is no longer on probation and isn't worried about losing her job. Her new-found control over her distractibility has given her a renewed sense of self-esteem that she hasn't experienced in many years. With her improved self-esteem Margaret has not felt anxious for at least a month and her mood has started to improve, "though I still have the blues sometimes." She continues to take the supplements, is not experiencing adverse effects, and has been following a healthy diet for almost 2 months. Dr. Janson praises her for her commitment to her health. "It sounds like you're doing an excellent job taking care of yourself and setting limits at work." Margaret sees this as an opportunity to tell Dr. Janson that she reduced her methylphenidate dose by half and started taking a product made from the bark of a pine tree soon after their first session. She learned about Pycnogenol from a German friend who told her that it is widely used to treat ADHD in Europe. "This is what they use to treat ADHD in Europe, and it's coming into the mainstream now. I was feeling so good with it that I didn't want to wait several more weeks to cut back on the Ritalin."

Margaret has been taking Pycnogenol for almost 1 month, together with a reduced dose of methylphenidate, and there are no apparent adverse effects or interactions between the herbal product, the methylphenidate, and the supplements. At half her previous dose of methylphenidate, her appetite has improved and she seldom "forgets" to eat meals. "I know it's always better to ask your doctor for advice on safety and so on, but I didn't want to wait. Anyway, I've been feeling fine—very clear inside. I think I've found the best medicine for my 'monkey mind.';thin" Dr. Janson nods. "It's usually better to first talk about changing medication doses or starting any new herbal or other natural product just to be sure it's safe. But I think you've done a nice job." He briefly reviews what he knows about Pycnogenol.

Evidence from anecdotal reports and one double-blind controlled study suggests that a standardized extract of the bark of the French maritime pine tree (*Pinus pinaster*) may be a safe and effective treatment of ADHD (Trebaticka et al., 2006), reducing symptoms of both hyperactivity and distractibility. To date the efficacy of Pycnogenol in ADHD has been evaluated in children only. Large controlled studies are needed to confirm that Pycnogenol is effective for ADHD in adults and establish optimal dosing.

In the final minutes of the session Dr. Janson and Margaret discuss the pros and cons of continuing with Margaret's current regimen versus stopping the methylphenidate while continuing the rest (Pycnogenol, supplements, EEG biofeedback, yoga, and improved nutrition). In view of Margaret's dramatic improvement and her strong commitment to an effective integrative treatment plan, Dr. Janson believes that discontinuing methylphenidate at this point will probably not place Margaret at significantly increased risk of recurring problems with distractibility, anxiety, or fatigue. He suggests that she wear off the remaining methylphenidate over 1 week while monitoring for signs of recurring symptoms and continuing the Pycnogenol. They agree to six more weekly sessions of EEG biofeedback therapy and review her treatment plan in its entirety, including the names and doses of supplements.

Second Follow-Up

Margaret has been off methylphenidate for 6 weeks and continues to feel "clear-headed." There have been no recurring symptoms of distractibility. She completed the last scheduled session of EEG biofeedback last week and uses the hand-held biofeedback device daily. Margaret continues to practice yoga and take the recommended supplements. There are no noticeable adverse effects. She continues to have "good energy" during the day and has not felt depressed in over a month. For the first time in years she is able to devote energy to a relationship: "I think it might really work this time." As the session ends, they schedule a follow-up appointment in 6 weeks.

Putting It All Together

Effective integrative management of ADHD starts with a complete history and should take into account the unique causes of the syndrome in every client, including genetic factors, perinatal insults or toxic exposure, early childhood neglect or abuse, food sensitivities, and others. When stimulants fail to result in significant reductions in symptom severity—as in this case—or when concerns about adverse effects, toxicities, or comorbid substance abuse preclude their use, EEG biofeedback should be considered as a first-line treatment of ADHD. Effective treatment of symptoms of distractibility generally requires regular EEG biofeedback training using a theta-suppression protocol over several weeks. The benefits of biofeedback training can be enhanced by portable biofeedback devices and the regular practice of yoga or other mind–body disciplines. Dietary changes, including improved overall nutrition and avoidance of high-sugar snacks, are a central part of effective integrative management in this case, which is complicated by the presence of depressed mood, fatigue, and anxiety. In this vignette the client has improved dramatically in response to an integrative treatment plan that includes dietary changes, a specific EEG biofeedback training protocol aimed at suppressing theta activity, a regular mind–body practice, omega-3 fatty acids, zinc, and folate. The adjunctive use of omega-3 essential fatty acids, zinc, and Pycnogenol may have improved Margaret's responsiveness to methylphenidate.

On the advice of a friend Margaret decides to use Pycnogenol in combination with methylphenidate without first discussing this with her physician. Fortunately, there are no adverse effects or toxic interactions, and Margaret's symptoms of distractibility further improve on this regimen. As noted several times in this book, before starting any natural product or conventional medication, it is always preferable for clients to be fully informed about risks and benefits by reviewing this information with a knowledgeable M.D. or naturopathic physician and giving informed consent to begin treatment. As the narrative ends Margaret's symptoms of distractibility, anxiety, and fatigue continue to be well controlled after the stimulant dose is reduced, and she has renewed self-confidence. At the same time her depressed mood has lessened, perhaps as a result of improved nutrition, an effective stress management plan, and improved self-esteem. She continues to improve with EEG biofeedback, yoga, Pycnogenol, and supplements, and a discussion with her physician about treatment alternatives concludes that little additional risk will result from discontinuing the stimulant in the context of regular follow-up appointments and ongoing EEG biofeedback training, yoga, improved nutrition, Pycnogenol, and other supplements. This is a reasonable strategy in view of emerging research findings suggesting that high doses of omega-3 fatty acids, zinc, and Pycnogenol are beneficial when used in the absence of stimulants.

∽

CHAPTER 8

Psychotic Symptoms and Schizophrenia

Evidence of psychosis is usually easy to find during a routine diagnostic interview. However, determining whether a specific psychotic disorder is present may require several sessions and the help of a client's relative or partner. People with schizophrenia may have consistently abnormal anatomical findings in specific brain regions, but findings on correlations between abnormal brain structure and schizophrenia are inconclusive, and brain imaging studies in this population are used for research purposes but not diagnostic assessment. Medical disorders such as brain tumors and hyperthyroidism sometimes manifest as psychotic symptoms, and stimulant abuse can result in a chronic syndrome that resembles schizophrenia. Because of this possibility, it is always important to inquire about substance abuse history when evaluating anyone who presents with auditory hallucinations, paranoia, or other psychotic symptoms. If you suspect that a new client who is psychotic—or a continuing client who suddenly develops symptoms of psychosis—has an undiagnosed or untreated medical problem or ongoing substance abuse, you should immediately refer him or her to an urgent care center or the nearest hospital emergency room for evaluation.

Nonconventional Approaches

Abnormally low blood levels of certain essential fatty acids may be biological markers of deficiency states that underlie schizophrenia and other psychotic disorders (Arvindakshan, 2003a). Many individuals who are chronically psychotic—especially with negative symptoms—have abnormally low serum folate levels (Goff, 2001). Low serum DHEA levels may correlate with increased vulnerability to schizophrenia in genetically predisposed individuals (Harris, 2001). Reductions in negative psychotic symptoms with treatment resulted in increased serum DHEA to normal levels (Strous, 2003).

Dysregulation of an enzyme that is linked to a genetic predisposition to develop schizophrenia results in the absence of a normal flushing response when people with schizophrenia are challenged with niacin (Tavares, 2003). Emerging research findings suggest that analysis of electrical brain activity using QEEG may help to predict response to conventional antipsychotics. Different kinds of abnormalities in brain electrical activity may correspond to different kinds of psychotic symptoms and reflect diverse causes of schizophrenia (John, 1994).

TREATMENT

Conventional Treatment

The majority of older "first-generation" antipsychotic medications are available in the form of inexpensive generics. These agents have serious adverse effects and may cause a permanent neurological syndrome that mimics Parkinson's disease. The newer so-called "atypical" antipsychotics are expensive and when first introduced were believed to be associated with fewer severe adverse effects. Unfortunately, the atypical agents are also associated with serious problems, including many of the same neurological syndromes caused by first-generation antipsychotics as well as the metabolic syndrome that can result in obesity, diabetes, and heart disease, as well as fatal cardiac arrhythmias. Typical doses of the newer antipsychotics, including risperidone (Risperdal), quetlapine (Seroquel), olanzapine (Zyprexa), and aripiprazole (Abilify) can cost $500–$600 monthly. Many insurances cover only a small portion of the cost of these medications, making them unaffordable for individuals who are not covered by health insurance or who live on a fixed income.

Recent studies suggest that the older antipsychotics and the newer atypical agents have roughly comparable efficacy against schizophrenia and other psychotic syndromes and may be associated with similar frequencies of adverse neurological effects (Geddes et al., 2000; Davis et al., 2003). This reality has sent many chronically psychotic patients back to less expensive generic medications. Depressed mood, anxiety, and cognitive impairment often occur together with psychotic symptoms, and conventional antipsychotics help many people who struggle with psychosis. However, a significant percentage of people with schizophrenia become symptomatic even while taking antipsychotics, and as many as one-fourth of people with schizophrenia do not take their medications as prescribed, resulting in a significant risk of relapse (Barbui et al., 2003). Individuals with schizophrenia frequently discontinue antipsychotics, against the advice of their psychiatrists, because of concerns about the serious side effects mentioned above (Rettenbacher et al., 2004). With a knowledge of emerging nonconventional treatments of psychosis, you can help your clients identify treatments that are both safe and beneficial.

Nonconventional Treatments

Eating fish and other foods rich in omega-3 essential fatty acids may be associated with reduced symptom severity in chronic schizophrenia (Emsley, 2003). There is some evidence that omega-3 fatty acids help improve response to conventional antipsychotics, but research findings are inconsistent. In one study, chronically psychotic patients experienced significant clinical improvements when treated with omega-3s (EPA and DHA) at 300 mg and antioxidant vitamins (Arvindakshan et al., 2003a, 2003b). In a larger placebo-controlled study, patients with schizophrenia who had failed to respond to conventional antipsychotics were randomized to different doses of purified EPA versus placebo together with their antipsychotic medications. Improvements were observed across the range of doses, but those receiving an intermediate dose of EPA (2 gm/day) improved most (Peet & Horrobin, 2002). A subsequent controlled trial failed to replicate these findings (Fenton et al., 2001). A subgroup of people with schizophrenia may benefit from large doses of niacin in the form of nicotinamide (3–8 gm/day) in the early stages of illness. However, research findings are inconsistent, the literature consists largely of case reports, few controlled studies have been published, and most studies were done in the 1960s (Wittenborn, 1974). Preliminary research findings suggest that chronically psychotic individuals who take high doses of folic acid (up to 15 mg/day) together with their conventional antipsychotic medications have fewer positive and negative psychotic symptoms and respond to treatment more rapidly than individuals who take antipsychotics alone (Procter, 1991; Godfrey et al., 1990). Large doses of thiamin (500 mg three times daily) taken in combination with conventional antipsychotics may lessen symptom severity in people with schizophrenia (Sacks et al., 1989). Glycine is another natural substance that shows promise as a treatment of psychosis. In a 6-week double-blind trial treatment-resistant patients with schizophrenia, randomized to high doses of glycine (up to 60 gm/day) versus placebo in addition to their conventional antipsychotic medication, experienced significant improvements in negative symptoms and global functioning (Heresco-Levy et al., 1999).

Taking a standardized ginkgo biloba extract with a conventional antipsychotic may improve negative and positive psychotic symptoms more than antipsychotics alone while reducing the risk of adverse neurological effects (Zhang et al., 2001). A few studies suggest that taking the hormone precursor DHEA with a conventional antipsychotic may improve response while reducing side effects (Strous et al., 2003, Strous, 2005). In a placebo-controlled study, hospitalized patients with schizophrenia treated with DHEA 100 mg/day, in addition to their regular antipsychotic medications, experienced significant improvements in negative psychotic symptoms, depressed mood, and anxiety (Strous, 2003). There were no improvements in auditory hallucinations, delusions, or other positive psychotic symptoms.

Certain herbals or compound herbal formulas used in Ayurveda and traditional Korean medicine show promise as treatments of schizophrenia and other chronic psychotic disorders. However, their appropriate and safe use requires great skill, and reliable sources of these herbal products are difficult to find in the United States and other Western countries (Chung et al., 1995; Ramu et al., 1992).

Findings of three small studies suggest that regular acupuncture treatment, using laser light to stimulate specific acupoints, may lessen the severity of auditory hallucinations and other positive psychotic symptoms and have efficacy comparable to conventional antipsychotics (Luo et al., 1986; Jia et al., 1987; Zhang, 1991).

The regular practice of yoga, qigong, or other mind–body practices can probably help some people with schizophrenia remain stable. Preliminary research findings suggest regular yoga practice reduces symptoms of agitation and anxiety in this population (Jordan, 1989). There is evidence that support groups that include a spiritual component and teach simple mindfulness skills can help people with schizophrenia remain grounded (Sageman, 2004). Table 8.1 summarizes nonconventional treatments of psychotic symptoms and schizophrenia.

TABLE 8.1 Nonconventional and Integrative Treatments of Psychotic Symptoms and Schizophrenia

More substantiated:

- There are no strongly substantiated nonconventional treatments of psychosis at the time of writing.

Less substantiated:

- Increasing consumption of foods rich in omega-3 essential fatty acids
- Taking concentrated omega-3 essential fatty acids with an antipsychotic
- Taking high doses of folate or thiamin with an antipsychotic
- Taking DHEA with an antipsychotic
- Taking Ginkgo biloba with an antipsychotic
- Taking high doses of niacin
- Taking high doses of glycine with an antipsychotic
- Taking certain Ayurvedic and Korean herbals
- Laser acupuncture
- Yoga (for agitation and anxiety caused by psychosis)
- Spiritually oriented support groups

CASE VIGNETTES

Moderate Psychosis

Intake

Pete is 25 years old, lives with his parents, and works part-time as a gardener. He has never been in a long-term relationship because "it's too hard to spend time with people." About a month ago, when working on a large landscaping project, he began to feel strange: "It was like colors were brighter, and the way I was seeing plants and rocks was different. It really scared me." Pete mentioned this experience to his mother, who encouraged him to see a psychiatrist. He found Dr. Stevenson's name in the Yellow Pages and made an appointment for the following week.

As he sits down across from Dr. Stevenson, he remarks, "My vision is changing . . . something weird is happening to me." In the ensuing hour Pete tries to describe recent changes in his senses and his mental life, but his words are unable to convey the subtlety of his changing perceptions. "Sometimes the colors are so vivid . . . it's like they're coming at me from the plants and rocks. What does this mean?" Pete has always been a loner, but during the past month he has been even more isolated than usual. "People might realize I'm different, and I know I'm different so I avoid them." Pete has never had a problem with depression or anxiety, and he does not drink or use drugs. He takes no medications or supplements and has no medical problems; however, he had a concussion with brief loss of consciousness when he was 12. He has never been evaluated or treated for a mental health problem. He denies hearing voices and does not believe people are following him or trying to harm him. He does not believe he receives messages from the radio or T.V. and has not had other "unusual experiences," such as telepathic communication with people or "spirits." "I know the spirits are out there, but I don't want to let them in. My Dad tells me not to let them in." Pete talks about his longstanding belief in the spirit world. He enjoys movies about ghosts and other supernatural themes. "I know that stuff is real. I'm trying to find a balance between that world and the world I live in. Sometimes I can almost see them, then my vision returns to normal and I know I won't see them." He has had experiences like this since he was 18 and believes his "encounters with the spirits" are becoming more frequent as he gets older. As a young man his father was diagnosed with schizophrenia and has been on medications since that time. "My father tells me how the visions were for him at first, before the medications." It is clear that Pete has insight into the general nature of his mental health problem and is seeking advice and treatment.

Assessment

Pete is a reliable historian and is able to tell his story clearly. A thorough structured interview is probably all that is needed to assess the nature and severity of his mental health problem. His voice is soft and barely audible, but he is articulate, appropriate, and stays on track throughout the interview, although he appears anxious and avoids direct eye contact. A history of head injury is the only possible indication for formal medical workup to rule out possible underlying neurological causes of psychosis. However, there is no evidence from his history that Pete's symptoms were caused by the head injury. Therefore, referral to a neurologist is unnecessary at this time and would probably not yield useful diagnostic information.

Formulation

Pete has never been able to achieve financial or emotional autonomy, tolerates social contact with difficulty, and has been able to make a successful living working as a gardener. Pete describes longstanding beliefs in spirits and psychic phenomena, but he does not hear voices or have visual hallucinations. He is not paranoid or delusional, but recent changes in his "vision" have resulted in ongoing feelings of anxiety. Pete has insight that he is mentally ill. Some of his magical beliefs appear to be more consistent with schizotypal personality than an evolving thought disorder. His recent experiences cannot be explained by substance abuse, a medical disorder, reaction to severe stress, or a preexisting psychiatric disorder. His father is has schizophrenia, experienced similar symptoms before starting treatment, and has been doing well on conventional medications. In view of known personal and family history, the progression of his symptoms, and his current level of functioning, a reasonable provisional diagnosis using DSM-IV criteria might be a psychotic disorder of moderate severity characterized by primarily negative symptoms. However, some of Pete's experiences may reflect longstanding magical beliefs and personality traits consistent with schizotypal personality disorder.

Treatment

Dr. Stevenson tells Pete that he isn't sure about his diagnosis yet but that "it might be similar to your father's problem." Pete nods his head, "I thought I was the same, but I don't see what happens to me as a problem . . . at least not all the time. My world is just different, but I want to find a balance between it and the world of other people."

Dr. Stevenson affirms this perspective. "I agree it's about finding the balance that works for you . . . so that you feel better, maybe feel safer around the visions."

Pete agrees. "One time I tried to do tai chi for balance. I think it helped."

"It's an ancient Chinese approach for balancing mind and body," replies Dr. Stevenson. "Doing tai chi every day might help you feel more grounded."

Note: Anecdotal reports suggest that individuals who have chronic psychotic disorders but are not having acute symptoms of psychosis may function at a higher level when they practice qigong or yoga on a regular basis. However, there are also reports of worsening psychosis following qigong, yoga, and other mind–body practices in individuals who are experiencing acute or severe symptoms. It is prudent to advise acutely psychotic individuals to wait until they are stabler before engaging in any kind of mind–body practice. Patients who have a history of psychosis but are currently stable may benefit from the regular practice of qigong under the supervision of a skilled instructor who is aware of particular exercises that may place the patient at risk of symptomatic worsening. Patients with schizophrenia or other psychotic disorders, including dissociative disorder and schizoaffective disorder, as well as severe personality disorders including borderline personality, risk an acute exacerbation of symptoms when practicing qigong, and should do so only under the supervision of a qualified instructor, and preferably a qigong master.

Dr. Stevenson then talks about antipsychotic medications as well as a few alternative and integrative therapies that might be beneficial for the psychotic symptoms of moderate severity that Pete is experiencing. In contrasting different treatment choices, Dr. Stevenson emphasizes that there is much more evidence for conventional antipsychotics than the nonconventional treatments.

When working with psychotic clients who have some insight into their illness, it is important to provide them with reliable information about the relative merits and limitations of available treatment choices. In general, the evidence for nonpharmacological therapies for psychotic symptoms is not very strong. Furthermore, a few herbal treatments used in other countries to treat psychosis and supported by promising research findings are not available in the United States, are associated with potentially serious safety issues, or require highly trained clinicians to properly administer (e.g., a Chinese medical practitioner, Ayurvedic physician, or traditional Korean herbal healer with advanced training).

"Your father takes an antipsychotic, and he seems to be doing well. Based on the evidence, I think the best approach at this time is to take a medication in combination with a few supplements that may help you get a better effect." Dr. Stevenson suggests starting with a low dose of an antipsychotic called perphenazine, and tells Pete about possible adverse effects.

All antipsychotics, including older ones and the newer so-called "atypical" antipsychotics, can cause neurological side effect that include tremors, akathisia (a condition that is experienced as restlessness throughout the body), and permanent serious movement disorders that continue even if the medication is stopped. All patients should be advised about these risks before deciding to take any conventional antipsychotic medication.

Dr. Stevenson remarks that the antipsychotic he is recommending seldom causes significant adverse effects at the dose Pete will be taking. In addition to taking perphenazine, Dr. Stevenson suggests three natural products: a specific essential fatty acid (EPA), DHEA, and niacin. "Taking these supplements can sometimes help you feel better than with an antipsychotic alone. They might also help the perphenazine work better even when you take it at a relatively low dose."

> Some research evidence suggests that taking 1–4 gm/day of the omega-3 essential fatty acid ecosapentanoic acid (EPA) with a conventional antipsychotic may be more effective than taking an antipsychotic alone, especially when symptoms are only beginning to occur. The prohormone DHEA occurs naturally in the body. Taking 100 mg of DHEA may help diminish the adverse effects of antipsychotics and may ameliorate some of the negative psychotic symptoms the client is experiencing. Finally, there is some evidence that taking a high dose (up to 8 gm/day) of the B-vitamin niacin with a conventional antipsychotic may be more effective than taking an antipsychotic alone.

Dr. Stevenson advises Pete about possible adverse effects of all three supplements and suggests the best times of day to take them to ensure optimum absorption and to reduce the risk of adverse effects.

> Essential fatty acids, including EPA, are absorbed best when taken with food. When taking doses as high as a few grams, it is reasonable to take them with every meal. Some people report upset stomach and diarrhea on high doses of omega-3s. DHEA and niacin can be activating and at the recommended doses can interfere with sleep if taken too close to bedtime. For this reason both supplements are usually taken in the morning. Niacin can cause flushing and at high doses it is best to take this B-vitamin as nicotinamide.

Dr. Stevenson writes down the names and doses of these supplements to ensure that Pete will find the most appropriate ones. He suggests obtaining them at a particular pharmacy that carries quality brands of these supplements. "It's important to get the best brand you can find when taking any supplement."

> There is enormous variation in the quality of commercially available supplements including herbals, vitamins, omega-3 essential fatty acids and others. For this reason it is helpful to guide clients when selecting supplements. Appendix B includes Web resources that will help you and your clients identify quality supplements.

A return appointment is scheduled for 2 weeks later.

Follow-Up
Pete has been taking the perphenazine and the supplements according to plan, but he stopped the niacin after a few days "because of all the itching." He reports feeling "clearer . . . and I don't get to the point where my vision starts to change as much as before." Since starting his integrative regimen of medications and supplements, Pete has not "felt as strange" and has noticed less anxiety when around people. Dr. Stevenson recommended taking perphenazine at a dose of 2 mg twice every day, but Pete has found that taking the medication only once each day "keeps me feeling solid." He is not having adverse effects from the perphenazine. He has started taking tai chi lessons and feels calmer when practicing the movements in his room. Dr. Stevenson compliments Pete on his rapid progress and his commitment to getting better. "It sounds like you've found a better balance than before." They agree to regular monthly appointments for the next 6 months "for fine-tuning."

Putting It All Together
In cases where psychotic symptoms are moderate and only beginning to emerge, it is reasonable to try an integrative strategy that includes both a conventional antipsychotic and select alternative therapies. For more severe or chronic psychotic symptoms this approach would not be appropriate, nor would it be in the client's best interest. In such cases (see following vignette) the initial treatment plan should emphasize aggressive management using conventional medications.

The natural supplements used as adjunctive therapies in this case may work synergistically with conventional antipsychotics, thereby potentially reducing effective doses of these drugs. When a lower dose of any antipsychotic results in adequate control of psychotic symptoms, the risks of adverse effects also diminish, and the likelihood that your client will continue taking the antipsychotic increases. This is a "win–win" situation for you and your client. Omega-3 essential fatty acids, DHEA, and niacin can be safely combined with antipsychotic medications. When a client who has had psychotic symptoms of moderate severity has been stable on a low dose of an antipsychotic and appropriate supplements for several months, it may be reasonable in some cases to consider further tapering or discontinuing the antipsychotic medication while continuing the supplements. To minimize the risk of relapse, this should be done only with the client's understanding of the risk of recurring psychosis, and only under the supervision of a psychiatrist. Most individuals who experience psychotic symptoms of moderate severity have insight that they are ill and can be motivated to follow a plan that will help them get better and remain stable. Doing tai chi, qigong, or another mind–body practice in the context of an individualized plan that includes appropriate medications and supplements will help your client remain stable by teaching him or her how to "center" in stressful situations, while encouraging frequent positive social contact.

Severe Psychosis

Intake

Lilly is 23, single, and unemployed. She was recently discharged from a 90-day stay at a residential facility that specializes in the care of individuals who have both a serious mental illness and a substance abuse problem (i.e., a program for "dual diagnosis" patients). Today is her first outpatient appointment since being discharged. Her mother chose Dr. Walsch, a community psychiatrist, because of his interest in integrative medicine. When scheduling the appointment, Lilly's mother expressed concerns about Lilly's "difficulties" with conventional treatment approaches, including the limited effectiveness of most antipsychotics and mood stabilizers and her long history of adverse effects, including weight gain, liver problems, neurological symptoms, and others, that had resulted in Lilly's decision to stop taking medications (against the advice of her psychiatrist). Lilly's "start–stop" approach to conventional medications had created a sporadic pattern of temporary improvement alternating with sudden worsening in her psychotic and mood symptoms, requiring repeated hospitalizations. Lilly describes frequent auditory hallucinations ongoing for approximately 3 years, which have commanded her to hurt herself for about a month now. She often has vivid disturbing dreams with images of "torture" that interrupt her sleep and result in chronic fatigue, poor concentration, and diminished desire to socialize with peers. During the same period she has been increasingly depressed, irritable, and anxious. She has not thought about suicide recently but feels "blank" and unmotivated and has little interest in pursuing former hobbies, including playing the guitar and painting. "I know it's the voices that want me to hurt myself . . . it's not me." Lilly is tense and hypervigilant throughout the interview and talks openly about concerns that "the government is monitoring me." She reports experiencing "faint whispers" during most of the intake interview but cannot make out words. She describes these auditory hallucinations as "always in the background" since her early teens. She has never had visual hallucinations. Her appetite is "too big," and she has gained about 10 pounds in the last month in spite of being on a strict vegan diet. The last time she experienced manic symptoms, including racing thoughts, overtalkativeness, euphoria, and diminished need for sleep was about 3 months ago.

Lilly's birth and early childhood history were unremarkable, except for her mother's report that she often preferred to be alone as a child. Lilly is the oldest of four children, none of whom has mental health problems. Her father abused alcohol as a young man and has been in recovery for over 20 years. Lilly attended public school and was an average student until about age 16, when she experienced her first manic episode for which she was hospitalized. She was diagnosed with bipolar disorder, started on a mood stabilizer and an antipsychotic, and followed in regular monthly sessions. She started to use marijuana soon after her first hospitalization and found that it "helped calm the demons." She soon developed a pattern of heavy marijuana abuse but denies other substance abuse. There has been only one subsequent episode of mania, and most of her five psychiatric hospitalizations since then have been for "adjusting medications" for the treatment of depression, auditory hallucinations, and paranoia. She often experiences auditory hallucinations and paranoia when her mood is stable, but these become worse when she is depressed. She has insight into the relationship between marijuana use and her mental health problems. "Weed helps me stay centered, but I think it messes with my mind."

Since adolescence, Lilly has had frequent headaches, which were recently diagnosed as migraines. There is no history of head injury or seizures. As the session ends, Dr. Walsch suggest running some tests on her blood to evaluate possible underlying biological causes of her symptoms and help identify the most appropriate conventional and alternative treatment approaches. He also suggests a simple procedure called the niacin challenge test to help clarify Lilly's diagnosis.

Emerging research findings suggest that individuals who have chronic psychotic syndromes may have abnormally low blood levels of a prohormone called dihydroxyepiandosterone (DHEA), as well as low levels of certain essential fatty acids. In some cases, chronic psychosis in women may be related to low levels of the hormone estradiol. These tests are now widely available and can provide useful information when advising chronically psychotic clients about reasonable treatment choices. The niacin challenge test is especially helpful when trying to differentiate a psychotic disorder from bipolar disorder. Most people with schizophrenia do not experience an uncomfortable flushing response when given a large dose of niacin (200 mg). In contrast, individuals who are bipolar or have another psychiatric disorder generally experience a strong flushing response.

Assessment

Lilly is disheveled and displays prominent slowing of speech and spontaneous movements. Her speech is sparse, and she frequently relies on her mother to provide historical information. Her affect is flat, and her mood is moderately anxious and depressed. She denies suicidal thoughts. Her comments about the government appear to reflect a delusional belief system. She experiences barely audible auditory hallucinations during the interview, reportedly at her chronic baseline, but does not appear to be distressed by the voices. Lilly correctly performs complex written instructions and provides a coherent abstract interpretation of a well-known proverb. Recent thyroid studies are within normal limits. There are no other known medical problems at the time of the intake. On formal mental status examination, Lilly is oriented to person, place, and time and understands the circumstances and purpose of the appointment. She is able to perform simple calculations and serial 7s to 51 without mistakes. Lilly suffers from frequent migraines but denies other symptoms possibly consistent with a primary neurological disorder. At this time there is no indication for a comprehensive neurological or medical assessment. Lilly has not previously been evaluated using functional testing of specific molecules in her blood or urine, and such testing might help to clarify possible metabolic or nutritional factors related to symptoms of psychosis, anxiety, and depressed mood. The niacin challenge test is a reasonable assessment tool in this case and will help to clarify Lilly's diagnosis and treatment plan.

Formulation

Like many cases of chronic psychosis, this case involves numerous complex factors, including the presence of both positive and negative psychotic symptoms and prominent mood symptoms beginning in adolescence, a documented history of severe manic episodes with psychosis, chronic marijuana abuse, poor responsiveness to conventional medications, and sporadic medication compliance due to adverse effects. Reasonable diagnostic possibilities include paranoid schizophrenia, bipolar disorder, and schizoaffective disorder. Her symptoms of anxiety and depression are probably caused by both a serious psychiatric disorder that has not yet been clearly established and chronic marijuana abuse. Persisting psychotic symptoms that occur when Lilly is not experiencing severe depressed mood or mood swings suggest a DSM-IV diagnosis of schizoaffective disorder. However, diagnosing a primary psychotic disorder cannot be done at this point because of a longstanding pattern of marijuana abuse. It is prudent to check blood levels of specific essential fatty acids, DHEA, and estradiol to evaluate the client for possible underlying nutritional or metabolic causes of symptoms. There is no indication that Lilly's symptoms result from an energetic imbalance.

Treatment

Over the past 4 years Lilly has tried virtually all of the older and more recently introduced (atypical) antipsychotics as well as mood stabilizers, many antidepressants, and combinations of these medications. Her typical pattern has been to discontinue a medication after a few days or weeks because of documented adverse effects or "because I didn't like the way it made me feel." Lilly and her parents are very health conscious and share a philosophy of taking medications only when needed and only when "the good effects outweigh their toxic effects." A brief trial on one atypical antipsychotic, aripiprazole (Abilify), resulted in diminished auditory hallucinations and "helped me feel more level for a while." However, Lilly discontinued that medication also "because I don't think I should need to take a medication for this problem."

Lilly is intelligent, articulate, and has strong negative feelings about conventional medicine. She is also hesitant about continuing to rely on conventional medications because of her disappointing and distressing experiences with them to date. "I've heard you know a lot about alternative medicine. Tell me about my choices other than pills in bottles."

It is already clear to Dr. Walsch that Lilly will not passively accept any treatment recommendation. "Sounds like almost everything you've tried hasn't worked, or in cases where you were feeling better, you chose not to take medication on principle. I respect your view, but my perspective is somewhat different. I try to find the best solution using both medications and alternative approaches. I think you need to take an antipsychotic to feel well, to get your life back to where you want to be. If you try other things together with the medication, you might be able to function better at a lower dose, do more of the things you want to do, and have fewer problems with side effects. I think of this approach as a kind of compromise between taking only prescription medications and taking only alternative therapies."

Lilly is listening intently. "I've never heard a doctor suggest anything like this before. I think I'm OK with this approach." After Lilly confirms that she was functioning well on the aripiprazole, Dr. Walsch encourages her to start taking it again. "You have anxiety, depression, and the psychotic symptoms. I'd like to work on the psychotic symptoms and go from there. I'd like you to make peace with the medication this time and to think of it as only one part of a broader plan." Dr. Walsch talks about the importance of stress management, good nutrition, a regular mind–body practice, and a support group for management of Lilly's mental health problems. He recommends taking a special form of an omega-3 essential fatty acid called EPA.

> There is some evidence from double-blind controlled studies that taking 2 mg/day of ethyl-ecosapentanoic acid (ethyl-EPA) together with an atypical antipsychotic is more beneficial than taking an antipsychotic alone.

Dr. Walsch also suggests taking a high-potency B-complex that includes folate, thiamin, and B-12, and vitamin C. "We're basically trying to optimize the environment of your brain. Taking these vitamins may give you more control over your symptoms even if you take a low dose of Abilify, and you'll probably function and feel better."

> Many psychotic individuals are deficient in folate and other B-vitamins because of chronic poor nutrition, the interfering effects of antipsychotics on absorption of vitamins in the gut, and possibly also genetic factors. Combining folate (up to 15 mg/day) with a conventional antipsychotic may be more effective than taking a medication alone. Taking thiamin (up to 500 mg three times daily) may also be beneficial. High doses of antioxidant vitamins, including C, E, and beta-carotene, may also reduce the severity of psychotic symptoms in some cases.

As the session comes to an end, Dr. Walsch decides to risk commenting on his concern about Lilly's longstanding marijuana use. "I need to tell you that I think there's a strong connection between the marijuana and your problem. In my opinion it's making your problem worse and probably harder to treat using any approach. I'd like you to think about backing away from the marijuana." Lilly nods tentatively, and they shake hands as she rises to leave.

First Follow-Up

Two weeks later Lilly appears less distracted, and her eyes are clearer. She has been taking aripiprazole at bedtime and the supplements in the morning. There are no noticeable adverse effects. Her level of anxiety is somewhat less and she no longer feels depressed. She has thought about her eating habits and realized that her appetite has been poor and she has been eating mainly fatty and sugary foods for months. "The marijuana was keeping my appetite down and then giving me the munchies." Dr. Walsch sees this as an invitation to talk about the connection between diet, anxiety, mood, and mental health in general.

Reducing saturated fats in the diet may reduce the severity of psychotic symptoms. Increasing consumption of foods rich in omega-3 fatty acids may also be beneficial for depressed mood and general cognitive functioning. Regulating sugar and caffeine intake can also significantly affect both depressed mood and anxiety.

They review the treatment plan, and Lilly is motivated to continue taking aripiprazole and the supplements. "I've been thinking about what you said about the marijuana, and it makes sense. I feel better now and I think I can stay 'even' most of the time without it." Lilly has heard about a support group for people with psychotic disorder. This group has a spiritual focus, and part of group time is spent in meditation and doing yoga stretches. She asks Dr. Walsch's opinion and he replies: "There's a lot to this approach. You'll get support from others who have the same problem, and you'll also learn how to balance your mind and body."

Individuals who struggle with psychotic disorders can benefit from a support group, but only if their symptoms are not severe. Several studies show that spiritually focused support groups improve self-esteem and help individuals function better in social contexts. Combining a mind–body practice such as yoga with a more conventional support group may be especially helpful for reducing anxiety symptoms and improving the overall level of functioning. Delusional individuals might become worse if they engage in any kind of spiritual or mind–body work and should be discouraged from engaging in these activities until they are stabler.

Second Follow-Up

Two weeks later Lilly continues to take the antipsychotic and the supplements. "I think the vitamins give me more energy, and my thinking is clearer." She has significantly reduced her use of marijuana and has found a part-time job as a server in a local cafe. "It's nice to be able to do something again." She has not experienced marijuana craving. She describes her frustration at being "derailed" for years. "It's been really, really hard and sometimes I think I've made it even harder by using so much weed and not staying with the treatment." Dr. Walsch affirms Lilly's choices and her new-found commitment to improving her health. "Well, you're certainly doing a great job now." She has been more mindful of her eating habits and has frequent conversations with a friend about nutrition and health. "I'm having a lot of fun, Doc. It's great to see that I can make such a difference to my brain by just eating better and staying off weed."

Lilly asks Dr. Walsch if it would be "safe" to stop taking the antipsychotic. "I feel fine now. I've really cleaned up my act, and I don't think I need it anymore." Dr. Walsch suggests a compromise: "You might be correct, but it hasn't been so long that you've been feeling well, and if you stop now it could send you into a tailspin. You might lose all the progress you've made and be back where you were a few short months ago. Would you agree to keep doing what you're doing for about 6 more months and then revisiting our options at that point?" He argues that continuing the current strategy—taking an antipsychotic with supplements, working on nutrition, and attending regular support groups, while abstaining from marijuana— for several months "will help solidify your gains." Lilly agrees. "I like this approach, Doc, and I like the way you listen to me. Let's do this." In closing, Dr. Walsch writes down the names of three psychotherapists. "I think you could get a lot out of some talk therapy at this point." They schedule a follow-up in 6 weeks.

Dr. Walsch hadn't heard from Lilly in over 8 months when he

received a call from her mother notifying him that Lilly had become manic and psychotic 2 weeks earlier and was now hospitalized on an involuntary hold as gravely disabled. A phone call confirmed that she had stopped psychotherapy several months earlier after only three appointments. Lilly had apparently continued taking the antipsychotic and the supplements recommended by Dr. Walsch for about 6 months after their final session. At that time she decided, for unclear reasons, to go off everything and had then started a special kind of laser acupuncture. Her mother remarked, "She wasn't having problems when she made the decision, but she thought she had been doing so well for so long that she didn't need to take them . . . then she read something about acupuncture and got excited."

> Evidence from research studies suggests that using a low-power laser to stimulate specific acupuncture points may lessen the severity of auditory hallucinations and other psychotic symptoms in chronic schizophrenia. One study done in China found that regular laser acupuncture treatments were as effective as a conventional antipsychotic. Large sham-controlled studies are needed to confirm that this specialized form of acupuncture has antipsychotic effects before this approach can be recommended to individuals afflicted with a psychotic disorder.

"This will be a difficult one to return from," Dr. Walsch commented. Lilly had apparently been picked up by the police when wandering down the middle of a busy street late one night. She was incoherent and disoriented and appeared to be responding to auditory hallucinations. She was brought to the emergency room, where her urine toxicology screen showed that she had been using marijuana.

Putting It All Together

Like many individuals afflicted with a chronic psychotic illness, Lilly has had a series of disappointing experiences with conventional medications, has strong negative feelings about Western medicine in general, and is at the point of rejecting all mainstream treatments of her mental health problems. Perhaps the single most skillful intervention in this case is the psychiatrist's successful "negotiation" of an integrative treatment plan that includes, but is not limited to, an antipsychotic medication that Lilly has previously tried and found effective. A discussion about the relevance of conventional treatment takes place in the context of an open-minded conversation about Lilly's general state of health and mental health in which her values and beliefs are acknowledged and respected. This naturally flows into a respectful but frank exchange about marijuana abuse in which conflict is avoided and therapist and client become allies. Psychiatrist and client collaborate to achieve a shared understanding of problems, treatment priorities, and a reasonable integrative plan that includes a conventional medication, appropriate natural products, basic lifestyle changes, and a spiritually oriented support group. Like many real-life cases, Lilly is initially motivated to pursue what she regards as a reasonable treatment plan. However, soon after making a commitment to her mental health she stops coming to appointments and at some point decides to stop taking the antipsychotic and the supplements. It isn't clear how long Lilly had been using marijuana when she began to have acute symptoms, and whether marijuana caused her problems or was being used, and self-treat symptoms of mania, anxiety, or psychosis.

This case underscores the importance of regular follow-up appointments for ongoing evaluation and making any necessary changes in treatment, even when a client appears to be stable and engaged in an effective treatment plan. This case also illustrates how tenuous mental health can be in someone who struggles with a psychotic disorder and a substance abuse problem at the same time.

CHAPTER 9

~

Mild Cognitive Impairment
and Dementia

WHEN evaluating any client who complains of memory loss, problems with reasoning, or other symptoms of cognitive impairment, your job is to find out how serious the problem is and how
impaired your client feels by the symptoms. Most people have problems with short-term memory as they age. The gradual decline in
one's ability to recall the day-to-day details of life, to learn with the
ease of a 20-year-old, or to make quick decisions do not *necessarily*
point to early Alzheimer's disease. Symptoms of mild cognitive
impairment do not constitute a disorder according to the DSM.
However, recent studies suggest that a significant percentage of individuals who are eventually diagnosed with Alzheimer's disease or
another form of dementia experienced progressive symptoms of cognitive impairment for several years before becoming profoundly
impaired (Petersen et al., 2001).

Conventional Approaches

When evaluating a cognitively impaired individual, conventionally
trained mental health professionals begin with a comprehensive
medical, social, and psychiatric history. A careful history clarifies the

course, severity, and type of cognitive impairment. Obviously, many cognitively impaired clients are unable to provide a reliable history. It then becomes necessary to obtain information from a partner, friend, or family member. If there is evidence that symptoms of cognitive impairment are related to an underlying medical problem, it is important to refer the client to the family physician. If a client does not currently have a physician, you should strongly encourage him or her to get one. Depending on the client's history and the nature of the medical problem, his or her physician may order brain imaging studies, diagnostic blood chemistries, or other laboratory tests to help clarify the causes of the memory loss or other cognitive symptoms. Studies that often provide useful information about underlying medical causes of cognitive impairment include thyroid hormone levels and blood tests that check for anemia and electrolyte levels. A brain scan can rapidly determine whether a tumor, or other serious disease process affecting the brain, may be contributing to cognitive impairment.

Chronic substance abuse is often associated with significant problems in memory and judgment, which may persist long after the substance abuse has ended. It is prudent to ask all clients who describe significant problems remembering or reasoning about their use of alcohol and drugs. This is especially important when evaluating someone who has a known history of alcohol or substance abuse. The basic structured interview that is most widely used for evaluating the severity and kind of cognitive impairment is the Folstein mini-mental status exam. The mini-mental exam reveals serious cognitive impairment but seldom provides useful information about mild symptoms that may be bothering your client.

Individuals who experience cognitive impairment frequently have other mental health problems that may or may *not* be related to their memory problem. For example, memory impairment to one degree or another often accompanies depressed mood, anxiety, and psychosis. Profoundly depressed individuals sometimes appear to be demented but regain normal cognitive functioning when their depressive mood symptoms lift. If clients describe increased difficulty remembering names or making decisions when they are more depressed or anxious, and no longer experience these problems when symptoms of depression or anxiety have improved, you can reasonably infer that their cognitive problem is directly related to an underlying psychiatric problem. In such cases, treating the primary mood or anxiety problem generally results in improved overall mental functioning.

Even with advanced brain imaging techniques and diagnostic tests of the blood, it is often difficult to confirm a biological cause of cognitive impairment. In the day-to-day practice of medicine a comprehensive neurological evaluation is seldom done and a diagnosis is made in the absence of definitive evidence. For this reason, many individuals are diagnosed with Alzheimer's disease even when a thorough medical workup has not been done. An incomplete medical evaluation can result in an incorrect understanding of the cause or causes of cognitive impairment, which, in turn, translates into inadequate and ineffective treatment.

Nonconventional Approaches

Emerging assessment approaches that are not presently used in mainstream clinical medicine may provide useful diagnostic information about possible underlying causes of cognitive impairment in some cases. Chronic malnutrition resulting in deficiencies of important nutrients can manifest as symptoms of cognitive impairment. Abnormally low blood levels of the omega-3 essential fatty acid DHA may be an indicator of the severity of cognitive impairment in malnourished or demented individuals (Tully et al., 2003). It has been suggested that low serum zinc levels might result in accelerated formation of amyloid plaques (Constantinidis, 1990). Testing for blood levels of DHA and zinc can provide useful diagnostic information, especially when there is a history of alcohol abuse or poor nutrition.

Brain mapping using quantitative electroencephalography (QEEG) is now used as a research tool in studies on dementia and other syndromes of severe cognitive impairment caused by head injury or stroke. QEEG brain mapping will probably emerge as a standard approach for differentiating cases of mild cognitive impairment from early cases of Alzheimer's disease (Benvenuto et al., 2002). As technology advances and the costs of equipment decrease, QEEG will probably become widely used by mental health professionals to evaluate clients who have problems with memory, abstract reasoning, and other areas of cognitive functioning. Virtual perform-ance testing and other virtual reality tools will permit earlier and more accurate assessment of cognitive impairment (Rizzo & Wieder-hold, 2000).

TREATMENT

Conventional treatment

Widely used conventional treatments of Alzheimer's disease work by interfering with the enzyme that breaks down acetylcholine—the neurotransmitter that is essential for learning and memory—resulting in relatively higher levels of this neurotransmitter in the brain. The cholinesterase inhibitors improve only some symptoms of dementia, are beneficial only in early or mild dementia, are fre-quently associated with adverse effects, and may cause liver damage.

Nonconventional Approaches

Changes in diet, certain herbals, vitamins, trace elements, and other natural products may have neuroprotective effects and help prevent or delay onset of dementia or reduce the severity of cognitive impair-ment caused by dementia or stroke (Ernst, 1999). Diets high in satu-rated fats are associated with increased risk of developing Alzheimer's disease, whereas diets high in fish are associated with relatively reduced risk (Grant, 1997; Kalmijn et al., 2004). Moderate wine consumption (one or two glasses/day) reduces the risk of Alzheimer's disease, but chronic alcohol abuse increases the risk of dementia (Orgogozo et al., 1997; Weuve et al., 2004).

Many studies have been done on the use of folate in people with dementia, but findings are inconsistent. Whereas some studies report positive findings (Passeri et al., 1993; Pelka & Leuchtgens, 1995), a systematic review of controlled studies found insufficient evidence to support use of folic acid (or B-12) as a treatment of dementia (Malouf & Areosa Sastre, 2004). Large doses (3–8 gm/day) of thiamin may reduce the severity of cognitive impairment in Alzheimer's patients (Mimori et al., 1996). Vitamins C and E are important free-radical scavengers and may slow progression of Alzheimer's disease and other neurodegenerative diseases. Individuals who take vitamin C and E supplements have a reduced risk of developing Alzheimer's disease (Englehart et al., 2002).

Considerable research has been done on the use of ginkgo biloba as a treatment in Alzheimer's disease, but findings are inconsistent. Early systematic reviews of placebo-controlled studies concluded that standardized preparations of ginkgo biloba (120–600 mg/day) improved memory, general cognitive functioning, and activities of daily living in mild Alzheimer's dementia, and multi-infarct dementia (Wong et al., 1998; Oken et al., 1998; Itil et al., 1998). However, a more recent systematic review questioned these conclusions on the basis of serious design flaws in many studies (Birks & Grimley, 2004). Standardized ginkgo preparations are also used to self-treat age-related declines in memory and problem solving, although recent research findings are inconsistent (Semlitsch et al., 1995; Cheuvront & Carter, 2003).

Huperzine-A is derived from an herbal formula used in Chinese medicine to treat dementia. This molecule is a naturally occurring cholinesterase inhibitor and may slow the rate of age-related cognitive decline (Zhao & Li, 2002). Placebo-controlled trials suggest that huperzine-A in doses between 200 and 400 micrograms/day improves cognitive performance in mildly impaired and demented individuals (Wang et al., 1994; Zucker, 1999).

Findings of a small open study suggest that a compound herbal formula used in traditional Japanese herbal medicine, called *kami-untan-to*, may significantly slow the rate of deterioration in individuals with dementia (Arai et al., 2000), and a standardized extract of lemon balm may significantly reduce the rate of global cognitive decline in individuals with dementia (Akhondzadeh et al., 2003). An Ayurvedic herbal called Ashwagondha may also improve global cognitive functioning in these individuals (Bhattacharya et al., 1995).

Phosphatidyl serine is an essential component of nerve cell membranes. Numerous placebo-controlled studies have shown that this natural substance improves cognitive functioning in mildly impaired individuals and those with dementia when dosed at 300 mg/day (Cenacchi et al., 1993; Crook et al., 1991).

The amino acid acetyl-L-carnitine (ALC) is beneficial for both cognitive impairment and depressed mood, which often go together in elderly clients with dementia. A systematic review of placebo-controlled studies of ALC in dementia found initial improvements in memory and global cognitive functioning after several weeks of treatment, which were not sustained with continued treatment (Hudson & Tabet, 2004). ALC at doses of 1.5–3.0 gm/day may reduce symptoms of age-related mild cognitive impairment in healthy elderly individuals (Bella et al., 1990). The beneficial effects of ALC may be enhanced when combined with alpha-lipoic acid, coenzyme Q10 (CoQ10), or omega-3 fatty acids (Di Donato et al., 1986; Lolic et al., 1997). The essential oils of lemon balm and lavender are calming when applied to the face and arms of agitated individuals with dementia (Ballard et al., 2002); however, aromatherapy using the same two volatilized essential oils is ineffective (Snow et al., 2004).

Regular physical activity reduces the risk of developing dementia but does not improve symptoms of cognitive impairment in individuals with dementia (Abbott et al., 2004; Weuve et al., 2004). Using weak electrical current (e.g., cranioelectrotherapy stimulation) to stimulate the brain may result in temporary improvements in word recall and face recognition in individuals with mild dementia (Cameron et al., 2004). Listening to relaxing music or getting a massage can have significant calming effects for agitated clients with dementia. A systematic review of studies on music therapy with this population concluded that singing and listening to music reduce agitation and anxiety, improve social interaction, and increase global cognitive functioning (Koger et al., 1999).

Regular healing touch therapy may reduce disruptive behaviors and improve emotional and cognitive functioning in individuals with severe dementia (Ostuni & Pietro, 2000, 2001). Individuals who received two therapeutic touch (TT) treatments daily for 3 days were significantly less restless and disruptive compared to patients who received mock TT (Woods et al., 2005). Lastly, remarkable anecdotal reports suggest that practicing qigong can slow or reverse the course of dementia (Manabu et al., 1996). Table 9.1 summarizes nonconventional treatments of mild cognitive impairment and dementia.

TABLE 9.1 Nonconventional and Integrative Treatments of Mild Cognitive Impairment and Dementia

More substantiated:

- Ginkgo biloba
- Huperzine-A

Less substantiated:

- Dietary modifications
- Certain vitamins (folate, thiamin, C, and E)
- Phosphatidyl serine
- Acetyl-L-carnitine
- Regular exercise
- Weak electrical currents (e.g., cranioelectrotherapy stimulation)
- Music (for agitation)
- Essential oils
- Ashwagondha
- Kami-untan-to
- Healing touch and therapeutic touch
- Qigong

CASE VIGNETTES

Moderate Cognitive Impairment

Intake

Mrs. Brown is a 75-year-old widow who lives in an upscale retirement home. She is brought to Dr. Persig's office by her daughter because of concerns that "she is getting more confused and hasn't been herself lately. We're here to find out if there is anything else that might help Mom besides the standard dementia drugs." Mrs. Brown stares at the floor for most of the interview and is unable to answer most of Dr. Persig's questions. Her daughter provides a thorough history. Mrs. Brown had been "enjoying life," functioning at her usual good level of mood and cognitive performance until about a year ago, when her daughter noticed that she had become more withdrawn, easily frustrated, and began to have problems finding her way around the small town where she lives. At about the same time she began to have difficulty doing simple chores and keeping her apartment tidy. Mrs. Brown comments, "I think I just haven't been myself for some time . . . I don't understand what is happening to me. I hate the idea that I have it . . . you know."

According to her daughter, Mrs. Brown has been "losing" days of the week, forgetting what month or season it is, and does not recognize many old friends. During the past few months she has felt more "restless—I don't know why," especially in the evening hours. More recently, she has had trouble sleeping through the night, and the night attendant has found her walking in her sleep in the common area. According to her daughter, she has felt depressed for several months; however, Mrs. Brown denies this. She has been taking an SSRI for approximately 6 months, but according to her daughter there has been little improvement in her mood. "It makes me feel like a zombie, and I don't have an appetite. I don't want to take it anymore." She does not have problems walking, and there have been no changes in coordination, balance, or vision. Her family physician started her on a cholinesterase inhibitor about a month ago, after confirming normal thyroid function and finding significant atrophy in the frontal cortex by both CT and MRI scans. Mrs. Brown takes both medications at bedtime because of their sedating effects, "but I don't think they're making any difference." She does not take vitamins or other supplements. Her daughter remarks that she has had fewer problems with agitation at night since starting the cholinesterase inhibitor, but there are no noticeable improvements in memory or mood. She has not experienced upset stomach, agitation, or other adverse effects.

Note: Most medications currently prescribed for dementia are cholinesterase inhibitors. Although they result in temporary improvement in memory and other symptoms of cognitive impairment in early or mild Alzheimer's disease, they have limited efficacy in more severe forms of dementia. They are nevertheless widely prescribed to individuals with dementia for reducing the agitated behavior that is often seen with dementia.

According to her daughter, Mrs. Brown has never had problems with her memory before, nor has she been diagnosed with major depressive disorder or other psychiatric disorders. There is no history of a head injury or seizure. Her daughter discloses that Mrs. Brown drank heavily for most of her adult life, and that she recently found a bottle of vodka in her mother's kitchen and is concerned that she still has a drinking problem. Mrs. Brown becomes agitated at her daughter's comments and angrily shakes her head. "Mom, you know we have to face this. It's become a real problem." Mrs. Brown began to notice hearing loss about 10 years ago, and she has some loss of sensation in her feet, but a recent evaluation by a neurologist found no evidence of a neurological disorder, including stroke. She has no other known medical problems, such as high blood pressure. She has not been physically active in years but used to enjoy walking and gardening. Mrs. Brown's weight is normal for her age, but she has been losing weight in recent months. Both Mrs. Brown's mother and older sister had Alzheimer's disease starting in their early 70s and passed away in their late 70s. "I'm scared I'll end like them," Mrs. Brown comments. Dr. Persig suggests a few specialized blood tests to check Mrs. Brown's general nutritional status.

Assessment

Mrs. Brown does not know the day of the week, date, month, or year. She thinks it is summer "because it's warm and sunny, so I know." She says the purpose of the appointment is to "talk about my memory." Mrs. Brown does not attempt to calculate serial 3s. She can repeat two of three words immediately but cannot recall any 5 minutes later. She provides a concrete interpretation of a well-known proverb and then laughs. "What kind of question is that, anyway?" Mrs. Brown's appetite has recently been poor. In view of probable ongoing alcohol abuse, general malnutrition may be a significant factor here. It is prudent to check blood levels of vitamins and a particular omega-3 essential fatty acid. Other appropriate medical and neurological tests have already been conducted.

Chronic alcohol abuse is frequently associated with malnutrition because of poor dietary habits and a malabsorption syndrome caused by the effects of alcohol on the intestines.

Alcoholics are especially susceptible to B-vitamin deficiencies, which can manifest as gait disturbances and impaired cognitive functioning. Chronically low levels of a particular omega-3 essential fatty acid—decosahexanoic acid (DHA)—caused by low dietary intake of foods rich in this omega-3 fatty acid, may increase the risk of developing Alzheimer's disease.

Formulation

In view of a known family history of dementia, the nature and progressive course of Mrs. Brown's symptoms, the absence of evidence consistent with a degenerative neurological disorder or other underlying medical causes of impaired memory and decline in global cognitive functioning, a reasonable provisional diagnosis is Alzheimer's disease. Chronic alcohol abuse is clearly a factor in this case, and it will be important to determine to what extent the client's global cognitive impairment is due to cumulative effects of chronic alcohol abuse versus the near-term effects of ongoing alcohol abuse.

Treatment

"We need to talk about the alcohol problem," Dr. Persig remarks in a firm but gentle voice.

"I don't see what the problem is if I have a drink for my nerves now and then," Mrs. Brown counters.

Dr. Persig replies, "The drinking might be your main problem. The only way to find out is to stop drinking. What do you think?" Mrs. Brown looks askance at her daughter who is intently staring at the floor, rocking, and angrily remarks, "Well, if it would help my daughter feel at ease and keep her from bothering me, I guess I could try, but I don't see the harm in it!"

Dr. Persig replies, "If you stop drinking, you might feel a lot better and you might not have all these problems that your daughter is worried about." Mrs. Brown agrees to let her daughter remove all alcohol from her apartment but she adamantly refuses to attend Alcoholics Anonymous (AA) meetings. "I'm not an alcoholic, I just like my drink now and then!"

Dr. Persig carefully summarizes his diagnostic impressions in language that Mrs. Brown can understand: "I think you have a serious problem with your memory and your thinking, but I'm not sure what's causing it. I think that not drinking and eating better could help a great deal." He then briefly reviews well-documented relationships between chronic alcohol abuse and the kinds of mood and memory problems Mrs. Brown is experiencing. He emphasizes the importance of abstinence from alcohol and the addition of good nutrition and vitamins.

> Malnutrition can result in deficiencies of vitamins, amino acids, essential fatty acids, and trace elements, including zinc and magnesium, that are essential for healthy brain functioning.

Dr. Persig suggests that Mrs. Brown take a few supplements with the goal of optimizing her brain functioning.

> Vitamins B-12 and folate are essential for normal mental functioning. Chronically low levels of these vitamins in the diet often result in severe symptoms of cognitive impairment because the neurotransmitters required for normal cognitive functioning are not being synthesized at the necessary rate. Taking a B-complex vitamin can significantly enhance overall cognitive performance in chronically malnourished individuals. Taking folate can also help with depressed mood and probably increase the efficacy of conventional antidepressants. Taking vitamins C and E on a regular basis may reduce the risk of developing Alzheimer's disease or slow its rate of progression.

In addition, Dr. Persig suggests that Mrs. Brown take an amino acid, acetyl-L-carnitine, starting at 500 mg/day for both the cognitive problems and depression.

Several studies have shown that acetyl-L-carnitine at a dose of 1–2 gm/day helps improve depressed mood, memory, and global cognitive functioning in elderly depressed individuals. Acetyl-L-carnitine also helps to diminish the severity of cognitive impairment that comes with normal aging. The mechanism of action probably involves increased production of acetylcholine, a neurotransmitter that is essential for memory and learning. Loss of neurons that produce this neurotransmitter is believed to be the primary cause of Alzheimer's disease.

Dr. Persig writes down the names and doses of the vitamins and other supplements. In closing, Dr. Persig suggests that Mrs. Brown spend more time outside of her apartment, especially in social activities. "I think you'd feel better for it," he remarks. Mrs. Brown agrees to get out more often and says she will follow Dr. Persig's recommendations, "but I'm not sure it will make any difference!" In the final moments of the session her daughter confirms that she understands the treatment plan and will bring Mrs. Brown to the community hospital for the recommended blood tests.

Follow-Up

One month later Mrs. Brown looks like a different person. Her appearance has changed dramatically, her gestures are more fluid, and she is more talkative. She is excited about being able to read again. "I can concentrate enough to read mysteries again. That's something I've always loved." She has been following Dr. Persig's recommendations carefully. "I think the vitamins and the other ones are really making a difference. I also think you were right about the vodka. I didn't realize how much I was drinking." She reports feeling better overall, more alert and more energetic since stopping drinking and "reforming" her diet, but she still has difficulty recalling some words and "forgetting people I should know." Her daughter persuaded her to start going to AA meetings, and after some initial resistance, she now attends meetings three times every week. "I have interesting conversations there, and I'm meeting some nice people. Now I know alcohol was a demon; it just got in the way of life." Mother and daughter are clearly on friendlier terms as they go over how they have been talking about Mrs. Brown's alcohol abuse problem for the first time in her life and have been working together on "Mom's new health program." Letting go of vodka was surprisingly easy for Mrs. Brown and has resulted in a rapid and marked increase in her appetite. Mrs. Brown has been enjoying dinners together with her daughter most evenings. Although she continues to have trouble feeling her toes, she has been walking more in recent weeks and enjoys casual encounters with people at the corner store. With her daughter's encouragement, Mrs. Brown has also been attending bingo night twice a week.

Dr. Persig reviews the laboratory findings, which confirm that Mrs. Brown was severely malnourished with low levels of most vitamins, trace minerals, and essential fatty acids. She and daughter are visabily relieved with this news. Almost immediately Mrs. Brown tells Dr. Persig she wishes to stop taking "those darn pills. They never helped and they make me feel bad anyway." Dr. Persig agrees: "I think it's reasonable to talk about a plan for going off the medications at this point." Dr. Persig recommends stopping the cholinesterase inhibitor first, then reducing and stopping the SSRI a few weeks later, assuming that Mrs. Brown's mood does not take a turn for the worse. They schedule a follow-up appointment 2 months later.

Putting It All Together

This case illustrates how severe cognitive impairment that has already been diagnosed as Alzheimer's disease and is being treated as dementia may not be dementia at all and may be reversible if caught early, evaluated thoroughly, and managed aggressively. Chronic alcohol abuse and chronically poor nutrition often go together and manifest as cognitive impairment, personality changes, and depressed mood. Complete abstinence from alcohol is fundamental, and regular attendance at AA or another abstinence-support program is an essential component of treatment. Improved nutrition along with an effective replenishment plan that includes vitamins, trace elements, and specialized nutrients known to have neuroprotective effects can result in rapid, dramatic improvement in cognitive functioning and mood. Remaining abstinent and engaging in regular social contact are keys to a successful outcome. When memory and mood symptoms respond dramatically to abstinence, improved nutrition, and supplements that enhance overall brain functioning, it is reasonable to consider discontinuing conventional pharmacological treatments under the supervision of a physician. Although the client is now functioning at a significantly higher level, periodic follow-ups should be made to assess changes in cognitive functioning and mood, to optimize the treatment plan, and to support the client's efforts to maintain sobriety.

Severe Cognitive Impairment

Intake

Frank is a 75-year-old retired architect. He enjoys golf and is well known as a community organizer. Five years ago he was in a serious car accident when returning from a day of golfing. His injuries included a severe concussion with loss of consciousness, whiplash, and three broken ribs. A CT of the head revealed no abnormal findings. He recovered rapidly with physical therapy and has been functioning at his usual baseline of good health, except for neck and upper back pain that sometimes wakes him up from a sound sleep. Frank walks daily and enjoys reading and gardening. He drinks moderately in social situations but has never abused alcohol or drugs. He was diagnosed with mild hypertension about 20 years ago, and his blood pressure has been well controlled on medications since then. He takes an over-the-counter pain medication and a prescription medication for an enlarged prostate. His wife Norma called Robin Stewart, Ph.D., last week out of concern that Frank "hasn't been himself recently." She had heard about Dr. Stewart's reputation as a good listener and an innovative therapist and thought it "would be good for Frank to have someone to talk with." Frank doesn't think he has any problems but agreed to see Dr. Stewart to allay his wife's concerns.

Dr. Stewart is highly regarded in the community as a skillful therapist. She is also an avid practitioner of qigong and yoga and frequently attends seminars on mind–body therapies, herbal medicine, and biofeedback, all of which she uses in her private practice. As Frank and Norma enter the waiting room, they notice the fragrance of lavender and the pleasing sound of a small fountain in the corner. Bookcases are filled with brochures and books about conventional and alternative therapies, and the walls are lined with photographs of beautiful mountain scenes.

"Nice waiting room, Doc," Frank comments, as Dr. Stewart shows Frank and Norma into her office. Dr. Stewart tells Frank that her work is to listen to whatever is on Frank's mind and then make observations or suggestions. Frank has never been in psychotherapy and is clearly feeling anxious at the prospect of talking about personal concerns. Norma offers, "He just hasn't been the same for some time. At first it was many little things, but I think it may be getting worse." Frank has been having problems remembering where things are around the house and sometimes asks his wife for help finding his reading glasses four or five times in the same day. He is often irritable and lately has been getting agitated for no apparent reason. Frank confirms that he has been feeling "blue" for several months and is aware of having more frequent arguments with Norma.

"I don't know why, but little things seem to get to me more these days." In the past few years he has been less active in the community, less interested in socializing, and sometimes sits alone for hours in his study staring out the window. Norma offers, "I don't know whether these changes are related to the accident. There were no problems immediately afterward, but Frank has been . . . different."

Frank eats a healthy diet and is physically active. He does not have problems with coordination, gait, strength, or vision. He enjoys reading the paper, but his wife has noticed that he often rereads the same paper two or three times. In his mid-30s Frank struggled with depression for several years during a very stressful period in his career. He did not seek treatment at that time and his mood eventually returned to normal. Norma believes he started to feel depressed again about 2 years ago. Frank's father had heart disease and died at the age of 79 from complications of Alzheimer's disease. Dr. Stewart suggests more thorough psychological testing and refers Frank to a neurologist who does a specialized kind of electroencephalography. "I think it would be useful to have another CT and get a specialized kind of brain map. He can also help you with your back pain and the mood problem you've been having."

Assessment

On the mental status exam Frank is oriented in all spheres, remembers what he had for breakfast 2 days ago, can perform simple calculations, and recalls two out of three words 5 minutes later. He easily reads instructions and performs a simple task. He can interpret a proverb abstractly. "I don't see why you're asking me these questions, Doctor. It's true that I'm having some memory problems, but I'm getting older. It's normal at my age. Anyway, I get along fine and I'm as healthy as ever. I guess I could be sleeping better." Dr. Stewart suggests more formal neuropsychological testing to determine whether Frank is experiencing problems with aspects of cognitive functioning that cannot be adequately evaluated using the mini-mental status exam.

The mini-mental status exam is a very general screening instrument consisting of 11 questions. It is a useful tool for evaluating individuals who are already profoundly cognitively impaired but does not provide clinically helpful information when evaluating mild dementia, early or unusual cases of cognitive impairment, or for differentiating cognitive problems due to head injury, psychiatric disorders, etc. In such cases more formal neuropsychological evaluation, including specialized tests of problem solving and abstract reasoning, can help clarify the nature and severity of cognitive impairment).

Although a CT of the head was normal in the hours following Frank's serious closed-head injury with loss of consciousness, it is possible that his brain sustained contusions and that his clinical picture of progressive personality change and cognitive decline is related to long-term consequences of that injury. A neurology consultation, including a formal neurological examination and a repeat CT scan, is indicated to rule out this possibility.

Quantitative electroencephalography (QEEG) is an established research tool and will soon become a valuable clinical tool in mainstream psychiatry. Emerging clinical applications include assessment of depressed or anxious individuals who do not respond to conventional medications and evaluation of cognitive impairment. QEEG and brain mapping can help differentiate cognitive impairment due to head injury, chronic substance abuse, depression, stroke, or dementia. Progressive deterioration in specific frequency ranges of brain electrical activity is an accurate predictor of Alzheimer's disease. QEEG analysis is especially useful in cases where the medical or psychiatric history is complicated and a diagnosis of dementia has not been clearly established.

Formulation

This 75-year-old man who does not drink, has a healthy diet, and is physically active has a history of one major depressive episode 30 years ago, a closed-head injury with loss of consciousness but normal CT 5 years ago, hypertension that is reportedly well controlled, and a family history of Alzheimer's disease. His sleep is frequently interrupted by pain, and he is chronically fatigued. During the past few years he has experienced progressive difficulty with short-term memory and reading. During the same time he has been withdrawn, irritable, and occasionally agitated. Findings on the mini-mental status exam are normal, but there is an evolving pattern of personality changes and deterioration in normal level of cognitive functioning. Formal neuropsychological testing and QEEG analysis are indicated. Diagnostic possibilities include recurring major depression with associated cognitive problems, memory and personality changes residual to head injury, multi-infarct dementia, and early Alzheimer's disease.

Treatment

Norma asks "So what is the problem, Doctor?" Dr. Stewart pauses. "At this point there are many possibilities. It's hard to say what's going on before we do some tests, but in the meantime there are many things we can do." Dr. Stewart talks about the relationship between depression and problems with memory, stating simply, "they often go together." She briefly outlines both conventional and alternative treatment choices. "I don't prescribe medications, but the neurologist can." Frank knows he is depressed and is amenable to taking an antidepressant. Dr. Stewart suggests that Norma and Frank "take notes" on Frank's behavior and memory problems. "Let's see if we can find some clues to work with." In closing, she suggests the use of soothing music at bedtime to help with sleep and a daily routine of exercise and relaxation. She also talks about the calming effects of aromatherapy, such as the essential oil of lavender.

> Research findings suggest that the essential oils of lavender and lemon balm may have general calming effects on agitated behavior in people with dementia when applied directly to the face and arms.

They schedule a follow-up in 1 month to go over new findings and discuss treatment options.

One-Month Follow-Up

One week after he saw Dr. Stewart, Frank went through a battery of cognitive and personality tests that revealed significant impairments in abstract reasoning, reading comprehension, and short-term memory, but no problems with long-term memory. These findings were interpreted as consistent with early Alzheimer's disease. Frank has also been seen by Dr. Cantor, the neurologist. A repeat CT scan showed areas of scarring on the left frontal and temporal lobes corresponding to the site of his head injury, as well as significant atrophy on both sides of the frontal and temporal cortex. A QEEG brain map showed abnormal findings in the theta frequency range (3.5–7.5 cycles per second) consistent with early Alzheimer's disease.

> Changes in brain electrical activity that can be detected using QEEG correspond to abnormal energy metabolism or cerebral blood flow, which are indicators of dementia and other progressive neurological disorders. This kind of information is often difficult to obtain using standard CT and MRI brain scans. Abnormal findings in theta activity are often found in the early stages of Alzheimer's disease and predict a gradually deteriorating course.

Dr. Cantor called Frank when the results came back, notified him that he is in the early stages of Alzheimer's disease, and recommended starting a cholinesterase inhibitor. Frank and Norma are discussing Dr. Cantor's recommendations but want to first explore alternative treatment options. Norma comments: "I've been reading about them, and I'm not sure how well they work. I'm also worried about the medication side effects." Frank's sleep and mood have both improved since Dr. Cantor started him on trazodone, a sedating antidepressant that he takes at night, which has lessened his back and neck pain in addition to helping him sleep. He is not having adverse effects. Norma and Frank present Dr. Stewart with a few pages of handwritten notes about Frank's symptoms and progress. "It looks like you're having more and more problems remembering things, Frank." Frank nods in agreement, barely holding back tears. "I'm working on accepting what is happening. It's hard." Norma holds Frank's hand, "We can do this together. There's a lot we can still do. We're not comfortable with the available antidementia drugs, Doctor. Tell us about our other options." Dr. Persig begins with ginkgo: "It's the most substantiated nonpharmacological treatment of dementia, but like the available conventional treatments, it's not perfect."

Ginkgo biloba is widely used in the United States and Europe to treat dementia. The cognitive-enhancing properties of this herbal in cases of early or mild Alzheimer's disease and vascular dementia have been validated by extensive research studies showing improvements in short-term memory, general cognitive functioning, and activities of daily living. Standardized preparations of ginkgo are generally taken in amounts of 120–to 600 mg/day divided into two or three doses. Beneficial effects are generally noticed 6 weeks to 2 months after the start of treatment. Some studies suggest that ginkgo may be as effective as cholinesterase inhibitors and other conventionally used treatments of Alzheimer's disease; however, other studies contradict these findings. The memory-enhancing effects of ginkgo may be greater when combined with ginseng (*Panax ginseng*) or other herbals used in Chinese medicine to treat dementia. There are few adverse effects or safety issues when ginkgo is taken alone, but there is a risk of bleeding when the herbal is taken together with an anticoagulant (e.g., aspirin or Coumadin).

Dr. Stewart briefly summarizes the evidence for three other non-conventional treatments that are sometimes effective for the kinds of cognitive problems that Frank is experiencing: huperzine-A, phosphatidyl serine, and golden root (*Rhodiola rosea*).

Huperzine-A is derived from a Chinese herbal medicine and may have a mechanism that is similar to conventional treatments of dementia. Preliminary findings suggest that at doses between 200 and 400 micrograms/day this naturally occurring compound may be more effective than synthetic cholinesterase inhibitors. Adverse effects of huperzine-A are uncommon but can include dizziness, nausea, and diarrhea.

Phosphatidyl serine occurs naturally in the brain and is necessary for maintaining the normal fluidity of nerve cell membranes. Controlled studies confirm that phosphatidyl serine 300 mg/day often improves memory and general functioning in patients with Alzheimer's disease.

Golden root is an herbal that is traditionally used in Siberia to promote health and longevity. It has been documented to increase brain levels of dopamine, serotonin, and norepinephrine and to improve memory while also providing a general calming effect. Preliminary findings suggest that 500 mg/day of golden root may result in more rapid recovery of normal cognitive functioning following closed head injury. This herbal may be highly stimulating and should not be taken by bipolar patients because of the risk of mania.

After discussing the pros and cons of all three alternative treatments, Frank says he would like to try huperzine. Dr. Stewart reminds Frank of possible adverse effects, suggests a reputable brand, and writes down the typical dosing strategy. Norma then asks, "Is there anything we can do about this other than taking pills and potions?" Dr. Stewart smiles, nods her head, and replies, "There are many other approaches that I believe can help Frank function better and feel more in control. Doing a regular mind–body practice can make a big difference in some cases, especially in the early stages of the illness." Dr. Stewart has been practicing qigong for years and has recently been involved in a study on qigong as a therapy for Alzheimer's disease.

> There have been remarkable case reports of dramatic improvement in severely cognitively impaired elderly individuals who engage in a regular qigong practice. In some cases previously abnormal EEG activity and cerebral circulation in the frontal lobes have reportedly returned to normal. Although such anecdotal reports are interesting, confirmation of the cognitive-enhancing effects of qigong in a population of individuals with dementia under the controlled conditions of a prospective study design must take place before qigong can be recommended as a general "treatment" of Alzheimer's disease or other kinds of dementia.

As the session ends, Dr. Stewart remarks on the importance of taking vitamins and following a healthy diet for slowing the progression of cognitive decline.

Six Months Later

Frank has continued to decline and now has problems recognizing familiar people. As he talks about his impressions of the last 6 months, he notes that he has gotten lost several times when out on simple errands, and that he always carries a list of tasks "to remind myself what I should be doing." He still reads the newspaper but realizes that "much of it just doesn't stick." His mood has improved since starting the antidepressant, and he sleeps well most nights. Norma confirms that Frank has not been irritable or agitated in recent months. "I rub some lavender oil on his wrists in the morning, and I think it soothes him." Frank has "thought about" qigong but hasn't tried it. He takes the B-vitamins some of the time but has not tried huperzine or the other supplements recommended by Dr. Stewart. "I just don't want to be taking pills all the time." Frank has been more social and makes a point of golfing at least three times every week. He continues to walk daily and has stayed on a healthy diet that frequently includes fish.

Ten minutes into the session Norma deliberately folds her arms on her lap. A tear flows down her left cheek. "Frank, I think you're not trying to fight this. You're letting things slip, and it's hurting us." Frank becomes restless, sighs deeply, and shifts his weight in the chair.

"Do you know what I have to deal with every day I wake up? My mind is gone a little bit more every morning, and . . . some mornings I don't even . . . remember this is . . ." Frank bends over and begins crying in a rocking motion.

"This is one of the hardest things that can happen in a marriage," Dr. Stewart acknowledges. "I know you're both doing everything you can, but it's still not working. It's hard for everyone. "I have a colleague whom I think can help you." She writes down the name of a social worker who specializes in therapy with couples in which one partner is becoming demented or going through a serious medical problem. "It's really about working with loss and finding balance between the day-to-day things and the big picture. I think you two could gain a great deal by seeing Joan. I'd also like you to think about some of the things you can do that might make this situation a little easier for both you and Norma. I mean trying the huperzine, the other supplements, and thinking about qigong. I think any one of these could make a difference."

Three-Month Follow-Up

Frank and Norma are sitting in the waiting room quietly holding hands. "Come on in, you two." As Frank sits in the chair he prefers, Dr. Stewart notices a change in his posture. "You know, the way you're walking and sitting is different, smoother."

"I think it's the qigong, Doctor. It's amazing how it makes me feel. I'm doing it all the time now," replies Frank. The qigong group meets twice weekly and is led by a qigong master who also teaches at the Academy of Chinese Medicine in town. "It's amazing stuff; don't know why I didn't try it before. And I figure since this works so well, why not try the Chinese medicine—you know, the hup . . ." Frank has been taking huperzine at the recommended dose for 2 months now. He and Norma have observed some changes they believe are related to the herbal, including fewer "emergencies" around Frank getting lost and his generally improved recall of the contents of that morning's newspaper. "I'm not sure if it's the qigong or the huperzine, Doctor, but I do feel better." He has continued to take B-vitamins in the morning—"They give me more energy"—and his sleep and mood continue the same as before. Frank has had a few episodes of agitation in recent months, but "we were able to talk our way out of them" using skills they learned in couple therapy. They just completed their eighth session with Joan and continue to practice empathic listening and clear communication skills almost daily. Norma comments: "I think we've needed a tune-up for a long time. It's made all the difference in the way we work together." They schedule a return appointment in 3 months and wrap up the session with hugs all around.

Putting It All Together

The early stages of dementia are often difficult to distinguish from the kinds of cognitive problems that come with normal aging or depressed mood. Changes in personality and day-to-day problems with short-term memory suggest an evolving picture of dementia; however, months or years may pass before the diagnosis becomes clear. Formal neuropsychological testing is indicated when a client who is cognitively impaired "looks normal" on a mini-mental status examination. When there is a history of head injury, hypertension, or other medical issues that may function as underlying factors, consultation with a neurologist, including brain imaging studies, is an important part of the workup. QEEG analysis and brain mapping can provide valuable information about the quality and severity of cognitive impairment.

Individuals who are beginning to experience cognitive decline are often in denial around their symptoms and are reluctant to begin treatment. Working together with their spouse or partner can provide an effective bridge to treatment and facilitate the establishment of a supportive relationship around their care plan.

No currently available conventional or alternative therapies "cure" dementia—that is, they do not interrupt or reverse the pathological changes in the brain that manifest as progressive cognitive deterioration. However, conventional medications and some natural substances may slow the rate of progression and improve general functioning in the early stages of Alzheimer's disease and other kinds of dementia. Reasonable integrative strategies include changes in diet, regular physical activity, meaningful social contact, a mind–body practice, supplements with known neuroprotective properties, and medications. The cognitive and behavioral symptoms of Alzheimer's disease continue to change as the illness progresses. Therefore, the most appropriate and effective treatment plan will also evolve over time.

~

CHAPTER 10

Alcohol and Substance Abuse

SUBSTANCE abuse and dependence can result from excessive use of alcohol, tobacco, certain prescription medications, illicit drugs, or a combination of two or more substances. Primary treatment issues involve management of ongoing abuse, acute intoxication, and withdrawal. Individuals who are intoxicated or in the acute stages of withdrawal often experience changes in mood, impaired judgment, and behavioral disturbances that interfere with their ability to function at work or in a relationship. Severe cases of intoxication or withdrawal can cause psychosis, severe anxiety, mood swings, cognitive impairment, insomnia, and other problems that are sometimes mistakenly interpreted as a primary psychiatric or medical disorder. For example, stimulant (cocaine and methamphetamine) abusers may become paranoid and agitated, with visual or auditory hallucinations, when acutely intoxicated and subsequently experience profound cognitive slowing or depressed mood when "crashing." Withdrawal from heroin can mimic a flu-like syndrome, with muscle aches, heavy perspiration, and general feelings of malaise. Acute intoxication with prescription sedative hypnotic drugs (e.g., clonazepam, lorazepam) often causes confusion and problems with balance. Acute withdrawal from these drugs generally causes confusion, anxiety, and insomnia. A significant percentage of depressed individuals are smokers and claim that smoking helps their mood. Alcohol abuse is commonly found among individuals diagnosed with bipolar disorder, and chronic marijuana use is frequent among individuals who have problems with anxiety or concentration.

The assessment of clients whom you suspect are abusing alcohol, an illicit drug, or a prescription medication begins with a thorough history and may proceed to referrals to their physician or an urgent care clinic for laboratory studies to check the urine or blood for substances. There are specific blood and urine tests for hallucinogens, heroin and other opiates, cocaine, and methamphetamine. There are many standardized screening tools for the assessment of substance abuse, but few are used in day-to-day clinical encounters. Chronic alcohol abuse results in liver damage, which causes elevations in the blood levels of several liver enzymes.

Nonconventional Approaches

In addition to these mainstream assessment approaches, measuring blood levels of certain nutrients or neurotransmitter metabolites can provide important clues about the severity or chronicity of alcohol abuse, which as noted previously, is frequently associated with malnourishment (McCauley et al., 1993). For example, people with chronic alcoholism frequently have abnormally low blood levels of vitamins A, B, and C, as well as deficiencies in the trace elements of zinc and magnesium and certain essential fatty acids. Chronic alcohol abuse also causes abnormally high serum homocysteine levels and associated increased risk of depressed mood and heart disease (Cravo et al., 1996). Quantitative electroencephalography (QEEG) findings in people who abuse alcohol or cocaine may provide useful information for planning biofeedback therapy that will increase chances of maintaining abstinence (Bauer & Hesselbrock, 1993). Analysis of the vascular autonomic signal (VAS), a technique used by many Chinese medical practitioners that may provide useful information about energetic imbalances associated with substance abuse, can help guide acupuncture therapy for managing acute intoxication or withdrawal.

TREATMENT

Conventional Treatments

Conventional treatment strategies for alcohol and other substance abuse and dependence problems emphasize the use of prescription pharmaceuticals for managing acute symptoms of intoxication or withdrawal, reducing craving, and maintaining abstinence (Finney & Moos, 2002). It should be noted that safely managing withdrawal from prescription sedative hypnotics sometimes requires hospitalization because of the risk of seizures. Support groups are frequently recommended for clients who are committed to staying clean and sober. However, relapse rates are very high for people who abuse alcohol as well as those who abuse narcotics, even among individuals who regularly attend group meetings. A great deal of attention has been focused on the role of spirituality and religion in maintaining abstinence. Twelve-step groups and other abstinence programs that include spirituality as a central component probably have higher abstinence rates than programs in which spirituality is not addressed. In spite of significant recent innovations in the pharmacological management of substance abuse and dependence, many alcoholics and narcotics abusers relapse while taking medications under the supervision of their physician and attending regular support groups (McLellan et al., 1992). Furthermore, cognitive–behavioral therapy and psychosocial approaches to relapse prevention are not very effective (Carroll, 1996). In response to the limited effectiveness of conventional treatments of substance abuse and dependence, recent efforts have been directed at developing optimal healing environments that incorporate conventional pharmacological treatments and alternative therapies in a supportive group context that emphasizes spirituality.

Nonconventional Treatments

Research findings suggest that improved nutrition, certain supplements, herbals, and other nonpharmacological therapies are beneficial for reducing craving, diminishing symptoms of withdrawal, and reducing relapse risk in people who abuse alcohol or narcotics. Most published studies have focused on alcohol abuse. A significant percentage of people with chronic alcoholism or drug addictions are malnourished; specifically, they are deficient in thiamin, folate, B-6, and important minerals (Gloria et al., 1997). Hypoglycemia is a frequent concomitant of chronic alcohol abuse and can manifest as confusion, anxiety, and impaired cognitive functioning. Studies suggest that people with alcoholism who improve their general nutrition maintain sobriety longer (Guenther, 1983). Reducing caffeine and sugar in the diet and increasing consumption of foods rich in omega-3 essential fatty acids reduces relapse in abstinent alcoholics.

Taking certain amino acids, including taurine and L-tryptophan, may reduce alcohol craving or consumption and diminish withdrawal symptoms. One study found that taurine in doses up to 3 gm/day significantly decreased alcohol withdrawal symptoms in hospitalized individuals undergoing acute detoxification (Ikeda, 1977). The amino acid SAMe in doses of 400–800 mg/day may reduce liver damage caused by chronic alcohol abuse and is also a reasonable treatment choice for depressed alcoholics (Lieber, 1997). Abstinent alcoholics who take the amino acid acetyl-L-carnitine (ALC) at 2 gm/day have fewer problems with routine cognitive tasks (Tempesta et al., 1990).

Chronic alcoholism frequently causes deficiencies in thiamin, folate, B-6, and B-12 because of the toxic effects of alcohol on the digestive system. Taking 2 gm of vitamin C 1 hour before drinking may reduce the toxic effects of alcohol on the liver and may also reduce the severity of hangovers (Chen et al., 1990). Low serum zinc levels caused by malnutrition can cause diffuse neuronal damage (Menzano & Carlen, 1994). People with chronic alcoholism who take magnesium (up to 1500 mg/day) and zinc (50 mg/day) may retain better overall cognitive functioning compared to those who do not take these trace elements (Thomson et al., 1988).

Kudzu (*Radix puerariae*), a traditionally used herbal in Chinese medicine, reduces alcohol craving and may also reduce relapse risk (Colombo et al., 1998). The herbals ashwagondha and ginseng diminish the severity of withdrawal in opiate abuse (Kulkarni & Ninan, 1997; Huong et al., 1996). Valerian (*Valeriana officinalis*) extract may lessen withdrawal symptoms following chronic benzodiazepine use and other conventional sedative hypnotics (Andreatini & Leite, 1994). Taking a controlled-release form of melatonin 2 mg at bedtime may make it easier to discontinue benzodiazepines (Garfinkel et al., 1999).

Certain EMG, thermal, and EEG biofeedback protocols reduce the risk of relapse in abstinent alcoholics (Sharp et al., 1997; Peniston & Kulkosky, 1989; Richard et al., 1995). Virtual environments are being used to stimulate alcohol, nicotine, or cocaine craving followed by desensitization using cognitive–behavioral techniques (Bordnick et al., 2008; Traylor et al., 2008; Saladin et al., 2006). A hand-held device that uses a weak electrical current to stimulate the brain (i.e., cranioelectrotherapy stimulation or CES) probably reduces the severity of withdrawal from alcohol and opiates. A long-term study of CES for craving reduction and relapse prevention in people with alcoholism or drug addiction concluded that regular use of CES resulted in diminished severity of withdrawal symptoms, rapid normalization of sleep, and reduced risk of relapse, compared to individuals taking conventional medications to prevent relapse but not receiving CES treatments (Patterson et al., 1984). In another study hospitalized cocaine abusers undergoing detoxification reported consistent improvements in mood, anxiety, and cognitive functioning following 1–3 weeks of daily CES treatments (Smith & Tyson, 1991).

Regular exercise, as well as practicing mindfulness or meditation, may reduce the relapse risk in abstinent alcoholics (Breslin et al., 2002; Palmer et al., 1995). The practice of yoga improves overall functioning and may reduce relapse risk in both alcoholics and drug addicts (Vedamurthachar, 2002; Shaffer et al., 1997). Preliminary findings suggest that energetic qigong treatments reduce withdrawal symptoms in those with heroin addiction (Li et al., 2002).

Research findings on the use of acupuncture for alcohol and substance abuse are highly inconsistent. A systematic review of sham-controlled studies concluded that regular manual acupuncture and electroacupuncture were ineffective for reducing symptoms of nicotine withdrawal and preventing relapse in cocaine addicts (D'Alberto, 2004). Specialized ear acupuncture protocols may reduce cocaine craving (Konefal et al., 1995; Margolin et al., 1993). Systematic reviews of sham-controlled studies found no benefit of actual acupuncture over sham acupuncture for smoking cessation (White et al., 1999, 2004). Findings on the use of acupuncture for relapse prevention in alcoholics are inconsistent, and certain acupuncture protocols are probably more effective than others (Bullock et al., 1989; Yankovskis, 2000). Many people with alcoholism report reduced craving with treatment but renewed craving and relapse soon after treatment is discontinued (Konefal et al., 1994; Richard et al., 1995). Table 10.1 summarizes the nonconventional treatments of alcohol and substance abuse.

Table 10.1 Nonconventional and Integrative Treatments of Alcohol and Substance Abuse

More substantiated:

- Micro-current stimulation of the brain reduces severity of alcohol and opiate withdrawal.

Less substantiated:

- Improved nutrition
- Taurine and L-tryptophan for alcohol craving
- High-dose vitamin C for hangovers
- Magnesium and zinc supplementation improves cognitive functioning in chronic alcoholics.
- Regular exercise may reduce relapse risk in abstinent alcoholics.
- Mindfulness training may reduce relapse risk in abstinent alcoholics.
- Yoga reduces relapse risk in alcoholics and narcotics addicts.
- EEG biofeedback may reduce relapse risk in abstinent alcoholics.
- Acupuncture reduces alcohol and cocaine withdrawal.
- Kudzu reduces alcohol craving and may reduce relapse risk.
- Ashwagondha and ginseng may reduce opiate withdrawal.

CASE VIGNETTES

Alcohol abuse

Intake
Cheryl has come to see Dr. Moran, a psychologist who specializes in the treatment of alcohol and substance abuse using Western-style

psychotherapy, herbs, and acupuncture. Cheryl is 50, recently separated from her spouse of 9 years, and has a high-stress job as a manager at a software firm. Her daughter, whom she describes as "my best friend," recently moved across the country to Vermont to start college. Cheryl recalls taking her first drink when she was 12 at a party at home. She continued to drink socially through college, with episodes of bingeing on weekends, and she realized she had a "drinking problem" in her 30s, which she ascribed to work-related stress. "My father and mother were both drunks and alcohol was easy to find at home. They acted like they thought alcohol would solve all of life's problems, but it destroyed their marriage." Cheryl's father was diagnosed with manic–depressive disorder but refused treatment. She cannot recall a time during childhood when her parents were not drunk or fighting. Her younger sister has been in recovery for 10 years. Cheryl was abstinent for almost 10 years until last December, when she relapsed at the company Christmas party. "I lost control . . . the next thing I remembered was waking up Saturday morning." Since then she has been attending AA meetings three times a week. She doesn't have a sponsor, but she's "looking for one."

Cheryl expresses deep feelings of embarrassment and regret about getting drunk at the company party. She has no memory of what she did or said but believes she was recently passed over for a promotion because of her behavior. She and her husband started arguing all the time after her relapse, and he asked for a separation about a month later. "I don't think he wants to go through this again," Cheryl commented. She recounts how Rick supported her over many years of alcohol abuse and during her 10 years of sobriety. "I guess he's just had enough of this . . . of me." She is visibly distressed and begins to cry.

Cheryl has a few close women friends to whom she confides about her drinking problem. One friend is also in recovery and attends AA meetings with her. Cheryl sometimes finds herself thinking about drinking and experiences moderate cravings. She does not smoke and has never abused illicit drugs. She has never experienced mood swings, including periods of euphoria or irritability (i.e., when not drinking), but has felt anxious and depressed for about a year and has experienced problems sleeping during the same period. She has never been in psychotherapy and has not been evaluated or treated by a mental health professional. "I think it's the job. It just doesn't end." In her 30s, she became very depressed after the birth of her second daughter. Her mood returned to normal after several months without treatment and remained "even" until last year.

Cheryl has lower back pain and is about 30 pounds overweight. She was recently diagnosed with mild hypertension and warned by her family doctor that she is at risk of developing diabetes if she does not lose weight. She has no other known medical problems and has never been hospitalized for medical or psychiatric reasons. She is in early menopause but does not take hormonal replacement therapy. Her thyroid has never been evaluated. She takes a blood pressure medication and a prescription sleep aid but does not take vitamins or other supplements. Cheryl leads a sedentary lifestyle and hasn't exercised in several years. Her diet often consists of fast foods and diet soda.

On completing the history, Dr. Moran suggests that she see her family physician to get a thyroid panel, do other blood tests to evaluate her nutritional status, and check her estrogen level. In addition to conventional psychological assessment tools, Dr. Moran recommends a specialized approach increasingly used by acupuncturists to evaluate clients for "energetic imbalances associated with substance abuse. Analysis of the vascular autonomic signal is believed to provide useful information for determining the most appropriate acupuncture or conventional treatment."

Assessment

Conventional blood tests are recommended to evaluate Cheryl's overall nutritional status, including blood levels of vitamins, trace elements, and other nutrients essential for normal mental functioning.

> *Note:* Deficiencies of several important vitamins, trace elements, and essential fatty acids commonly occur with chronic alcohol abuse because alcohol damages the lining of the intestines, impairing normal absorption of nutrients. Furthermore, chronic alcoholics frequently obtain most of their calories from alcohol and—as in this case—have nutrient-poor diets. Alcohol abuse is "the great mimic," and chronic

alcohol-related deficiencies of vitamins A, C, folate, thiamin, and other B-vitamins; zinc, magnesium, and other trace elements; and amino acids and essential fatty acids can result in general malaise, fatigue, impaired memory and judgment, depressed mood, and anxiety.

A thorough medical assessment in this case should also include tests of anemia and thyroid function.

Both anemia and hypothyroidism can manifest as chronic fatigue and feelings of malaise. The anemia of chronic alcohol abuse can be a result of vitamin-B deficiency, a general malabsorption syndrome, or in advanced cases, alcohol-induced suppression of the bone marrow's ability to produce healthy red blood cells. Evaluation of thyroid function is a good idea for any client who has a history of recent weight gain and a mood problem.

In addition to the above conventional medical tests, Dr. Moran decides to evaluate the client on an energetic level to find out whether energetic deficiencies or imbalances, according to Chinese medical theory, are associated with chronic alcohol abuse.

Analysis of the vascular autonomic signal (VAS) reflex is widely used by practitioners of ear acupuncture (auriculotherapy) to determine the most effective acupuncture points to stimulate when managing withdrawal in people who abuse alcohol or narcotics and for identifying nutrients required to return clients to a healthy energetic balance.

Formulation

Cheryl has been drinking since adolescence, abused alcohol heavily for 20 years, and recently relapsed after a prolonged period of sobriety. There is a strong history of alcohol abuse on both sides of the family, and she is probably genetically predisposed to have a high tolerance for alcohol. In view of her father's bipolar disorder, she may be self-treating an undiagnosed mood disorder with alcohol; however, her history does not appear to be consistent with this diagnosis. She has experienced blackouts but so far has avoided serious medical consequences of alcohol withdrawal, including delirium tremens. High blood pressure and being overweight are probably consequences of chronic stress, poor diet (related to chronic alcohol abuse), and lack of exercise. She does not report craving. Her recent relapse and ongoing symptoms of anxiety and insomnia are probably related to chronic work stress. It is unclear from her history whether Cheryl's anxiety is also related to the hormonal changes of menopause or an undiagnosed medical problem (including possibly hypothyroidism or a metabolic problem). Her circumstances are further complicated by acute distress over separation from her spouse and her daughter's recent move—both of which need to be addressed in psychotherapy as serious relapse risks. Finally, there is a question of an underlying energetic imbalance that may be associated with a longstanding pattern of alcohol abuse or malnutrition. Cheryl has a close friend who is supportive and also in recovery.

Treatment

As they begin to discuss the treatment plan, Dr. Moran emphasizes the importance of lifestyle changes, including improved nutrition, regular exercise, and stress management.

> The effects of malnutrition seen in chronic alcohol abuse include hypoglycemia, serious deficiencies in amino acids and vitamins required for the synthesis of neurotransmitters, and associated longterm changes in mental functioning, including anxiety, impaired memory, and depressed mood. Generally improved nutrition, including quality sources of protein and complex carbohydrates and omega-3 fatty acids, together with reduced intake of refined sugar and caffeine, probably reduces the risk of relapse in abstinent alcoholics. Numerous studies show that regular vigorous physical activity enhances mood in depressed alcoholics who are in recovery.

Dr. Moran encourages Cheryl to set limits around her work hours and to take time away from work during lunch. Cheryl previously enjoyed running and working out at a fitness center during lunch breaks but has been too tired to "do much of anything" for years. Dr. Moran talks about the priority of managing Cheryl's alcohol cravings to reduce the risk of relapse. He suggests an herbal called kudzu.

> The medicinal herbal kudzu (*Radix puerariae*) is traditionally used in Chinese medicine to treat alcohol abuse. Recent research findings suggest that taking this herb on a regular basis substantially reduces the intensity of alcohol craving.

Cheryl has been anxious, irritable, and moderately depressed. She describes her major problem as severe physical and mental fatigue. Dr. Moran encourages Cheryl to make an appointment with her family doctor as soon as possible to evaluate her general nutritional status, rule out an anemia, check her estrogen level, and make sure there isn't a primary problem at the level of her thyroid. He advises her to take a high-potency B-complex and a multivitamin starting immediately after her blood tests are taken.

> As noted above, people with chronic alcoholism are deficient in many important vitamins and trace elements. Supplementation with thiamin probably diminishes alcohol craving and reduces the severity of withdrawal. Taking a large dose of vitamin C before drinking may mitigate the injurious effects of alcohol on the liver. There is evidence that magnesium and zinc supplementation improves cognitive deficits caused by chronic alcohol abuse.

Dr. Moran describes an emerging diagnostic approach based on Chinese medical theory for evaluating the energetic state of the body (above) and gives Cheryl a handout describing the theory behind the VAS reflex. Cheryl has always been interested in Chinese medicine and is very intrigued by this idea. They agree to try this procedure during the next appointment. As the session ends, Dr. Moran strongly recommends that Cheryl find a suitable abstinence support group, preferably one that encourages spiritual work or incorporates a mind–body practice.

There is an inverse relationship between the degree of affiliation with a religious or spiritual group and the risk of developing substance abuse. Successful support group strategies include cognitive skills training for relapse prevention and stress management. Important spiritual themes of 12-step meetings include self-acceptance, forgiveness, humility, and acknowledging a higher power. Mindfulness training using Kabat-Zinn's mindfulness-based stress reduction model, Christian prayer, or Eastern meditation practices are increasingly used in abstinence support groups. Innovative group support programs that incorporate yoga may further reduce the risk of relapse.

Two Week Follow-Up

Cheryl appears more energetic. She had all the recommended tests done and then started taking the vitamins Dr. Moran recommended, as well as the kudzu. The blood tests revealed consistently low levels of several vitamins but normal estrogen levels and normal thyroid function. She has been working on improving her nutrition: "I think it's really making a difference in my energy level." She has been attending a 12-step meeting in the basement of a church that includes 10 minutes of meditation at the beginning of every meeting. "The meditation helps me feel centered . . . safe." She recounts to Dr. Moran how she approached her supervisor and confided in her about her drinking problem. "It was amazing. She really listened to me and then we cried together. It turns out that she is also in recovery."

Since then she and her new friend have been going out to lunch several times each week to talk about their shared journey in recovery: "we're really being there for each other." Cheryl does not have a sponsor yet but has someone in mind to ask in the coming weeks. She attributes a significant reduction in alcohol craving to "eating better and the kudzu" but continues to feel anxious and depressed much of the time. Her insomnia has not improved. Dr. Moran briefly goes over reasons for using the VAS technique, then carefully examines her pulses and takes notes on his findings.

Analysis of the VAS in this case may provide clinically useful information about the nature and causes of nutritional deficiencies and energetic imbalances resulting from chronic alcohol abuse that manifest as chronic fatigue, mood changes, and insomnia. It may also help clarify the most effective acupuncture treatment protocol.

The VAS findings suggest that a particular ear acupuncture treatment protocol will help Cheryl return to a more "balanced" energetic state, control alcohol craving, and improve general feelings of vitality.

Numerous studies have confirmed that the benefits of acupuncture in abstinent alcoholics cannot be explained on the basis of placebo effects. Stimulation of specific acupoints on the ears, hands, and neck may be especially effective for reducing alcohol craving. However, research findings for the use of acupuncture in relapse prevention for abstinent alcoholics are more ambiguous. Numerous studies suggest that the efficacy of acupuncture for reducing craving, managing withdrawal, and promoting abstinence in alcohol and drug abuse varies in relationship to specific points treated, the kind of acupuncture employed (manual vs. electoacupuncture vs. laser acupuncture), frequency and duration of sessions, and total number of treatments administered.

Although Dr. Moran has some training in Chinese medicine, he decides to refer Cheryl to someone who is more experienced in this specialized kind of acupuncture. Dr. Moran briefly reviews both conventional and alternative treatments of anxiety, depression, and insomnia, including the use of SSRIs, amino acid therapies, and mind–body practices. Cheryl replies that she does not want "to take something I might become dependent on to replace something I've been dependent on" and instead wishes to try "the nonprescription approach to life's problems." The discussion soon narrows to a review of the evidence for specific amino acids that may address Cheryl's mood symptoms and insomnia while also reducing alcohol craving and helping her maintain abstinence.

The amino acid L-tryptophan may reduce alcohol craving, and the amino acid SAMe improves liver function, increases energy, and enhances mood in depressed alcoholics. 5-HTP, the immediate precursor of serotonin, is important for normal mood regulation and is often deficient in chronic alcoholics. Taking small doses of 5-HTP (e.g., 25–50mg two to three times daily) can help help reduce moderate symptoms of anxiety. When taken at higher doses at bedtime (200–300 mg), 5-HTP is an effective treatment of insomnia.

Dr. Moran goes over the basic principles of sleep hygiene and suggests using a relaxing guided imagery script before bedtime. In the final minutes of the session, Dr. Moran praises Cheryl for her rapid progress, encourages her to continue attending AA meetings, and emphasizes the importance of good nutrition and regular exercise.

Four-Week Follow-Up

Cheryl has had four acupuncture treatments in the ensuing month. "I feel calmer afterward, and I think the effect carries over into the next day," she reports. She takes the recommended vitamins, minerals, and omega-3 fatty acids, and has also been taking recommended doses of 5-HTP during the day and at bedtime. There are no adverse effects. She attends AA meetings four times weekly and now has a sponsor. Most of Cheryl's lunchtimes are now spent walking with her new friend, and she recently joined a fitness center that offers yoga classes. She feels optimistic about losing 5 pounds. Her mood is markedly improved—"I think it's the 5-HTP, but it could be just from not drinking"—and she sleeps well most of the time. "I think at this point I need to work on some old stuff." Dr. Moran agrees that Cheryl would likely benefit from ongoing psychotherapy and offers her weekly sessions to explore dynamic issues related to her history of alcohol abuse, to process the loss of her marriage, and to examine codependence issues in her relationship with her daughter.

Putting it all together

This case illustrates the complex social, relational, psychological, and biological factors that are often present in alcohol abuse. Treatment is initially focused on identifying and correcting nutritional deficiencies to improved Cheryl's general state of health and mental functioning while aggressively addressing alcohol craving and relapse prevention. Group support is a fundamental component of relapse prevention. Groups that incorporate meditation or other mind–body practices are probably more effective than conventionally structured 12-step groups. Assessment of underlying energetic imbalances, using analysis of the VAS reflex, results in a specific ear acupuncture treatment plan that helps improve Cheryl's feelings of vitality, reduce her general level of arousal, and control alcohol cravings. Sleep hygiene and guided imagery are introduced for management of insomnia. Amino acid therapy targets residual symptoms of anxiety, depressed mood, and insomnia. Long-term insight-oriented psychotherapy core dynamic issues from childhood and will help Cheryl maintain abstinence.

Narcotic Abuse: Methamphetamine and Cocaine

Intake

Jake is 32, unemployed, and finished his most recent prison sentence about 3 months ago. He is required to have weekly urine toxicology screens as a condition of probation. Jake started drinking when he was 13, started smoking marijuana when he was 15, and had progressed to regular use of crystal meth (methamphetamine or "speed") by age 16. He went on to cocaine, mushrooms, and PCP (but hallucinogens "made me feel too out of control"), and speed became his drug of choice: "It gave me the high I was working for and my head felt clearer." He tried IV heroin a few times, then stopped, because "I couldn't see risking getting AIDS." Although he was a good student, Jake dropped out of high school at age 17. "It was a waste of my f***ing time. All the teachers had this attitude. I couldn't concentrate enough to finish anything." He soon became adept at shoplifting, which became an easy way for him to support his habit without working.

His first felony arrest for narcotics possession was at age 18 and his second was at age 20 for grand theft auto. Since that time Jake has spent about one-third of his life behinds bars, homeless, or in residential rehabilitation programs, where most of the time "I could get whatever I needed there anyway." After several failed attempts in expensive residential rehabilitation programs, Jake's parents gave him an ultimatum: "Next time you relapse, you're on your own." Jake was able to stay clean for only 1 month when he ran into a dealer at a party. He relapsed and continued to use heavily until his next arrest at age 23. Since then he has been completely out of touch with his parents. "That was it, they couldn't take my behavior after that."

At age 26, during a 6-month residential treatment program in the mountains outside Tucson, Jake realized that he was profoundly depressed. He was diagnosed with major depressive disorder and attention-deficit disorder (ADD) and started on medications.

> A significant percentage of stimulant abusers have undiagnosed depression, bipolar disorder, or ADD/ADHD. Accurate diagnosis and appropriate treatment can be transformative, however, as seen in this case. Stimulant medications such as methylphenidate (Ritalin), mixed amphetamine salts (Adderall), and dextroamphetamine (Dexadrin) often become substances of abuse in this population. Consultation with a psychiatrist is important for selecting medications with the lowest abuse potential and monitoring the client's symptoms and behavior to ensure that the medications are effective and being used appropriately. It is often difficult to know when someone is abusing narcotics; indeed, many individuals continue to use methamphetamine or cocaine while attending NA meetings and keeping regular appointments with their physician or therapist.

"It turned my world upside down. I finally got the idea I had been taking drugs to fix this big hole in my head." From that time until now, Jake has continued to use cocaine and speed sporadically between brief periods of abstinence. "I think the speed helps the Ritalin work better." He works as a day laborer for a local contractor and barely earns enough to share a house with two other "crack heads," one of whom is his principle supplier. His last relationship, "with a woman who ripped me off," ended 4 years ago, and he has not been in a relationship since then. He has been in treatment with a psychiatrist for 3 years, but "nothing I've tried really helps my mood stay even, and I keep going up and down anyway, so I keep using to balance myself out. I'm starting to get scared that my life is always going to be like this—prison and drugs and no real life."

The last time Jake free-based cocaine was about 2 weeks ago and he has been experiencing intense cravings for the past week. In addition to an SSRI prescribed by his psychiatrist, Jake gets lorazepam (Ativan) from a dealer "to smooth me out when I'm too high or coming down," but his psychiatrist is not aware that he takes 4–6 mg/day of that potent sedative hypnotic.

> Abuse of prescription sedative hypnotics, including the benzodiazepines lorazepam and clonazepam, is widespread in Western countries. Many alcoholics and narcotics abusers become polysubstance abusers in that they also use inappropriately large doses of prescription sedative hypnotics concurrently.

Jake's sister recently had a baby, and he has noticed that "it would be great to have something nice like that in my life." During a recent NA meeting Jake heard about the opening of the Center for the Whole Person in Santa Barbara, a clinic specializing in the integrative treatment of substance abuse that includes psychotherapy, conventional medication management, NA and AA group meetings, nutrition counseling, EEG biofeedback, and virtual reality exposure therapy. Jake was intrigued by the comprehensive treatment program available at the clinic and for the first time in years felt hopeful. Later that day he called his parents, and after describing the program and pleading with them, they eventually agreed to cover the costs of evaluation and treatment.

As he finishes filling out the intake form in the waiting room, Jake notices how relaxed he feels because of the music and the "cool energy" of the large aquarium with tropical fish and sea anemones. He goes over to the aquarium, sits down, and watches the colorful fish, a tiny striped shrimp and the slow waving movements of a green sea anemone. He is quietly sitting in front of the aquarium as Janet Paterson, a licensed clinical social worker, approaches him. "Looks like you've discovered the aquarium. Hi, Jake, I'm Janet Paterson. Here we specialize in the holistic treatment of substance abuse. We don't just deal with substance abuse. We treat the whole body and the whole mind here." As they walk together down a corridor to Janet's office, Jake can still hear the same soothing music that was playing in the waiting room. Inside Janet's office Jake notices the calming fragrance of lemon. In addition to her graduate school diploma, paintings of pastoral scenes are hanging on the walls. Two pole lamps provide a soft light that diffuses into the corner of her office. An open window looks onto a courtyard where birds are singing. "It's nice here . . . relaxing."

"I noticed how much you enjoyed the aquarium. That's the kind of feeling I want you to learn how to create inside your head without using drugs," remarks Janet. As the interview progresses, Jake talks about intense feelings of isolation and despair and discloses that he has been experiencing cravings for about 2 weeks. He tells Janet that has never had a serious relationship. "I think I would be happier and could stay clean if I could just figure out how to be in a good relationship." He talks about feeling disconnected from "my family . . . everything good in life." As he reveals feelings of despair, hopelessness, and demoralization, he begins to cry. Janet hands Jake a box of tissues. "Sounds like you're way down on the bottom, Jake."

Jake goes over a long list of antidepressants, sedatives, and drugs for craving reduction he has tried over the years. "Sometimes they work, but I take them like candy or I'm afraid I'll get addicted to them and I just stop taking them—then I start using again." Jake clearly has insight into the cyclic nature of his addiction to many drugs and how he uses prescription drugs the same way he uses speed and cocaine. Although he has been attending NA meetings for several years, "it feels mechanical . . . it doesn't really motivate me to do anything . . . everyone knows that we're still using when we're not in the meetings . . . it feels like lying to myself."

Further questioning reveals that Jake has probably been experiencing periods of hypomania alternating with depression when not using cocaine or speed. Jake nods in agreement. "My psychiatrist told me it's depression, but I've always thought my mood was all over the place." He was diagnosed with major depressive disorder several years ago, and there has been no further consideration of other possibilities since then. For several years Jake saw a psychiatrist every 6 months for medication management. "He always asked me the same five questions, then just refilled my prescription and sent me on my way." Jake has taken many antidepressants but has never tried a mood stabilizer. For many years his pattern has been to stop taking his antidepressant "when I'm feeling too good" and resume it the next time he is depressed. "My psychiatrist thought my ups and downs were always due to the cocaine, but I'm not sure that's true." Jake has never been checked for a thyroid problem or other medical problems, and the physicians who worked with him when in prison and residential rehab programs assumed all of his mental health problems were related to cocaine abuse.

> In this case it is reasonable to assume that the client's mental health problems are probably related to chronic abuse of cocaine or other narcotics. However, a careful review of history points to probable bipolar disorder and cycles of repeated narcotics abuse in an effort to self-treat alternating manic and depressive mood swings. Jake has already disclosed using his prescription stimulant medication together with street drugs to get a better high. Furthermore, there is evidence that antidepressants prescribed by his psychiatrist have been working at cross-purposes, possibly resulting in manic episodes that the client has managed with (nonprescription) benzodiazepines obtained from a dealer. Before recommending any kind of treatment, it is important to determine whether a psychiatric disorder other than substance abuse is present, clarify the nature and severity of that disorder, and rule out any medical problems that may be affecting the client's mental health, interfering with response to treatment, or increasing the risk of relapse.

"I think you could really benefit from spending some time here." Janet describes the unique NA groups held daily at the center, which begin with 10 minutes of meditation and end with 20 minutes of yoga stretches.

> Practicing yoga helps recovering alcoholics and addicts manage stress and may reduce the chance of relapse.

"It's about integrating the body and mind. First I want you to talk with our psychiatrist, Dr. Patterson, and I think you should have a brain map so we can get a better sense of what is going on in your brain that is related to your substance use and your mood problems." Janet tells Jake about a colleague at the center who does a specialized kind of brain mapping, called quantitative electroencephalography—QEEG for short—to help clarify the diagnosis and provide direction for treatment planning. "Stewart is our high-tech guru. He does brain maps, EEG biofeedback, and also has a virtual reality machine that I think could help you with the cravings. The other part of our program is acupuncture."

Assessment

A complete history is of fundamental importance for clarifying the psychiatric diagnosis when evaluating any client who is abusing narcotics. A careful review of history and mood symptoms reveals a probable discrepancy between the client's symptoms and history and his current psychiatric diagnosis and treatment plan. Serial random urine toxicology screens, as required by the terms of probation, are important for evaluating whether the client is able to maintain abstinence. Conventional blood tests, including a complete blood count, anemia panel, and blood vitamin levels, are important for ruling out nutritional deficiencies or undiagnosed medical problems that may be consequences of chronic substance abuse or causes of Jakes's mood or attention problems. QEEG may be a valuable adjunct in this case for clarifying the diagnosis of a mood disorder and helping plan the most appropriate treatment for both his substance abuse disorder and his mood disorder.

QEEG analysis is increasingly used in outpatient settings to help distinguish between psychiatric disorders that are sometimes difficult to diagnose on the basis of history alone. Specific patterns of abnormal electrical brain activity are found in unipolar depression, bipolar disorder, and other psychiatric disorders. Furthermore, abnormal QEEG findings can help identify the most effective pharmacological treatment or biofeedback protocol. There is emerging evidence that QEEG analysis of narcotics abusers can also help identify the most effective EEG biofeedback protocols to use for craving reduction and relapse prevention.

Formulation

Jake has a history of chronic polysubstance abuse. His drugs of choice are the stimulants methamphetamine and cocaine. He last used about 3 weeks ago, is having cravings, and is at significant risk of relapsing. He previously abused alcohol and marijuana, and briefly tried IV heroin and hallucinogens, but he does not currently abuse these substances. He has been diagnosed with unipolar depression and ADD and treated with prescription antidepressants and stimulant medications that failed to stabilize his mood. Although Jake may have ADD, for which prescription stimulants are often beneficial, use of stimulant medications is problematic in his case because of their high abuse potential in the context of an established history of cocaine and methamphetamine abuse. Furthermore, Jake is using his prescription stimulant medication inappropriately in combination with methamphetamine while attending NA meetings and without the awareness of his psychiatrist. Jake reports mood swings during prolonged periods of abstinence that are not a consequence of substance abuse and which are probably consistent with a primary diagnosis of bipolar disorder. His apparent pattern of abuse entails taking stimulants alternating with benzodiazepines to self-treat manic and depressive episodes, respectively. There is no family history of substance abuse or mental illness, and no known medical problems are driving his pattern of substance abuse or mood swings. Jake's history suggests that some manic episodes were probably precipitated by antidepressants. His long criminal record, difficulty adapting to life outside of prison, and failed relationships point to low self-esteem and antisocial behavior that may be consistent with antisocial personality, although Jake has never committed violent crimes, and most arrests were for charges of narcotics possession or thefts committed to finance his addiction.

Treatment

At the end of Janet's interview with Jake, they walk over to Dr. Stevenson's office. After reviewing her notes and asking about specific medication trials and adverse effects, Dr. Stevenson instructs Jake to taper and discontinue his SSRI antidepressant over the next few days and gives him a prescription for lithium carbonate, starting at 150 mg and increasing to 600 mg at bedtime. He gives Jake a lab slip for checking his lithium level and another slip for blood tests to evaluate his thyroid and general nutritional status. He prescribes a medication called naltrexone to address Jake's cravings and briefly reviews common side effects of both medications.

> Lithium carbonate is a commonly used mood stabilizer. Adverse effects include tremor, weight gain, and increased urination. Naltrexone acts at the site of brain opioid receptors and can help reduce cravings of cocaine, methamphetamine, and other narcotics. Naltrexone also diminishes the intensity of "highs" if narcotics are used when it is being taken. Naltrexone is generally well tolerated.

"I know you have to get a urine tox every week, so we don't have to repeat that here." Dr. Patterson takes a few more minutes to talk about brain mapping, emphasizes the importance of taking the medications on a regular basis, and invites Jake to call him if he has problems with adverse effects. Janet walks Jake back through the common waiting room area. She schedules a session for the brain mapping procedure, a follow-up session with herself for psychotherapy and training in relaxation skills, and a brief appointment with Dr. Patterson for medication management. "This is all about finding your path, and you've just received the tools you need to do that." Jake smiles, shakes Janet's hand, and walks out of the clinic into a bright summer afternoon in Santa Barbara.

First Follow-Up

Jake has been attending daily NA meetings at the center and is enjoying meditating and doing yoga stretches. His labs, including thyroid studies, returned within normal ranges, except for low levels of several vitamins and essential fatty acids, and abnormally high levels of three liver enzymes. He has been attending talks on nutrition after most NA meetings and is more conscientious about food preferences. He started taking a multivitamin and an omega-3 fatty acid supplement. He talks about meeting others in the NA groups who have also bottomed out and—like himself—are committing themselves to staying clean.

He has been thinking about his new diagnosis of bipolar disorder and viewing his addiction problem in that context. "It really makes sense that I've been using drugs to treat my mood cycles." Jake has been taking the lithium and naltrexone but doesn't like the tremor caused by lithium. "It really gets in the way; my hands are shaking all the time. Is there something else I could try?"

Jack reports a significant reduction in craving with naltrexone. He had the QEEG last week and the blood work done the following day. It has now been about 5 weeks since he last used cocaine or methamphetamine, and he reports feeling less "speedy." He describes his mood as "more even" and his sleep has improved. He continues to use lorazepam (Ativan) for sleep most nights and has not disclosed this fact to Janet or Dr. Patterson. He has been walking every day, which helps him feel calmer. Jake called his father last week and they cried together for the first time in years. "I told him the way I'm doing it this time feels different. Maybe I can make it this time. I think he believes I'm serious this time, and he's going to help me out with the financing."

Janet runs Jake through a guided imagery exercise in which he is instructed to visualize himself on a white sandy beach. After 10 minutes Janet checks in with him and Jake confirms that he was able to experience vivid imagery and achieve a deeply relaxed state. "This is something I want you to do several times a day. Think of it as one of your medicines." The balance of the session is divided between psychotherapy and a guided imagery script. Janet walks with Jake to Dr. Patterson's office for a 15-minute appointment focusing on medication issues. Jake tells Dr. Patterson how upset he is over the tremors caused by lithium, and they review other medication options, including valproic acid and different atypical antipsychotics. Jake is given a prescription for an atypical antipsychotic called quetiapine (Seroquel) for managing bipolar symptoms and is instructed to take the medication before bedtime because of its highly sedating properties. Afterward he has a brief appointment with Stewart Wilson, who introduces Jake to the principles of neurotherapy and virtual reality exposure therapy. They agree to a schedule of two weekly sessions for neurotherapy and, on alternating days, two sessions for VRGET. The first session is scheduled for the following Monday.

First Neurotherapy Session

Jake feels anxious as he arrives at Stewart's office for his first neurotherapy session. "I'm just not sure about all this technological stuff, putting electricity into my brain waves . . . going into virtual environments . . . it's kind of spooky." Stewart reassures him that EEG biofeedback does not involve putting electricity into the brain, that the therapy will be very relaxing and safe, and that after several sessions he will be able to achieve a clear and calm state of consciousness without the machine. Stewart explains the basic concepts behind EEG biofeedback: "This is a machine that will help you train your brain so that you can go into a quiet safe place any time, anywhere you choose." He then reviews the findings of Jake's QEEG brain map, which suggest that a specific EEG biofeedback protocol aimed at rebalancing alpha and theta waves will probably be most beneficial for Jake's overall mental and emotional state, help reduce his general level of arousal, and possibly help control cocaine cravings. Several times during the 30-minute session Stewart records Jake's brain-wave activity for his archive and asks him about his general arousal level. Jake finds the experience of neurotherapy exactly as Stewart described it and reports feeling extremely "calm and centered" afterward. In the final minutes of the session Stewart gives Jake advice on achieving the same "inner state" on his own, between neurotherapy sessions, and recommends an inexpensive computer game that incorporates a simple biofeedback routine for use at home. "This is basically a machine that trains the brain to achieve greater flexibility. After several sessions you'll be able to do this on your own." Jake smiles and feels reassured.

Second Follow-Up

Jake has been consistently sleeping through the night for 3 weeks, has not experienced strong cravings for most of that time, and his mood is more even. Although he feels "a little spacy" on his new medications, he has better control of his mood overall. He is drinking several cups of coffee every day as well as energy drinks "just to feel more up." Dr. Patterson explains that this is a common experience in individuals who have used cocaine or methamphetamine for long periods of time and advises Jake on how to maintain his energy without relying on "the legal stimulants."

> Chronic stimulant abuse can result in abnormally low levels of dopamine and other neurotransmitters required for mood regulation and maintaining a sense of general well-being. Sustained abstinence, improved nutrition, and regular use of supplements that restore deficient neurotransmitters will gradually restore the overall level of vitality.

Dr. Patterson reassures Jake that he will gradually feel better and experience increased vitality over several weeks. He suggests that Jake drink green tea instead of coffee because of its calming effects.

> Green tea contains caffeine and is rich in the amino acid L-theanine, the precursor of the brain's primary inhibitory neurotransmitter GABA. Drinking green tea or taking a concentrated green tea extract can enhance overall energy level while also increasing feelings of calm. Taking coenzyme Q-10 (CoQ10) or ginseng tea also enhances feelings of vitality and restores energy without the "highs" usually associated with stimulant narcotics.)

Dr. Patterson also encourages Jake to continue doing yoga and following a healthy diet, both of which will help increase his energy level but not stimulate him. He remarks that acupuncture and Chinese herbs may be helpful for increasing Jake's general energy level and increasing feelings of well-being.

> Numerous studies show that conventional manual acupuncture and electroacupuncture help diminish cocaine craving, promote feelings of increased calmness, and reduce the risk of relapse in abstinent narcotics addicts. The stimulation of specific points on the ears may be especially effective for reducing craving, promoting abstinence, and improving mood in cocaine addicts. The mechanism is not completely

understood but probably involves stimulation of the brain's own morphine-like molecules.

Finally, Dr. Patterson suggests that Jake take a natural substance called CoQ10 for energy.

CoQ10 is a molecule that helps boost energy production at the level of the mitochondria that are naturally present in the body and are fundamentally important for healthy cardiac function and several other important biological processes involved in maintaining good health. Individuals who are chronically fatigued often experience significantly increased energy with CoQ10, which generally does not result in subjective feelings of stimulation.

Jake schedules an appointment for the following week with Michael, the clinic's Chinese medical practitioner. Dr. Patterson notices that Jake appears anxious and asks "Is there anything else going on?" Jake discloses that he has been taking Ativan all along and manipulating his urine screens but now feels confident that he will be able to sleep and control his mood symptoms without it. He asks Dr. Patterson for advice on how to get off the Ativan and continue to get good sleep. Dr. Patterson uses this as an opportunity to tell Jake about melatonin, explaining that taking melatonin or valerian extract before sleep can replace the sleep-inducing effects of Ativan and other sedative hypnotics. He also encourages Jake to try a few relaxation techniques just before going to bed.

Simple relaxation practices, including deep breathing and guided imagery, can reduce the overall level of stress and arousal and reduce the severity of withdrawal symptoms when sedative hypnotic drugs are discontinued. Taking melatonin (2 mg) at bedtime helps improve the quality of sleep after conventional sedative hypnotic drugs are discontinued. Valerian at doses of 600–900 mg improves sleep quality, is not addictive, and may be as effective as conventional sedative hypnotics for the management of insomnia. Taking valerian extract on a regular basis may also be an effective way for chronic users of sedative hypnotics to gradually taper and discontinue these highly addictive drugs without disrupting their sleep.

Two Days Later

Two days later Jake has his first VRGET session. Stewart brings Jake into a room that is dedicated to VRGET and shows him the monitor, the head-mounted display, and other hardware. They walk through a simulation and Jake selects a scenario: a virtual crack house intended to stimulate craving.

> Innovative software programs incorporating virtual reality graded exposure therapy (VRGET) have been developed to lessen cravings for cocaine, other narcotics, and nicotine. The goal of this high-tech exposure therapy is to evoke the subjective experience of craving under controlled conditions in the presence of a skilled clinician, who then guides the client through cognitive therapy strategies and relaxation exercises that gradually reduce craving in a virtual environment that simulates situations in which drugs may be available in the client's life. Research has shown that repeated VRGET sessions can significantly reduce craving in real-life situations.

The 30-minute session begins with an ordinary street scene and gradually progresses to a meeting with a cocaine dealer in a dingy warehouse. Jake is aware of his increasing level of arousal as the virtual scene shifts to an interaction with a drug dealer. Stewart monitors his pulse and respirations and talks him through these stressful moments, instructing him to take deep breaths and stay focused in the moment. Following the session Jake comments that he was surprised that he had not experienced intense cravings in the virtual world.

Ongoing Therapy

Jake has now been at the clinic for over 2 months and has participated in almost daily NA groups with yoga and meditation, individual psychotherapy, neurotherapy, and VRGET therapy. He moved into a studio apartment about a month ago and no longer has conflicts with housemates who continue to abuse narcotics. He continues to take quetiapine at bedtime but has reduced the dose. He no longer takes lorazepam and has been sleeping well using recommended doses of melatonin and valerian. His mood is stable. He has not experienced significant craving for over a month, which he attributes to the naltexone, the VRGET, and his meditation practice. During a recent family weekend he made a breakthrough around "old trust issues" with his mother and father, and they continue to talk about "the big picture" in a constructive way. The intensive outpatient program will continue for a total of 6 months and include regular EEG biofeedback training, VRGET, NA groups, individual therapy, yoga, meditation, and nutritional counseling. Jake has started seeing the center's social worker to identify job opportunities in the area.

Putting It All Together

Chronic narcotics abuse is perhaps the most complex and difficult mental health problem to assess and treat. Several skilled therapists working together may be required to adequately mange symptoms of withdrawal and craving and to assist the client in developing an effective plan for maintaining abstinence. Stimulant narcotics abuse frequently coexists with a primary psychiatric disorder, in this case, bipolar disorder. An essential initial task of the therapist is to determine whether a major psychiatric disorder is also present and whether it is related to the pattern of substance abuse. The misdiagnosis of major depressive disorder led to inappropriate treatment with an antidepressant, exacerbation of the client's symptoms, and sporadic use of cocaine and nonprescription benzodiazepines in an effort to self-treat manic and depressive episodes. Misdiagnosis can result in inappropriate treatment, exacerbation of symptoms and—as in this case—worsening of both substance abuse and the primary psychiatric disorder.

Initial assessment priorities include evaluation of nutritional status and routine blood work to rule out medical problems that may be consequences of chronic narcotics abuse. In this case assessment also includes QEEG analysis to determine whether abnormal brain electrical activity is associated with chronic narcotics abuse or bipolar disorder and to clarify pharmacological treatment options and EEG biofeedback protocols that will most likely prove beneficial. In the early stages of abstinence, conventional pharmacological treatment is frequently the most prudent and effective option. Ongoing individual psychotherapy is important for helping the narcotics addict achieve insight about longstanding dynamic issues that reinforce abuse patterns, for facilitating exploration of self-defeating patterns, and for teaching stress reduction strategies aimed at reducing the risk of relapse. Group therapy following a 12-step model is an essential part of recovery and is probably more effective when there is a spiritual component or a mind–body practice. VRGET is emerging as a clinically practical adjunctive approach for the management of narcotics craving. Lastly, stimulation of specific acupuncture points can improve general feelings of vitality, diminish craving, and reduce relapse risk.

CHAPTER 11

~

Insomnia and Daytime Sleepiness

DISTURBANCES of sleep or wakefulness can occur in isolation or as a consequence of a medical or psychiatric problem. Insomnia is a common problem in Western countries where a significant percentage of the population is affected by chronic stress (Ohayon, 2002). Insomnia is often reported by individuals who do shift work in which the normal rhythm of sleep and wakefulness is reversed. Disturbances of nighttime sleep or daytime wakefulness are associated with many psychiatric and medical disorders and are common adverse effects of numerous conventional medications—including psychotropic drugs—as well as natural substances (Buysse et al., 1994; Foley et al., 2004). Insomnia is frequently seen in chronic alcohol or narcotics abuse. The severity of mental illness is directly related to the probability of developing insomnia, and severely anxious, depressed, or demented individuals are especially susceptible to sleep disturbances. It has been estimated that 50% of people with alcoholism experience chronic insomnia (Brower, 2003).

When evaluating a client who complains of insomnia, the initial work is to accurately assess underlying medical or psychiatric causes.

Such an assessment involves a thorough medical history and a list of all medications and supplements, including doses and times of day they are taken. Having clients keep a sleep diary can help clarify the pattern and severity of insomnia or daytime somnolence, including middle-of-the-night awakenings, early waking, naps, and stimulant use. Conventional sleep studies using EEG can help determine whether abnormal brain electrical activity is causing the insomnia or daytime somnolence.

Nonconventional Approaches

Individuals who are chronically sleep deprived often have low blood levels of several vitamins and minerals. Abnormally low serum levels of vitamins C, E, thiamin, folic acid, pantothenic acid, and B-12 may cause daytime sleepiness (Tahiliani & Beinlich, 1991). Excessive daytime fatigue can also be caused by dietary deficiencies in iron, folic acid, and B-12 (Higgins, 1995). In addition, low serum levels of magnesium and zinc may manifest as daytime fatigue and difficulty falling asleep (Durlach et al., 1994; Bakan, 1990). Preliminary findings suggest that excessive daytime fatigue is caused by abnormal daytime levels of specific immune factors that regulate sleep and wakefulness (Vgontzas et al., 2002). Because a common medical cause of insomnia and daytime fatigue is hypoglycemia, every client who complains of insomnia or chronic fatigue should be asked about his or her diet and whether symptoms of intense daytime sleepiness or insomnia are related to food preferences or the timing of meals. Chinese pulse diagnosis can point to a specific energetic imbalance manifesting as daytime somnolence or difficulty sleeping at night (Flaws & Lake, 2001).

TREATMENT

Conventional Treatments

Good sleep hygiene consists of following a routine schedule for going to sleep and waking up, avoiding alcohol and large meals late at night, minimizing stressful activities, and practicing relaxation, meditating, or listening to soothing music before bedtime. Sedative hypnotics and certain antidepressants and atypical antipsychotics that have adverse sedating effect profiles are frequently prescribed for management of insomnia. Physicians may prescribe stimulating medications, including methylphenidate, dextroamphetamine, and others to increase the overall energy level of individuals who complain of severe daytime fatigue or sleepiness. Certain antidepressants that have stimulating properties are also widely prescribed for the management of daytime fatigue or sleepiness.

Benzodiazepines are the most widely prescribed class of sedative hypnotics for the management of insomnia. However, there are growing concerns that these potent drugs are frequently prescribed at inappropriately high doses, resulting in their widespread abuse (Dollman et al., 2003). Consequences of the long-term use of benzodiazepines include chronic fatigue, impairments in short-term memory and other areas of cognitive functioning, and increased risk of falling in the elderly (Mant et al., 1995). Use of benzodiazepines for insomnia is especially problematic in people who abuse alcohol or narcotics because of potentially life-threatening interactions. Antidepressants that have sedating properties are commonly prescribed for insomnia, but these medications frequently cause adverse effects, such as dry mouth and weight gain, and may also cause residual daytime drowsiness (Riemann et al., 2002). Although prescription medications are probably more effective than relaxation or behavioral strategies for the management of moderately severe insomnia, many studies have shown that cognitive–behavioral interventions work better overall (Holbrook et al., 2000).

Nonconventional Treatments

Simple changes in nutrition, including restricting caffeine and sugar consumption, can improve the quality of sleep and reduce daytime fatigue. Supplementation with folate 10 mg/day and thiamin 10 mg/day may significantly reduce symptoms of daytime fatigue and sleepiness (Botez et al., 1979; Smidt et al., 1991). Iron supplementation in individuals who are iron deficient and anemic significantly reduces fatigue (Ballin et al., 1992). Dietary magnesium or potassium deficiency can cause insomnia, which improves with supplementation (Davis & Ziady, 1976; Drennan, et al., 1991).

Melatonin is especially effective for management of insomnia caused by disruption of circadian rhythms, as in jetlag or shift work. A systematic review of placebo-controlled studies concluded that melatonin, at doses between 0.3 and 3.0 mg, decreases the time needed to fall asleep and increases total sleep time (Brzezinski et al., 2005). Sustained-release preparations are most effective for increasing the duration of sleep, whereas immediate-release formulations are most effective for individuals who have difficulty falling asleep. Melatonin at doses of 0.5–5.0 mg is an effective treatment of sleep disturbances and wakefulness caused by jetlag (Herxheimer & Petrie, 2004). Controlled-release melatonin 2 mg can help individuals discontinue conventional sedative hypnotics following chronic use (Garfinkel et al., 1999).

Valerian root extract is widely used to self-treat insomnia. A systematic review of placebo-controlled studies of valerian extract for insomnia concluded that 600–900 mg taken at bedtime improves the quality of sleep and has few adverse effects (Krystal & Ressler, 2002). A large study found that valerian extract 600 mg was as effective as a widely prescribed sedative hypnotic for the treatment of chronic insomnia (Ziegler et al., 2002). Research findings suggest that adding a standardized ginkgo biloba extract (240 mg/day) to conventional antidepressants improves sleep quality in agitated, depressed individuals (Hemmeter et al., 2001). Depressed individuals who respond to St. John's wort (*Hypericum perforatum*) often experience improved sleep (Holsboer-Trachsler, 2000). Ashwagondha (*Withania somnifera*) and compound herbal formulas used in Ayurvedic medicine probably improve sleep quality (Rani & Naidu, 1998; Vaidya, 1997). Standardized ginseng extracts at doses of 200–600 mg/day significantly improve daytime wakefulness and sleep quality (Marasco et al., 1996).

The amino acids L-tryptophan and 5-hydroxytryptophan (5-HTP) are sedating at certain doses and are widely used by naturopaths to treat situational insomnia. L-tryptophan, dosed between 1 and 15 gm at bedtime, is often effective in cases of situational insomnia (Schneider-Helmert & Spinweber, 1986). Combining L-tryptophan 2 gm with certain conventional antidepressants does not increase the risk of adverse effects and has been found to improve the overall quality of sleep (Levitan et al., 2000). 5-HTP at doses between 100 and 300 mg is often effective in cases of situational insomnia (Birdsall, 1998).

Taking a sauna or hot bath before bedtime can significantly improve the quality and duration of sleep (Dorsey et al., 1996). Regular exercise enhances sleep quality and improves overall quality of life (Montgomery & Dennis, 2004). Two systematic reviews concluded that progressive muscle relaxation and other mind–body therapies result in more sustained improvements in sleep quality and are more cost-effective than conventional pharmacological treatments (Murtagh & Greenwood, 1995; Morin et al., 1994).

Sleeping with white noise in the background may reduce episodes of middle-of-the-night awakening in chronic insomnia (Lopez et al., 2002). Early morning bright light exposure therapy is especially effective for insomnia related to a disturbance in the body's normal circadian rhythms and also helps to improve the daytime energy level. Carefully timed bright light exposure suppresses melatonin production and improves daytime wakefulness and nighttime sleep in jetlag but is not an effective treatment of situational insomnia (Campbell et al., 1995). Research findings suggest that exposure to pulsed magnetic fields over several weeks may improve insomnia (Pelka et al., 2001).

A special kind of EEG biofeedback that employs alpha–theta training and provides feedback in the form of an individual's unique "brain music" may be a more effective treatment of situational insomnia than progressive muscle relaxation (Morin et al., 1998). Cranioelectrotherapy stimulation (CES) is widely used to self-treat insomnia; however, studies were done almost 30 years ago and findings are inconsistent (Cartwright & Weiss, 1975; Courtsey et al., 1980).

Different acupuncture protocols are used to treat insomnia, depending on the energetic imbalance that is interfering with normal sleep. Numerous case reports and a systematic review of studies on body acupuncture for insomnia suggest that many acupuncture procedures improve sleep quality and duration (Sok et al., 2003; Xu, 1997). Acupuncture also improves sleep quality when individuals diagnosed with schizophrenia or generalized anxiety respond to treatment (Shi & Tan, 1986). In addition, specific auricular acupuncture protocols improve sleep quality and duration (Suen et al., 2003).

When done on a regular basis, meditation, mindfulness-based stress reduction (MBSR), guided imagery, and progressive muscle relaxation are also effective treatments of insomnia. Regular practice of certain yogic postures and breathing techniques can significantly improve sleep quality in people with insomniac and may reduce the need for sedative hypnotics (Cohen et al., 2004). Table 11.1 summarizes the nonconventional treatments of insomnia and daytime sleepiness.

TABLE 11.1 Nonconventional and Integrative Treatments of Insomnia and Daytime Sleepiness

---

More substantiated:

- Dietary changes
- Supplementation with folate, thiamin, and iron (if iron deficient) for daytime fatigue; magnesium for insomnia
- Melatonin for insomnia caused by jetlag or shift work
- Early morning bright light exposure for both
- Acupuncture (including auriculotherapy)
- Valerian extract

Less substantiated:

- Ginkgo biloba, St. John's wort, and ashwagondha
- L-tryptophan
- 5-HTP
- Mindfulness-based stress reduction
- Sauna or hot bath
- Guided imagery
- Progressive muscle relaxation
- Meditation
- Yoga

CASE VIGNETTES

Moderate Insomnia

Intake

Matthew is a 26-year-old fireman who works on a rotating shift schedule. He has experienced severe daytime somnolence, headaches, and moderately depressed mood for about 5 years since being on this schedule. When he returns home after working the graveyard shift, he is often unable to sleep because of the noise out-side his house. He is appropriately concerned about the strain his work schedule is causing in his family life with his wife and two young sons. "I'm always wiped out and irritable, or just sleeping through the day when they want me around."

Over the years his family physician has treated him with various benzodiazepines, a short-acting nonbenzodiazepine sedative hyp-notic, and a sedating antidepressant. Although each of these medica-tions helped him sleep, Matthew discontinued all of them after brief trials because of excessive grogginess when on duty, which interfered with his capacity to focus and perform his work. He has been repri-manded three times for "not holding my own" when on duty, and he believes he has been passed over twice for promotions because of "my inability to stay awake when I need to be alert" during graveyard shifts. Last month he was given an ultimatum to "take care of my sleep problem or find another job."

Matthew never had problems with insomnia before being required to do shift work, and he has never had serious mental health problems of any kind, such as episodes of mania or major depression. He is in perfect health and does not smoke, drink, or use drugs. There is no family history of depression, bipolar disor-der, or other psychiatric disorders. His family physician referred him to Dr. Taplett, a psychiatrist in the community, for consulta-tion and recommendation of nonpharmacological options for man-aging both his insomnia during the daytime (i.e., when he needs to sleep to prepare for the next p.m. or graveyard shift) and excessive sleepiness during his on-duty time (i.e., late-night or early-morning hours).

Dr. Taplett introduces himself as an integrative psychiatrist and describes his practice as including psychotherapy, medication management, and advising clients about a range of alternative modalities. Matthew explains that because of his history of disciplinary action in the city fire department, he has not been able to transfer to a daytime work schedule and therefore his only option is to adapt to his assigned schedule of alternating late p.m. and graveyard shifts. Matthew has not tried alternative therapies to assist with sleep, nor has he tried therapies that promote wakefulness during time periods when he is required to be alert and functioning at a high level of proficiency.

After thoroughly reviewing his history, Dr. Taplett establishes that Matthew has a primary sleep disorder, is moderately depressed, and has a problem with severe daytime somnolence which is probably a direct result of chronically disrupted sleep due to shift work. Dr. Taplett briefly summarizes the evidence for melatonin and valerian, two naturopathic treatments widely used to treat insomnia.

> Melatonin is a hormone that is naturally present in the brain and is integrally involved in sleep regulation. It has been extensively researched as a sleep aid. Melatonin at doses between 0.5 and 5.0 mg is effective for improving both the quality and duration of sleep in chronic insomnia and reducing the severity of insomnia symptoms associated with jetlag and shift work. Taking melatonin—especially a controlled-release form—together with a conventional sedative hypnotic often helps improve both sleep quality and duration and does not result in excessive sedation on waking.

> Valerian is a widely used and effective treatment of insomnia when taken at doses between 600 and 900 mg just before bedtime, and it does not cause residual daytime grogginess. Numerous studies show that valerian extract is probably as effective as conventional sedative hypnotics for moderately severe insomnia, and it avoids problems of addiction associated with medications in this class. For this reason valerian extract is often recommended to individuals who wish to discontinue conventional prescription sleep medications. It is important to

advise all clients using valerian extract that this herbal preparation should not be taken with a conventional sedative hypnotic
or with alcohol and that doing so could result in excessive sedation with potentially life-threatening consequences.

In addition to these two widely used naturopathic treatments of
insomnia, Dr. Taplett briefly reviews the evidence for early morning
bright light exposure therapy in insomnia associated with circadian
rhythm disturbances related to jetlag or shift work and comments on
the combined use of bright light and melatonin for Matthew's sleep
problem.

Numerous studies have validated the effectiveness of early
morning bright light exposure for the management of insomnia and excessive daytime somnolence, especially when these
problems are related to circadian rhythm disturbances
caused by jetlag or shift work. Because Matthew's active part
of the day is required to be in the late night or early morning
(i.e., between midnight and 8 a.m.), he has a "phase delay"
circadian disturbance of sleep. However, because of his job
requirements the goal of treatment is not to correct the phase
delay but to use bright light exposure in a way that will permit
him to sleep more effectively *out of synch* with his normal circadian rhythms. Thus, instead of recommending bright light
exposure in the early morning hours (which would help him
"reset" his biological clock), Matthew is advised to use bright
light exposure in the late afternoon (corresponding to early
morning in relation to his phase-advanced circadian
rhythms). An effective and safe integrative strategy for
improved sleep and diminished daytime somnolence involves
combining bright light exposure therapy in the early morning
(i.e., relative to the client's sleep schedule) and taking a
sustained-release form of melatonin before bedtime.

Dr. Taplett also mentions approaches that are used to increase
alertness and diminish somnolence during Matthew's "day" (i.e., the
period of time in Matthew's schedule that is the active part of his 24-
hour circadian cycle; in this case, the period between midnight and

8:00 a.m.). These include certain vitamins and minerals as well as the medicinal herbal ginseng.

> Many individuals who experience chronic daytime fatigue or somnolence are deficient in the vitamins B, C, and E and sometimes the minerals zinc and magnesium. A high-potency vitamin and mineral supplement taken at the beginning of the client's day (i.e., in relation to his or her circadian rhythm) can significantly reduce feelings of fatigue and sleepiness associated with chronic insomnia. Ginseng taken as a standardized extract is widely used to treat daytime fatigue and sleepiness.

Matthew is encouraged by Dr. Taplett's comments that the supplements will help improve both the quality of his sleep and his energy level when on duty and that he may not need to take prescription medications, thereby avoiding the performance problems he has had in the past with conventional sedative hypnotic drugs. As the session ends, Dr. Taplett comments on the importance of regular exercise during Matthew's "daytime" for increased wakefulness, reviews basic principles of sleep hygiene, and suggests a regular relaxation program before sleep. He talks about the evidence that simple mind–body practices improve both quality of sleep and mental clarity when awake and prescribes a simple progressive muscle relaxation routine together with a guided imagery scenario designed to help Matthew improve his sleep quality.

> Mind–body practices such as meditation, progressive muscle relaxation, massage, and others can improve the quality and duration of sleep in people with chronic insomnia. Over the long term, mind–body practices may be more effective, safer, and more affordable than conventional sedative hypnotic drugs. Individuals with chronic insomnia generally improve more when they combine a conventional sedative hypnotic with relaxation or a mind–body practice.

Matthew is relieved that he will not be taking another prescription medication that might interfere with his ability to work the graveyard shift. The next possible date Matthew can schedule a follow-up appointment is 3 weeks later.

Assessment

In view of the client's excellent health and benign medical and psychiatric history, no laboratory studies or other tests are indicated. A structured diagnostic interview is all that is required in this case to assess his complaint and plan treatment.

Formulation

Except for chronic insomnia and difficulty staying awake and alert during his active duty shifts due to shift work, this 26-year-old man is in excellent health, has no significant medical or psychiatric history, no significant family history, does not abuse alcohol, tobacco, or drugs and is not having symptoms consistent with mania or mood swings. He has tried numerous conventional sedative hypnotics and sedating antidepressants, but the adverse effects of those treatments proved more detrimental than beneficial. His complaints of moderately depressed mood and irritability when off duty and difficulties focusing and remaining alert when on duty can be attributed to a primary sleep disturbance caused by phase advance of his circadian rhythm, which, unfortunately, is a required condition of his employment.

Treatment

For 3 weeks Matthew has been taking melatonin in the early morning (just before his bedtime, which is appropriate given his reversed circadian rhythm), after spending an hour of quality time with his boys and wife before their day begins. After they have gone to school he enjoys a small meal and sits in a darkened room listening to soothing classical music. Once he begins to feel groggy from the effects of melatonin, he listens to a guided imagery CD designed to put him into a deeply relaxed state while going through a simple progressive muscle relaxation routine for about 20 minutes. He then puts on eye shades, inserts ear plugs, sets the alarm for 9 hours later, and lets himself drift off to sleep. When he wakes up, it is about 5:00 p.m. He opens the blinds and sits at the dining room table, where he enjoys a light "breakfast" with his wife and his sons. He takes a multivitamin as well as C, B-complex, and ginseng supplements with his "morning" meal. Afterward he goes to his study where he sits in front of a bright light box while reading the morning paper for about 30 minutes, until "I feel awake and mentally clear." He then goes on a brisk walk around the neighborhood with his sons and wife and enjoys the balance of the evening with his family until he has to drive to the fire station at 10:30 p.m. to begin his shift.

In the 3 weeks since starting this simple routine, Matthew has noticed significant and sustained improvements in sleep "when I need to sleep" and alertness and attention "when I need to be focused on my work." There is no residual grogginess from the melatonin, he feels clear and awake during his on-duty shifts with the help of the vitamins and ginseng, his mood is noticeably lighter, and he hasn't been irritable or "short" with his wife and boys for about 2 weeks (since his sleep has been consistently better). Matthew reports feeling more confident at work and has recently been complimented by the unit chief for his impressive performance during an emergency. He no longer feels estranged from his wife and sons, and there is a renewed sense of joy in their time spent together. Matthew tells Dr. Taplett that he is determined to continue the new approach to managing his problems of sleep and fatigue for 1 more month and then plans to apply for transfer to the day shift "so I won't have to do this insane shift-work routine much longer." As they shake hands at the end of the appointment, Matthew assures Dr. Taplett that he will call to schedule another appointment sometime in the next few months.

Putting It All Together

Effective management of insomnia and fatigue that are related to clearly identifiable stressors and unavoidable circumstances in the absence of complicating medical or psychiatric problems can often be achieved through simple strategies: improved sleep hygiene; regular exercise; the consistent and skillful practice of simple relaxation routines, including guided imagery or progressive muscle relaxation; and use of melatonin, valerian extract, and other supplements at appropriate times in the client's sleep–wake cycle for the purpose of improving the quality and duration of sleep while also diminishing symptoms of fatigue and somnolence during the active, awake period of their day.

Severe Insomnia

Intake

Jennifer is a 52-year-old stockbroker who often works 14 hour days and is constantly stressed. She frequently eats fast food, has gained 25 pounds in the last 2 years, and seldom exercises. She has been treated for anxiety by her family physician for approximately 10 years and takes an SSRI together with a prescription sedative hypnotic medication every day to manage her symptoms. After noticing that the sedative hypnotic wasn't "keeping me calm," she increased the dose to 1 mg four times daily, but has not disclosed this to her physician. She has felt increasingly depressed for at least 6 months but has not sought treatment.

Her medical history is significant for a diagnosis of hepatitis C about 15 years ago, for which she is taking an antiviral medication. Her liver enzymes are chronically elevated, but she has no other symptoms of hepatitis, including chronic fatigue or jaundice. She has no other serious medical problems but has experienced increasing difficulty focusing and remembering "all the details at work" in the past several months. Jennifer drinks three or four glasses of wine most nights and has recently noticed that she is "drinking more and sleeping less." Sometimes she tops off her night with a martini "to take the edge off" before going to sleep.

Her firm recently changed hands in a hostile takeover and many coworkers were laid off or forced to take early retirement. Although Jennifer has been ambivalent about her work for several years, she is not in a financial position to retire. She has been married 15 years and has no children—"My work substitutes for children." Last year her husband was diagnosed with lung cancer; he is on medical disability and is currently receiving radiation therapy. His prognosis is poor, and he may have less than a year to live. Taking care of medical bills has placed an enormous strain on Jennifer and her husband. She has no close friends and is estranged from her siblings and parents. There is a history of depression and alcohol abuse on her father's side. Last week she had an upsetting conversation with her husband, who expressed concern about her stress level, her drinking, and her increasing problems with insomnia and depression.

She soon found a psychologist who specializes in integrative mental health care. Today is Jennifer's first appointment with Dr. Rush, who directs the sleep disorders clinic at the local medical school and has a part-time private practice. Dr. Rush obtains a detailed social, psychiatric, and medical history, focusing on Jennifer's insomnia, depression, and alcohol abuse. He asks questions about her husband's health situation and work-related stressors, confirms that Jennifer has been drinking more heavily over the past few months, and learns that she has never had cyclic mood changes. Furthermore, Jennifer's hepatitis has remained stable on her antiviral medication. He briefly describes how a conventional sleep study is done and schedules this procedure for the following week. He explains how drinking at night is at first sedating but rapidly leads to a pattern of interrupted sleep a few hours later, and he urges Jennifer to actively work on moderating her drinking and to start attending regular AA meetings.

As the session ends, he directs Jennifer to Dr. Thompson, an internist specializing in sleep disorders, who screens new patients for medical problems and prescribes medications. Dr. Thompson meets briefly with Jennifer, then suggests several lab studies to evaluate the health of her liver and her general medical status. He also suggests that she get a blood alcohol level "to give us a sense of how serious your drinking problem is." Dr. Thompson prescribes a sedating antidepressant to be taken only at night, reviews basic sleep hygiene practices, and encourages Jennifer to start taking a multivitamin and a high-potency B-complex in the morning. Jennifer agrees to all recommended tests, and they schedule a follow-up appointment in 2 weeks.

Assessment

Sleep polysomnography is an important initial component of evaluating any chronic sleep disturbance. This procedure requires the client to stay overnight in a special clinic where electrical brain activity and vital signs are monitored to determine whether insomnia is caused by partial obstruction of the airways or abnormal brain activity during sleep. An urgent part of assessment in this case is determination of the severity of depressed mood, including questions about suicidal thoughts. It is equally important to ask about anxiety symptoms and to find out whether there is a relationship between anxiety and insomnia. In view of the client's drinking history, it is prudent to check her blood alcohol level. Other conventional laboratory studies that will help clarify whether medical problems are related to her insomnia, anxiety, or depression include a repeat hepatitis panel, a thyroid panel, an anemia panel, liver enzymes, and blood levels of important vitamins and other nutrients.

Formulation

Jennifer's sleep disturbance is apparently related to many factors, including chronic severe stressors (chronic work-related stress, her tenuous employment situation, her spouse's terminal illness), alcohol abuse (complicated by hepatitis C with elevated liver enzymes), prescription sedative hypnotic dependence (possibly including partial withdrawl when sleeping), poor nutrition, and lack of exercise. In addition, Jennifer's sleep disturbance may be directly related to a primary anxiety disorder (which she may be self-medicating with alcohol), and she may fulfill criteria for a diagnosis of major depressive disorder, which could further exacerbate her symptoms of insomnia. Her increasing use of alcohol in recent months is probably manifesting as rebound insomnia. Because of her weight problem it is important to rule out sleep apnea.

Treatment

Three weeks after the intake Jennifer's blood alcohol level was found to be in the moderate range. Her liver enzymes are elevated and confirm that her hepatitis C is not progressing. Blood levels of several vitamins, minerals, and essential fatty acids are in the low-normal range. The findings of the sleep polysomnography study confirm that she has obstructive sleep apnea, which is probably related to her weight. She has moderated her consumption of wine but continues to drink two or three glasses daily. She is taking trazodone at bedtime, has improved overall sleep quality and fewer middle-of-the-night awakenings, but sometimes feels groggy until the late morning hours. She has made an effort to attend AA meetings two times weekly. There has been no change in her work stress, her husband's prognosis remains guarded, and Jennifer's level of distress and anxiety remain very high. She continues to take lorazepam 1 mg four times daily for anxiety, "and I sometimes need to take more."

Dr. Thompson explains the principles of continuous positive airway pressure (CPAP), the conventional treatment for obstructive sleep apnea, and Jennifer agrees to try the approach. During the remaining minutes of the session Jennifer talks about her despair and fear over her husband's cancer. "How can I expect to feel better or sleep better when my husband is dying?" Dr. Rush listens to Jennifer, offering consolation. "If I were you, I would feel as anxious and depressed as you do. I can't take this burden from you, but I can help you sleep better and learn how to manage stress. If you can do these things—even if your husband's situation does not improve—at least you will be more resilient. I think drinking is interfering with your goals. It will make sleep, anxiety, depression—everything you're dealing with—even harder to manage." Dr. Rush also mentions nonaddictive alternatives to lorazepam for anxiety, including kava, 5-HTP, and L-theanine.

> Kava is an herbal, 5-HTP and L-theanine are amino acids. All three natural therapies are widely used to treat generalized anxiety. (See Chapter 6 for a discussion of their appropriate uses and a review of potential adverse effects.)

"It's not just about taking pills. I think you could also benefit from relaxation techniques for both the insomnia and anxiety." They agree on 5-HTP and discuss a plan to titrate the dose for both daytime and bedtime use. Dr. Rush suggests a quality brand of 5-HTP. He then goes over the evidence for mind–body practices that are beneficial for both anxiety and improved sleep, including mindfulness-based stress reduction, guided imagery, and yoga. In the closing minutes of the session, Dr. Rush suggests couple therapy for Jennifer and husband and writes the names of two therapists to whom he often refers clients. "I know we need to do this work together," Jennifer whispers through her tears, "it's just too hard to imagine."

First Follow-Up Session

Jennifer is noticeably brighter and less anxious. She has been sleeping better and has further reduced her alcohol use to about one glass of wine with dinner. She continues to attend AA meetings. She and her husband Paul have attended three therapy sessions together "and we just cried and held each other and talked about our fears for the first time in over a year." Jennifer describes the enormous sense of relief she and Paul share since beginning couple work. "We're talking about life—and death—in an open, honest way, and we're facing our fears together." She is able to achieve consistently more restful sleep using the CPAP machine. She is taking 5-HTP twice every day (50 mg) for anxiety and a higher dose (200 mg) at bedtime together with the trazodone. Her overall anxiety level has been lower since starting therapy and using the CPAP machine. Because of this reduction, she has been able to reduce her use of lorazepam to two or three doses daily. She has been taking the recommended vitamins and other supplements and feels more awake, focused and resilient in the face of continued work stress. She and her husband have worked together on improving diet and health and she has lost about 5 pounds since her first appointment with Dr. Rush. She has been doing simple yoga stretches in the morning and at night.

Dr. Rush describes an approach that will permit Jennifer to gradually substitute 5-HTP for lorazepam. He also talks about the evidence for the use of micro-current stimulation for management of both anxiety and insomnia. He loans Jennifer a small portable unit and shows her the settings known to be effective for anxiety reduction and improved sleep.

Second Follow-Up

Jennifer continues to sleep better as the weeks pass, and she has lowered her bedtime dose of trazodone to one half the prescribed amount. She now takes 5-HTP 300 mg at bedtime and 50 mg in the morning and afternoon. She continues to moderate her consumption of wine. She does yoga stretches daily and attends couple therapy but no longer goes to AA meetings ("I don't think I need those at this point"). She has lost another 5 pounds since the previous session and stopped using the CPAP machine a few weeks ago. She uses the micro-current stimulator for about 30 minutes before bedtime, 15 minutes before going to work, and during her lunch break. She attributes improvements in her sleep and the reduction in her overall stress and anxiety level to the yoga, the supplements, improved nutrition, and the portable stimulator. In a recent meeting with her supervisor, Jennifer "took control . . . really set limits on what I should be expected to do." She also requested and received approval for a leave-of-absence to spend more time with Paul. "I've been learning how to take better care of myself and to set healthier limits around work. What is most important now is my journey with Paul."

Putting It All Together

The evaluation of chronic severe insomnia often reveals multiple underlying causes, exacerbating factors, or serious mental health problems. In this case there are undercurrents of chronic work stress, anxiety over a serious medical illness of the client's spouse, alcohol abuse, obstructive sleep apnea (caused by being overweight, which in turn is probably related to poor eating habits and chronic stress), depression, and possibly also the psychiatric consequences of hepatitis C. Routine laboratory studies are done to evaluate the client's general health and nutritional status, liver function, and the status of her hepatitis C. Improved nutrition is achieved through basic changes in diet and high-potency supplements. A realistic plan for moderating alcohol consumption, including regular AA meetings, is an essential part of treatment in this case. A conventional antidepressant with a sedating side effect profile is prescribed to treat both depression and insomnia. 5-HTP is a logical adjunct to conventional psychotropic medications for management of both the sleep disturbance and daytime anxiety, while helping the client achieve her goal of gradually tapering her doses of both the antidepressant and the sedative hypnotic. Together with the medications and the 5-HTP, improved sleep hygiene, relaxation training, and yoga constitute an effective integrative strategy for managing insomnia, stress, and anxiety. The prognosis of Jennifer's husband remains very poor. However, couple therapy is an important intervention to help Jennifer and her spouse process intense feelings of despair, grief, anger, and loss of control over their lives—factors that are certainly affecting her insomnia as well as her general anxiety level and mood.

~

Suggested Reading

Baker, S. (2005). *Textbook of functional medicine.* Boulder, CO: Johnson Printing.

Bloomfield, H. (1998). *Healing anxiety with herbs.* New York: HarperCollins.

Brown, R. (2005). *The Rhodiola revolution.* New York: Rodale Books.

Brown, R., Gerberg, P., & Muskin, P. (2009). *How to use herbs, nutrients, and yoga in mental health care.* New York: Norton.

Cass, H., & Holford, P. (2002). *Natural highs: Supplements, nutrition, and mind–body techniques to help you feel good all the time.* New York: Avery.

Cohen, M. (2006). *Legal issues in alternative medicine: A guide for clinicians, hospitals, and patients.* Victoria, British Columbia: Trafford Publishing.

Demos, J. (2004). *Getting started in neurofeedback.* New York: Norton.

Dossey, L. (2000). *Reinventing medicine: Beyond mind–body to a new era of healing.* New York: HarperOne.

Fetrow, C., & Avila, J. (2003). *Professional's handbook of complementary and alternative medicine.* Philadelphia: Lippincott, Williams & Wilkins.

Flaws, B., & Lake, J. (2001). *Chinese medical psychiatry: A textbook and clinical manual.* Boulder, CO: Blue Poppy Press.

Harison, L. (2004). *Healing depression naturally.* New York: Kensington.

HealthGate Data Corporation & Mosby. (2002). *Mosby's handbook of herbs and supplements and their therapeutic uses.* New York: Mosby.

HealthGate Data Corporation & Mosby. (2002). *Mosby's handbook of drug–herb and drug–supplement interactions.* New York: Mosby.

Hobbs, C. (1992). *Foundations of health: Healing with herbs and foods.* Capitola, CA: Botanica Press.

Jackson, G. (2005). *Rethinking psychiatric drugs: A guide for informed consent.* Bloomington, IN: AuthorHouse.

Kligler, B., & Lee, R. (2004). *Integrative medicine: Principles for practice.* New York: McGraw-Hill.

Khalsa, D., & Stauth, C. (1999). *Brain longevity: The breakthrough medical program that improves your mind and memory.* New York: Grand Central Publishing.

Knaster, M. (1996). *Discovering the body's wisdom.* New York: Bantam.

Lake, J. (2006). *Textbook of integrative mental health care.* New York: Thieme.

Lake, J., & Spiegel, D. (2007). Complementary and Alternative Treatments in Mental Health. Arlington, VA: American Psychiatric Publishing, Inc.

Lee, M. Y., Chan, C., Ng, S. M., & Leung, P. (2009). *Evidence-based integrative body–mind–spirit social work: An Eastern holistic approach toward transformation and change.* New York: Oxford University Press.

Lewith, G., Jonas, W., & Walach, H. (2002). *Clinical research in complementary therapies: Principles, problems, and solutions.* New York: Churchill Livingstone.

Logan, A. (2007). *The brain diet: The connection between nutrition, mental health, and intelligence.* Nashville, TN: Cumberland House Publishing.

Oschmann, J. (2000). *Energy medicine: The scientific basis.* New York: Churchill Livingstone.

Nathan, P., & Gorman, J. (2007). *A guide to treatments that work.* New York: Oxford University Press.

Pizzorno, J. (2007). *The clinician's handbook of natural medicine.* New York: Churchill Livingstone.

Shannon, S. (2002). *Handbook of complementary and alternative therapies in mental health.* San Diego, CA: Academic Press.

Stoll, A. (2002). *The omega-3 connection: The groundbreaking antidepression diet and brain program.* New York: Free Press.

Walker, L., Brown, E., & Corcoran, D. (1998). *The Alternative Pharmacy.* New York, NY: Prentice Hall.

Werbach, M. (2002). *Case studies in natural medicine.* Tazana, CA Third Line Press.

Werbach, M. (1991). *Nutritional influences on mental illness.* Tazana, CA: Third Line Press.

Ullman, R., & Ullman, J. (2002). *Prozac free.* Berkeley, CA: North Atlantic Books.

◁～◁

Web Resources

CLINICAL PRACTICE GUIDELINES FOR THE CONVEN-TIONAL TREATMENT OF MENTAL HEALTH PROBLEMS

www.library.nhs.uk/mentalhealth. This is the Web site of the National Electronic Library for Health of the U.K.'s National Health Service. This site is intended to provide comprehensive information on the range of conventional treatments for mental health problems. There is no fee. There are also links to patient resources. The site includes guidelines and treatment appraisals, Cochrane systematic reviews, and a compendium of best practice articles (including clinical evidence chapters and WHO guidelines for mental health in primary care).

www.psychguides.com. This site contains Expert Consensus Guidelines for the conventional treatment of common mental health problems. These clinical recommendations are based on a survey of expert opinions in both research and clinical domains. Although the guidelines are comprehensive they emphasize medications over psychotherapy and other conventional treatments.

http://www.psych.org/psych_pract/treatg/pg/prac_guide.cfm. This site is sponsored by the American Psychiatric Association and includes full text of many (but not all) of the practice guidelines developed by this organization. Topics include Psychiatric Evaluation of Adults, Bipolar Disorder, Major Depressive Disorder in Adults, Eating Disorders, Substance Use Disorders (Alcohol, Cocaine, Opioids), Alzheimer's Disease and Other Dementias of Late Life, Schizophrenia, and Nicotine Dependence.

GENERAL RESOURCES ON NONCONVENTIONAL MEDICINE

http://www.pitt.edu/~cbw/database.html. This is the site of the Alternative Medicine Homepage, a project coordinated by the staff of the Falk Library of Health Sciences, University of Pittsburgh, Pennsylvania. The site provides extensive links to reviewed web sites on professional associations, centers of excellence where nonconventional medical care is available, and databases on many nonconventional treatments. The site also includes links to professional e-bulletin boards and e-journals in many areas of nonconventional medicine.

http://nccam.nih.gov/ This is the official site of the National Center for Complementary and Alternative Medicine (NCCAM). The National Center for Complementary and Alternative Medicine (NCCAM) is 1 of the 27 institutes and centers that comprise the National Institutes of Health (NIH). The NIH is one of eight agencies under the Public Health Service (PHS) in the Department of Health and Human Services (DHHS). NCCAM is dedicated to (1) exploring complementary and alternative healing practices in the context of rigorous science, (2) training complementary and alternative medicine (CAM) researchers, and (3) disseminating authoritative information to the public and professionals. The NCCAM citation index contains over 200,000 citations of studies on all areas of nonconventional medicine indexed in the National Library of Medicine, beginning in 1966. The four primary focus areas are research, career development, outreach, and integration of nonconventional and conventional approaches.

http://www.naturalstandard.com/ This is the home page for Natural Standard Database and is an excellent resource covering the range of non-conventional biological modalities. Natural Standard is an international research collaboration that aggregates and synthesizes data on nonconventional therapies and therefore is an excellent resource covering the range of nonconventional modalities. The goal of this collaboration is to provide objective, reliable information that aids clinicians, patients, and health care institutions in making more informed and safer therapeutic decisions.

http://www.embase.com/ The EMBASE Web site is a gateway to biomedical and pharmacological information pertaining to both conventional and nonconventional treatments. The site includes, but is not limited to, Medline entries. Approximately 2,000 records are added daily, and 600,000 articles are added annually. It includes many search tools that quickly facilitate rapid identification of relevant clinical or research information, and the user can generate table-of-content alerts to keep up to date with significant emerging findings.

http://micromedix.com/products/healthcare/cam/ This is the gateway to five databases on nonconventional and integrative medicine that cover herbal medicines and supplements, clinical information on integrative approaches, patient education information, a database on herb–drug and supplement–drug interactions, and referenced monographs on herbal medicinals.

http://www.thefacts.org/ The FACTs-Home is the Web site for the Friends of Alternative and Complementary Therapies Society. The goal of this society of healers and patients is to create "a repository of health information that is factual, accessible, credible and ethical." Information included in the web site comes from different traditions of medicine and different cultures. FACT is an Associate Member of the Canadian Health Network.

http://www.texshare.edu/bridge/tutorial/alt_health_watch.html Alt Health Watch provides a gateway to full text searches of over 100 serials on all major nonconventional medical approaches. The list is maintained by EBSCO Publishing, a leading provider of popular secondary databases such as MLA International Bibliography, CINAHL(r), PsycINFO,(r) and others. Extensive use of linking enables users to access full text information from virtually all library holdings.

http://www.medicinescomplete.com/journals/fact/current/ This site contains a quarterly review journal that aims to present the evidence on complementary and alternative medicine (CAM) in an analytical and impartial manner. With increasing interest and growing research in nonconventional medicine, there are dozens of specific complementary medicine journals and thousands of general medical journals that present articles and research findings in this area. Realizing that it is impossible to scan all pertinent publications, FACT systematically searches the world literature to uncover key articles in CAM research. The most important factual papers found worldwide are summarized and then critically appraised in FACT. They are followed by an expert commentary written by a member of FACT's international editorial board and include a reply from the author of the original paper. All FACT summaries and commentaries are evidence-based, reporting clinical trials, systematic reviews or meta-analyses, and compiling, interpreting, and disseminating the up-to-date evidence for or against complementary medicine.

MONITORING RESEARCH IN CONVENTIONAL AND NONCONVENTIONAL TREATMENTS

www.clinicaltrials.gov. This site covers mostly government-sponsored studies and is the most comprehensive clinical trials directory on the Internet. The site provides regularly updated information about federally funded and some privately supported human clinical trials that are currently in progress, and it encompasses studies on nonconventional modalities. Data include the purpose of the study, who may participate, locations, and phone numbers for more details.

EVALUATING NATURAL PRODUCTS AND SELECTING BRANDS

www.naturaldatabase.com (subscription fee). This Web site is a valuable resource for both practitioners and patients. The Natural Medicines Comprehensive Database was released in September 1999 and is updated daily. The mission of the research and editorial team at Therapeutic Research Center is to critically evaluate the literature to produce an objective, evidence-based resource designed for health care professionals. This database provides a comprehensive listing of brand-name natural product ingredients, and these ingredients are linked to particular monographs. Clinically relevant information is presented in a user-friendly format. Thousands of new references are added each year, and new interactions and safety concerns are added as soon as they are recognized. Effectiveness ratings are raised or lowered based on emerging research findings. An interface permits identification of potential interactions between a specified natural product, other natural products, and conventional drugs. A new database and web site have recently been created specifically for patients, with the goal of providing patient-friendly wording on natural medicines. Sections of the patient database can be printed for patients during sessions.

http://www.consumerlab.com (subscription fee). ConsumerLab.com, LLC ("CL") provides independent test results and information to help consumers and health care professionals evaluate health, wellness, and nutrition products. It publishes results on its Web site, in published form in an annually updated book (*ConsumerLab.com's Guide to Buying Vitamins and Supplements*), and in technical reports covering a range of supplements. ConsumerLab is a certification company that enables companies of all sizes to submit their products voluntarily for testing and potential inclusion in its list of Approved Quality products. Such products also bear its seal of approval. In the past five years, CL has tested more than 1,200 products. Products tested and rated include herbal products, vitamins and minerals, other natural product supplements, sports and energy products, functional foods, foods and beverages, and personal hygiene products.

http://www.usp.org. The United States Pharmacopeia (USP) is the official public-standards-setting authority for all prescription and over-the-counter medicines, dietary supplements, and other health care products manufactured and sold in the United States. USP is an independent, science-based, public health organization that sets standards for the quality of these products and works with health care providers to help them reach the standards. USP's standards are also recognized and used in many other countries outside the United States. Prescription and over-the-counter medicines available in the United States must, by federal law, meet USP's public standards, where such standards exist. USP disseminates its standards to pharmaceutical manufacturers, pharmacists, and other users through publications, official USP Reference Standards materials, and courses. USP also conducts verification programs for dietary supplement ingredients and products. These programs involve independent testing and review to verify ingredient and product integrity, purity, and potency for manufacturers who choose to participate.

IDENTIFYING QUALIFIED PRACTITIONERS OF NON-CONVENTIONAL THERAPIES

http://www.pitt.edu/~cbw/prac.html. This is a section of the Alternative Medicine Homepage (see above) that contains links to directories of practitioners in many areas of nonconventional medicine, including Chinese medicine, naturopathy, homeopathy, mind–body practices, and others. The site can be used to identify qualified nonconventional practitioners when referring patients.

http://www.byregionnetwork.net lists registered alternative medical practitioners by practice area and geographic region. This site is a useful tool for identifying practitioners who use a range of nonconventional approaches.

http://www.naturopathic.org. The official Web site of the American Association of Naturopathic Physicians, this site includes a search engine for identifying naturopathic physicians by specified geographic location or city.

http://www.holisticmedicine.org. The official Web site for the American Holistic Medicine Association (AHMA), the major organization for physicians who practice holistic medicine, this site includes a search engine for identifying AHMA members when looking for appropriate referrals in your area.

Note that appropriate referrals to nonconventional practitioners can also be identified through many Web sites included in the following sections.

BIOLOGICAL THERAPIES

http://www.bastyr.edu/library/resources/researchguide/cammedline.asp. This site provides a user-friendly gateway to the medical library at Bastyr College of Naturopathic Medicine, where searches can be done on the range of nonconventional biological therapies, including herbs and other natural products used as medicine, foods, aromatherapy, and many others.

http://ods.od.nih.gov/Health_Information/IBIDS.aspx. The IBIDS Database (subscription fee) is the official Web site of the Office of Dietary Supplements, National Institutes of Health. The IBIDS database provides access to bibliographic citations and abstracts from published, international, and scientific literature on the range of dietary supplements. Users can search the full IBIDS database, a subset of Consumer Citations Only or Peer Reviewed Citations Only.

http://www.functionalmedicine.org/ is the Web site of the Institute of Functional Medicine, whose mission is to improve patient outcomes through prevention, early assessment, and comprehensive management of complex, chronic disease. This objective is accomplished via developing the functional medicine knowledge base as a bridge between research and clinical practice; teaching physicians and other health care providers the basic science and clinical applications of functional medicine; and working with policy makers, practitioners, educators, researchers, and the public to disseminate the functional medicine knowledge base more widely.

http://www.pitt.edu/~cbw/herb.html. This is part of the Alternative Medicine Homepage (see above) and is a valuable gateway to the official web sites of numerous professional associations concerned with all aspects of herbal medicine.

http://www.herbs.org/. This is the Web site of the Herb Research Foundation (subscription fee) and includes expert compilations on specific herbals that contain carefully selected articles, studies, and/or discussions by experts that are available as downloads or in print form. The work of the Herb Research Foundation is based on its dedicated holdings of more than 300,000 scientific articles on thousands of herbs.

http://abc.herbalgram.org/site/PageServer?pagename=Homepage_2009. The American Botanical Council (subscription fee) is the leading independent, non-profit, international member-based organization providing education using science-based and traditional information to promote the responsible use of herbal medicine. Depending on the level of membership, the site includes data-bases on safety, use conditions for specific herbals, and searchable monographs.

http://ijca.net/ This is the site of the International Journal of Aromatherapy, which covers the uses of aromatherapy for mental, emotional, and physical com-plaints. Subjects include the use of natural, aromatic plant oils and essential oils for massage and touch therapy.

SOMATIC AND MIND–BODY APPROACHES

http://www.federationmbs.org/members.html. This is the Web site of the federa-tion of massage, body work and somatic practice organizations, a non-profit membership organization in the massage, bodywork and somatic practice field. The site is a gateway to other web sites of organizations related to different somatic approaches, including massage, rolfing, Feldenkrais, the Alexander technique, and others.

http://www6.miami.edu/touch-research/ This is the Web site of the Touch Research Institutes, which are dedicated to studying the effects of touch ther-apy. The TRIs have researched the effects of massage therapy at all stages of life, from newborns to senior citizens. The site includes summaries of studies conducted through the TRI as well as abstracts of studies on tai chi, yoga, and acupuncture.

http://www.pitt.edu/~cbw/manual.html This section of the Alternative Medicine Homepage (see above) is on manual therapies and provides valuable links to official web sites of numerous professional associations concerned with a broad range of somatic therapies.

http://www.wmin.ac.uk/sih/page-300. This site provides access to the electronic version of Journal of Bodywork and Movement Therapies, which covers thera-peutic advances using bodywork, including the Alexander technique, chiroprac-tic, cranial therapy, dance, Feldenkrais, massage therapy, osteopathy, shiatsu and tuina massage, tai chi, qigong, and yoga.

http://www.pitt.edu/~cbw/mind.html This part of the Alternative Medicine Homepage provides a valuable gateway to numerous web sites pertaining to the range of mind–body practices. Note that this site also includes links to many web sites on somatic approaches and therapies based on subtle energy.

http://www.massagetherapyfoundation.org/. This is the Web site of the Massage Therapy Foundation and the Massage Therapy Research Database. The mission of the foundation is to chart an agenda for research on health benefits of massage therapy. The initial version of the database was compiled in 2000 and is updated quarterly. There are currently more than 4,700 citations of articles and books about massage therapy.

ENERGY-INFORMATION THERAPIES VALIDATED BY CURRENT WESTERN SCIENCE

http://www.musictherapy.org/research.html The mission of the American Music Therapy Association is to advance public awareness of the benefits of music therapy and increase access to quality music therapy services in a rapidly changing world.

http://www.musictherapy.org/research.html. The Biofeedback Network provides extensive links to societies and research groups that study various applications of biofeedback.

http://www.appliedneuroscience.com/Articles.htm. This site contains the research library for Applied Neuroscience Inc. and includes research articles on emerging clinical applications of QEEG and EEG biofeedback in mental healthcare.

http://vrlab.epfl.ch/~bhbn/psy/index-VR-Psychology.html. This site is an excellent resource for mental health practitioners who are considering using VR exposure therapy. The mission of the site developers is to develop an accessible global knowledge base on emerging clinical applications of virtual reality exposure therapy.

APPROACHES BASED ON FORMS OF ENERGY-INFORMATION NOT VALIDATED BY CURRENT WESTERN SCIENCE

http://www.siib.org/default.asp. This is the web site of the Samueli Institute. A central goal of the Institute is to promote and support scientifically credible research on spiritual and energy healing including testing the impact of healing energy on patients, and exploring mechanisms of healing energy in the laboratory. Development of objective and clinically relevant measures is a key focus of the research program.

http://asianmedcom.site.securepod.com/research/tibet/projects/page7.htm. This site provides extensive links to Web sites on traditional Asian systems of medicine including Chinese medicine, Ayurveda, Tibetan medicine, and others. Centre members edit a Wellcome series publishing fine editions of classical texts in their own language. This Web site also aims to introduce key areas in the history of Asian medicine and focuses on current Centre work in the field.

http://www.cintcm.com/index.htm. This resource is a gateway to over 20 online databases on Chinese medicine, most of which are in Chinese but some of which are in English. Databases cover Chinese herbal medicine, Tibetan medicine, clinical indications for Chinese medical treatments, services available in thousands of Chinese hospitals, newspaper articles on Chinese medicine (ie, in

China) and others. This web site is a valuable research tool for individuals interested in the practice of Chinese medicine and Tibetan medicine in Asian countries.

http://acudetox.com/ This is the official Web site of the National Acupuncture Detoxification Association (NADA). The mission of the site is to promote improved understanding of the principles of both Chinese medicine and chemical dependency. The site includes NADA protocols that have been carefully developed and extensively tested. More than 500 clinical sites in the United States, Europe, Australia, and the Caribbean currently utilize these protocols for the management of detoxification in alcohol and drug abuse. The protocols are promoted through public education about acupuncture as a recovery tool, training and certification of professionals in use of the techniques, consultation with local organizations in setting up treatment sites, and the distribution of NADA-approved literature, audiotapes, and videotapes.

http://www.neurology.emory.edu/CAM/index.html. This is the Web site of Emory University's Center on Complementary and Alternative Medicine in Neurodegenerative Diseases, whose mission is to rigorously study promising nonconventional interventions that preserve or enhance function and quality of life among individuals with neurodegenerative disorders. The center was started in 2000 under a 5-year National Institutes of Health grant. Ongoing pilot studies include the investigation of nonconventional treatments of insomnia in patients with Parkinson's disease, the investigation of qigong and tai chi on movement symptoms in Parkinson's disease, the putative role of sex hormone therapy as neuroprotective agents in transgenic mice with Huntington's disease, and investigation of the effects of neuromuscular massage therapy in Parkinson's disease.

http://hominform.soutron.com/ This Web site is the home of the British Homeopathic Library, an information service dedicated to the research and practice of homeopathy. Library services include a database of over 25,000 article and book references on homeopathy, and access to Hom-Inform, a search and query service on homeopathy. Both services are available free of charge.

http://www.healingtouch.net/. Home page of Healing Touch International, whose mission is to disseminate information about healing touch while supporting member practitioners. The site is a gateway to three large professional organizations of healing touch practitioners: Healing Touch International, the Colorado Center for Healing Touch, and Healing Touch International Foundation. The site for Healing Touch International includes an extensive bibliography of studies on healing touch in all areas of medicine and descriptions of ongoing research.

http://www.issseem.org. Home page of the International Society for the Study of Subtle Energies and Energy Medicine. ISSSEEM was established to explore the application of subtle energies to the experience of consciousness, healing, and human potential and is designed as a bridging organization for scientists, clinicians, therapists, healers, and laypeople. ISSSEEM encourages open-minded exploration of phenomena associated with the practice of energy healing. The site includes abstracts and contents of the *Subtle Energies and Energy Medicine Journal*. Links to conferences on subtle energy healing, shamanic healing, and consciousness research are provided.

http://www.csh.umn.edu/ The Center for Spirituality and Healing was established in 1995 at the University of Minnesota. The Center has the goal of integrating biomedical, complementary, cross-cultural, and spiritual care. The center provides interdisciplinary education, clinical care, and outreach, while integrating evidence-based research to renew, enhance, and transform health care practice, health sciences education, and clinical care.

MISCELLANEOUS RESOURCES

www.APACAM.org. This is the dedicated Web site of the Caucus on Complementary, Alternative, and Integrative Approaches in Mental Health Care of the American Psychiatric Association. There is no subscription fee, but you must be a psychiatrist to be a full member of the caucus. The site is evolving rapidly and includes online forums that are useful for networking with other psychiatrists regarding a range of nonconventional treatments. The site includes a library and links to related sites reviewed by caucus members.

www.IntegrativeMentalHealth.net. This is my Web site. Several of my conference presentations and recent journal publications are posted on the site. You can also contact me through the site.

References

Abbot N. Healing as a therapy for human disease: A systematic review. *Journal of Alternative and Complementary Medicine.* 2004;6(2): 159–169.

Abbott R, White L, Ross W, Masaki K, Curb D, Petrovitch H. Walking and dementia in physically capable elderly men. *Journal of the American Medical Association.* 2004;292(12):1447–1453.

Achterberg J, Cooke K, Richards T, Standish LJ, Kozak L, Lake J. Evidence for correlations between distant intentionality and brain function in recipients: A functional magnetic resonance imaging analysis. *Journal of Alternative and Complementary Medicine.* 2005;6:965–971.

Ackerman J.A The biophysics of the vascular autonomic signal and healing. *Frontier Perspectives.* 2001;10(2):9–15.

Ackerman JA Study of device technology based on acupuncture meridians and chi energy. In *Proceedings of the Conference on Energy Fields in Medicine.* Kalamazoo, MI: John E. Fetzer Foundation; 1989:156.

Akhondzadeh S, Mohammadi MR, Khademi M. Zinc sulfate as an adjunct to methylphenidate for the treatment of attention deficit hyperactivity disorder in children: A double blind and randomized trial. *Bmc Psychiatry.* 2004;4(1)1:9.

Akhondzadeh S, Naghavi HR, Vazirian M, Shayeganpour A, Rashidi H, Khani, M. Passion flower in the treatment of generalized anxiety: A pilot double-blind randomized controlled trial with oxazepam. *Journal of Clinical Pharmacy and Therapeutics.* 2001:26(5):363–367.

Akhondzadeh S, Noroozian M, Mohammadi M. *Melissa officinalis* extract in the treatment of patients with mild to moderate Alzheimer's disease: A double blind, randomized placebo controlled trial. *Journal of Neurology, Neurosurgery, and Psychiatry.* 2003;74:863–866.

Anderson J, Anderson L, Felsenthal G. Pastoral needs for support within an inpatient rehabilitation unit. *Archives of Physical Medicine and Rehabilitation.* 1993;74:574–578.

Andreatini R, Leite, JR. Effect of valepotriates on the behavior of rats in the elevated plus-maze during diazepam withdrawal. *Eur J Pharm.* 260(2–3);233–235.

Arai H, Suzuki T, Sasaki H, Hanawa T, Toriizuka K, Yamada H. A new interventional strategy for Alzheimer's disease by Japanese herbal medicine. (Article in Japanese) *Nippon Ronen Igakkai Zasshi.* 37(3):212–15.

Arnold LE, Bozzolo H, Hollway J, et al. Serum zinc correlates with parent- and teacher-rated inattention in children with attention-deficit/hyperactivity disorder. *Child Adolesc Psychopharmacol.* 2005 Aug;15(4):628–36.

Arnold LE, DiSilvestro RA. Zinc in attention-deficit/hyperactivity disorder. *Child Adolesc Psychopharmacol.* 2005 Aug;15(4):619–27.

Arvindakshan M, Ghate M, Ranjekar PK, Evans DR, Mahadik SP. Supplementation with a combination of omega-3 fatty acids and antioxidants (vitamins E and C) improves the outcome of schizophrenia. *Schizophr Res.* 2003b;62(3):195–204.

Arvindakshan M, Sitasawad S, Debsikday V, et al. Essential polyunsaturated fatty acid and lipid peroxide levels in never-medicated and medicated schizophrenic patients. *Biol Psychiatry* 2003a;53:56–64.

Astin J, Harkness E, Ernst E. The efficacy of "Distant Healing": A systematic review of randomized trials. *Annals of Internal Medicine* 2000;13(11):903–910.

Atwater F. *The Hemi-Sync Process.* Faber, VA: Research Division, The Monroe Institute; 1999.

Baehr E, Rosenfeld JP. Mood disorders. In: Moss D, McGrady A, Davies T, Wickramasekera I, eds. *Handbook of Mind Body Medicine for Primary Care.* Thousand Oaks, CA: Sage; 2003:377–392.

Baehr E, Rosenfeld JP, Baehr R. Clinical use of an Alpha asymmetry neurofeedback protocol in the treatment of mood disorders: Follow-up study one to five years post therapy. *Journal of Neurotherapy.* 2001; 4(3):11–18.

Bagby R, Gyder A, Schuller D, Marshall M. The Hamilton depression rating scale: has the gold standard become a lead weight? *Am Jour Psychiatry.* 2004 Dec;161:2163–2177

Bakan P. Confusion, lethargy and leukonychia *J Orthomol Med.* 1990;5(4):198–202.

Ballard CG, O'Brien JT, Reichelt K, et al. Aromatherapy as a safe and effective treatment for the management of agitation in severe dementia: the results of a double-blind, placebo-controlled trial with Melissa. *J Clin Psychiatry.* 2002;63(7):553–558

Ballin A, Berar M, Rubinstein U, et al. Iron state in female adolescents *Am J Dis Child.* 1992;146(7):803–805.

Barbui N, Gray R, et al. Clinical interventions for treatment non-adherence in psychosis: meta-analysis. *Br J Psychiatry.* 2003;183:197–206.

Bares M, Brunovsky M, Kopecek M, Stopkova P, et al. Changes in QEEG prefrontal cordance as a predictor of response to antidepressants in patients with treatment resistant depressive disorder: a pilot study. *J Psychiatr Res.* 2007 Apr–Jun;41(3–4):319–25.

Barkley RA. *Attention-deficit Hyperactivity Disorder: A Handbook for Diagnosis and Treatment.* 2nd Ed. New York, NY: Guilford Press, 1998.

Barnes P, Powell-Griner E, McFann K, Nahin R. Complementary and alternative medicine use among adults: United States, 2002. *Seminars in Integrative Medicine.* 2004;22:54–71.

Bauer L, Hesselbrock V. EEG autonomic and subjective correlates of the risk for alcoholism. *J Stud Alcohol.* 1993;54:577–589.

Bell I, Caspi O, Schwartz G, et al. Integrative medicine and systemic outcomes research: issues in the emergence of a new model for primary health care. *Arch Intern Med.* 2002;162(2):133–40.

Bella R, Biondi R, Raffaele R, Bennisi G. Effect of acetyl-L-carnitine on geriatric patients suffering from dysthymic disorders. *Int J Clin Pharmacol Rese.* 1990;10:355–60.

Bender K. Study to reveal drug study reforms. *Psychiatric Times.* 2004 Dec;p. 1.

Benedetti F, Colombo C, Pontiggia A, Bernasconi A, Florita M, Smeraldi E. Morning light treatment hastens the antidepressant effect of citalopram: a placebo-controlled trial. J Clin Psychiatry 2003;64(6):648–653.

Benor D. *Spiritual Healing: Scientific Validation of a Healing Revolution.* Professional Supplement, Healing Research. Vol. 1. Southfield, MI: Vision Publications; 2002.

Benvenuto J, Jin Y, Casale M, Lynch G, Granger R. Identification of diagnostic evoked response potential segments in Alzheimer's disease. *Experimental Neurology.* 2002;176(2):269–76.

Berrios G, Markova I. Assessment and measurement in neuropsychiatry: a conceptual history. *Seminars in clinical neuropsychiatry.* 2002;7(1):3–10.

Bhandari M, Busse JW, Jackowski D. Association between industry funding and statistically significant pro-industry findings in medical and surgical randomized trials. *CMAJ.* 2004 Feb 17;170(4):481–3.

Bhattacharya SK, Kumar A, Ghosal S. Effects of glycowithanolides from Withania somnifera on an animal model of Alzheimer's disease and perturbed central cholinergic markers of cognition in rats. *Phytotherapy Res.* 1995;9(2):110–113.

Bilici M, Yildirim F, Kandil S, et al. Double-blind, placebo-controlled study of zinc sulfate in the treatment of attention deficit hyperactivity disorder. *Prog Neuropsychopharmacol Biol Psychiatry.* 2004;28(1):181–190.

Birch S. Clinical research on acupuncture: Part 2, controlled clinical trials, an overview of their methods. *JACM.* 2004;10(3):481–498.

Birdsall TC. 5-Hydroxytryptophan: a clinically-effective serotonin precursor. *Altern Med Rev.* 1998 Aug;3(4):271–280.

Birks J, Grimley E. Ginkgo biloba for cognitive impairment and dementia (Cochrane Review) In: *The Cochrane Library*, Issue 2. Chichester, U.K.: John Wiley & Sons, Ltd; 2004.

Bland J. New functional medicine paradigm: dysfunctional intercellular communication. *Int Jour Integrative Medicine.* 1999 July/Aug;1(4):11–16.

Blumenthal JA, Babyak MA, Moore KA, et al. Effects of exercise training on older patients with major depression. *Arch Intern Med.* 1999 Oct 25;159(19):2349–2356.

Bocchetta A, Chillotti C, Carboni G, Oi A, Ponti M, Del Zompo M. Association of personal and *familial suicide risk with low serum cholesterol concentration in male lithium patients. Acta Psychiatr Scand.* 2001 Jul;104(1):37–41

Boerner RJ, Sommer H, Berger W, Kuhn U, Schmidt U, Mannel M. Kava-Kava extract LI 150 is as effective as Opipramol and Buspirone in Generalised Anxiety Disorder—an 8-week randomized, double-blind multi-centre clinical trial in 129 out-patients. *Phytomedicine.* 2003;10 Suppl 4; 38–49.

Bordnick PS, Traylor A, Copp HL, et al. Assessing reactivity to virtual reality alcohol based cues. *Addict Behav.* 2008 Jun;33(6):743–56.

Boschert S. Evidence-based treatment largely ignored in bipolar disorder. *Clinical Psychiatry News.* 2004 Jun;1.

Botez M, Botez T, Leveille J, et al. Neuropsychological correlates of folic acid deficiency: facts and hypotheses. In: Botex MI, Reynolds EH, eds. *Folic Acid in Neurology, Psychiatry and Internal Medicine.* New York NY: Raven Press; 1979;435–61.

Bottiglieri T. Folate, Vitamin B12, and neuropsychiatric disorders. *Nutr Rev.* 1996;54:382–90.

Bratman S, Girman AM. *Mosby's Handbook of Herbs and Supplements and their Therapeutic Uses.* St. Louis, MO: Mosby, Inc; 2003.

Bradway, C. *The Effects of Healing Touch on Depression.* Healing Touch Research Summary; 2003.

Breslin, FC, Zack M, McMain S. An Information-Processing Analysis of Mindfulness: Implications for Relapse Prevention in the Treatment of Substance Abuse. *Clinical Psychology: Science & Practice.* 2002 Fall;9(3):275–299.

British Acupuncture Council. Depression, anxiety and acupuncture: the evidence for effectiveness. *Briefing paper no. 9.* 2002 Feb.

Brower K. insomnia, alcoholism and relapse. *Sleep Med Rev* 2003;7(6):523–539.

Brown R, Gerbarg P. *The Rhodiola Revolution: Transform Your Health with the Herbal Breakthrough of the 21st Century.* New York, NY: Rodale; 2004.

Brzezinski A, Vangel M, Wurtman R, et al. Effects of exogenous melatonin on sleep: a meta-analysis. *Sleep Medicine Reviews.* 2005;9:41–50

Bullock M, Culliton P, Olander R. Controlled trial of acupuncture for severe recidivist alcoholism. *Lancet* 1989;1(8652):1435–1439.

Butnik SM. Neurofeedback in adolescents and adults with attention deficit hyperactivity disorder. *J Clin Psychol.* 2005;61(5):621–625.

Buysse D, Reynolds C, Hauri P, et al. Diagnostic concordance for DSM-IV sleep disorders: A report from the APA/NIMH DSM-IV field trial. *Am J Psychiatry.* 1994;151(9):1351–1360.

Cameron M, Lonergan E, Lee H. Transcutaneous electrical nerve stimulation (TENS) for dementia (Cochrane Review). In: *The Cochrane Library.* Issue 2. Chichester, U.K.: John Wiley & Sons, Ltd; 2004.

Campbell S, Eastman C, Terman M, Lewy A, Boulus Z, Dijk D. Light treatment for sleep disorders. *Jour of biological rhythms.* 1995 Jun;10(2):105–109.

Cartwright R, Weiss M. The effects of electro-sleep on insomnia revisited. *Jour Nerv and Mental Dis.* 1975;161(2):134–137.

Carroll K. Relapse prevention as a psychosocial treatment: A review of controlled clinical trials. *Exp Clin Psychopharmacol.* 1996;4(1):46–54.

Beckner W, Berman B. *Complementary therapies on the Internet.* St. Louis, MO: Churchill Livingstone; 2003.

Casacalenda N, Perry C, Looper K. Remission in major depressive disorder: A comparison of pharmacotherapy, psychotherapy and control conditions. *Am J Psychi.* 2002 Aug;159:1354–1360.

Castanon N, Leonard BE, Neveu PJ, Yirmiya R. Effects of antidepressants on cytokine production and actions. *Brain Behav Immun.* 2002 Oct; 16(5):569–574.

Cenacchi T, Bertoldin T, Farina C, et al. Cognitive decline in the elderly: A double-blind placebo-controlled multicenter study on efficacy of phosphatidylserine administration. *Aging Clin Exp Res.* 1993;5:123–133.

Chan E, Rappaport LA, Kemper KJ. Complementary and alternative therapies in childhood attention and hyperactivity problems. *J Dev Behav Pediatr.* 2003;24(1):4–8.

Chaudhary AK, Bhatnagar HN, Bhatnagar LK, et al. Comparative study of the effect of drugs and relaxation exercise (yoga shavasan) in hypertension. *J Assoc Physicians India.* 1988;36(12):721–723.

Chen M, et al. Effect of ascorbic acid on plasma alcohol clearance. *J Am Coll Nutr.* 1990;9(3):185–189.

Cheuvront SN, Carter R. Ginkgo and memory. *JAMA.* 2003;289(5):547–548.

Chung I, Kim Y, Ahn J, et al. Pharmacologic profile of natural products used to treat psychotic illnesses. *Psychopharmacology Bulletin.* 1995;31:139–145.

Cohen L, Warneke C, Fouladi R, et al. Psychological adjustment and sleep quality in a randomized trial of the effects of a Tibetan yoga intervention in patients with lymphoma. *Cancer.* 2004;100:2253–2260.

Cohen M. *Legal Issues in Alternative Medicine.* Trafford Publishing; 2003.

Colombo G, Agabio R, Lobina C, et al. From medicinal plants promising treatments for alcoholism. *Fitoterapia.* Vol 69, Suppl. 5. 1998; 20.

Constantinidis J. Alzheimer's disease and the zinc theory. [in French] *Encephale.* 1990;4:231–239.

Coppen A, Bailey J. Enhancement of the antidepressant action of fluoxetine by folic acid: A randomized, placebo controlled trial. *J Affect Disord.* 2000;(60):121–130.

Courtsey R, Frankel B, Gaarder K, Mott D. A comparison of relaxation techniques with electrosleep therapy for chronic sleep-onset insomnia: A sleep-EEG study. *Biofeedback and self-regulation.* 1980;5(1):7–73.

Cravo M, Gloria L, Selhum J, et al. Hyperhomocysteinemia in chronic alcoholism: Correlation with folate, vitamin B-12 and vitamin B-6 status. *Am J Clin Nutr.* 63:220–4, 1996.

Crook T, Tinklenberg J, Yesavage J, et al. Effects of phosphatidylserine in age-associated memory impairment. *Neurology.* 1991;41:644–649.

D'Alberto A. Auricular acupuncture in the treatment of cocaine/crack abuse: A review of the efficacy, the use of the National acupuncture detoxification association protocol, and the selection of sham points. *Jour Alt Comp Med.* 2004;10(6):985–1000.

Dantzer R, Wollman E, Vitkovic L, Yirmiya R. Cytokines and depression: Fortuitous or causative association? *Molecular Psychiatry.* 1999;4:328–332.

Davidson J, Hypericum Depression Trial Study Group. Effect of Hypericum perforatum (St John's Wort) in major depressive disorder: A randomized controlled trial. *JAMA.* 2002;287:1807–1814.

Davis J, Chen N, Glick I. A meta-analysis of the efficacy of second-generation antipsychotics. *Arch Gen Psychiatry.* 2003;60(6):553–564.

DeFelice, E. Cranial electrotherapy stimulation (CES) in the treatment of anxiety and other stress-related disorders: A review of controlled clinical trials. *Stress Medicine.* 1997;13:31–42.

Delgado PL, Moreno FA. Role of norepinephrine in depression. *J Clin Psychiatry.* 2000;61 Suppl 1:5–12.

Deslandes A, Veiga H, Cagy M, Fiszman A, Piedade R, Ribeiro P. Quantitative electroencephalography (qEEG) to discriminate primary degenerative dementia from major depressive disorder (depression).*Arq Neuropsiquiatr.* 2004 Mar;62(1):44–50.

Didonna F, ed. *Clinical Handbook of Mindfulness.* New York: Springer-Verlag; 2009.

Diego MA, Jones NA, Field T, et al. Aromatherapy positively affects mood, EEG patterns of alertness and math computations. *Int J Neurosci.* 1998 Dec;96(3–4):217–24.

Dixon M, Sweeney K. *The Human Effect in Medicine: Theory, Research and Practice.* Oxford, UK: Radcliffe Medical Press; 2000.

Dollman W, Le Blanc V, Roughhead E. Managing insomnia in the elderly—what prevents us using non-drug options. *J Clin Pharm Ther.* 2003;28(6):485–491.

Dorsey CM, Lukas SE, Teicher MH, et al. Effects of passive body heating on the sleep of older female insomniacs. *Journal of Geriatric Psychiatry and Neurology.* 1996;9(2):83–90.

Dossey L. *Healing Words: The Power of Prayer and the Practice of Medicine.* New York, NY: Harper Collins; 1997.

Dragull K, Yoshida WY, Tang CS. Piperidine alkaloids from Piper methysticum. *Phytochemistry.* 2003;6(2):193–198.

Drennan M, Kripke D, Klemfuss H, Moore J. Potassium affects actigraph-identified sleep. *Sleep.* 1991;14(4):357–360.

Drohan M. From myth to reality: How music changes matter. *Alternative Health Practitioner.* 1999 Spring;5(1):25–33.

Druss BG, Rosenheck RA. Use of practitioner-based complementary therapies by persons reporting mental conditions in the United States. *Arch Gen Psychiatry.* 2000;57(7):708–14.

Durlach J, Durlach V, Bac P, et al. Magnesium and therapeutics. *Magnes Res.* 1994;7(3/4):313–328.

Effects of Omega-3 Fatty Acids on Mental Health. *Evidence Report/Technology Assessment No. 116. Agency for Healthcare Research and Quality Publication No. 05-E022-2.* 2005 July.

Eisenberg D, Davis R, Ettner S, et al. Trends in alternative medicine use in the United States, 1990–1997: Results of a follow-up national survey. *JAMA.* 1998 Nov 11;280(18):1569–1575.

Elkins G, HRajab MH, Marcus J. Complementary and alternative medicine use by psychiatric inpatients. *Psychol Rep.* 2005;96(1):163–166.

Emsley R, Oosthuizen P, van Rensburg SJ. Clinical potential of Omega-3 fatty acids in the treatment of schizophrenia. *CNS Drugs.* 2003;17(15):1081–1091.

Engebretson J, Wardell DW. Energy-based modalities. *Nurs Clin North Am.* 2007 Jun; 42(2):243–59.

Engelhart MJ, Geerlings MI, Ruitenberg A, et al. Diet and risk of dementia: Does fat matter?: The Rotterdam study. *Neurology.* 2002;59(12):1915–1921.

Ernst E. Complementary medicine: The facts. *Phys Ther Rev.* 1997;2:49–57.

Ernst E. Diet and dementia, is there a link? A systematic review. *Nutritional Nuero-science.* 1999;2:1–6.

Ernst E, Hentschel C. Diagnostic methods in complementary medicine: Which craft is witchcraft? *Int Jour Risk and Safety in Medicine.* 1995;7:55–63.

Ernst E, Resch K. Clinical trials of homeopathy: A re-analysis of a published review. *Forsch Komplementarmed.* 1996;3:85–90.

Eskinazi D. Policy perspectives: Factors that shape alternative medicine. *JAMA.* 1998 Nov 11;280(18):1621–1623.

Even C, Schröder CM, Friedman S, Rouillon F. Efficacy of light therapy in nonseasonal depression: A systematic review. *J Affect Disord.* 2008 May;108(1–2):11–23.

Faraone SV, Wilens T. Does stimulant treatment lead to substance use disorders? *J Clin Psychiatry.* 2003;64 Suppl 11:9–13.

Feingold, B. *Why Your Child is Hyperactive.* New York, NY: Random House; 1975.

Fenton WS, Dickerson F, Boronow J, Hibbeln J, Knable M. A placebo-controlled trial of omega-3 fatty acid (ethyl eicosapentaenoic acid) supplementation for residual symptoms and cognitive impairment in schizophrenia. *Am. J. Psychiatry.* 2001 Dec;158(12):2071–2073.

Finney J, Moos R. Psychosocial treatments for alcohol use disorders. In: Nathan P, Gorman J, eds. *A Guide to Treatments that Work.* 2nd ed. New York, NY: Oxford University Press; 2002: 157–168.

Flaws B, Lake J. *Chinese Medical Psychiatry.* Boulder, CO: Blue Poppy Press; 2001.

Foley D, Ancoli-Israel S, Britz P, Walsh J. Sleep disturbances and chronic disease in older adults: Results of the 2003 National Sleep Foundation Sleep in America survey. *J. Psychosom Res.* 2004;56(5):497–502.

Folstein M, Liu T, Peter I, et al. The homocysteine hypothesis of depression. *Am J Psychiatry.* 2007 Jun;164(6):861–867.

Forbes MA, Rust R, Becker GJ. Surface electromyography (EMG) apparatus as a measurement device for biofield research: Results from a single case. *Journal of Alternative and Complementary Medicine.* 2004;10(4):617–626.

Freeman MP, Hibbeln JR, Wisner KL, et al. Omega-3 fatty acids: Evidence basis for treatment and future research in psychiatry [American Psychiatric Association Subcommittee Report]. *J Clin Psychiatry.* 2006;67:1954–1967.

Frei H, Everts R, von Ammon K, et al. Randomised controlled trials of homeopathy in hyperactive children: Treatment procedure leads to an unconventional study design. Experience with open-label homeopathic treatment preceding the Swiss ADHD placebo controlled, randomized, double-blind, cross-over trial. *Homeopathy.* 2007 Jan;96(1):35–41.

Gallinat J, Bottlender R, Juckel G, et al. The loudness dependency of the auditory evoked N1/P2-component as a predictor of the acute SSRI response in depression. *Psychopharmacology.* 2000;148(4):404–411.

Gallo F. *Energy Psychology: Explorations at the Interface of Energy, Cognition, Behavior, and Health.* Boca Raton, FL: CRC Press; 1999.

Garakani A, Martinez JM, Aaronson CJ, Voustianiouk A, Kaufmann H, Gorman JM. Effect of medication and psychotherapy on heart rate variability in panic disorder. *Depress Anxiety.* 2008 Oct 6.

Garfinkel D, Zisapel N, Wainstein J, Laudon M. Facilitation of benzodiazepine discontinuation by melatonin: A new clinical approach [comment]. *Arch Intern Med.* 1999 Nov 8;159(20):2393–2395.

Gartner J, Larson D, Allen G. Religious commitment and mental health: A review of the empirical literature. *Jour Psychol and Theol.* 1991;19:6–25.

Gaylord S, Davidson J. The constitution: Views from homeopathy and psychiatry. *British Homeopathic Jour.* 1998 Jul; 87:148–153.

Geddes J, Freemantle N, Harrison P, Bebbington P. Atypical antipsychotics in the treatment of schizophrenia: Systematic overview and meta-regression analysis. *BMJ.* 2000;32(1):72–73, 1371–1376.

Geddes JR, Game D, Jenkins NE, et al. What proportion of primary psychiatric interventions are based on evidence from randomized controlled trials? *Qual Health Care.* 1996;5:215–217.

Gibbons R, Hur K, Bhaumik D, Mann J. The relationship between antidepressant medication use and rate of suicide. *Arch Gen Psychiatry.* 2005 Feb;62(2):165–172.

Gijsman HJ, Scarna A, Harmer CJ, et al. A dose-finding study on the effects of branch chain amino acids on surrogate markers of brain dopamine function. *Psychpharmacology.* 2002 Mar 16;2:192–197.

Glória L, Cravo M, Camillo ME, et al. Nutritional deficiencies in chronic alcoholics: Relation to dietary intake and alcohol consumption. *Am J Gastroenterol.* 1997;92:485–489.

Godfrey P, Toone B, Carney M, et al. Enhancement of recovery from psychiatric illness by methylfolate. *Lancet.* 1990;336:392–395.

Gloria L, Cravo M, Camilo ME, et al. Nutritional deficiencies in chronic alcoholics: Relation to dietary intake and alcohol consumption. *Am J Gastroenterol.* 1997;92(3):458–459.

Goel N, Terman M, Terman JS, Macchi MM, Stewart JW. Controlled trial of bright light and negative air ions for chronic depression. *Psychol Med.* 2005 Jul;35(7):945–955.

Golden RN, Gaynes BN, Ekstrom RD, et al. The efficacy of light therapy in the treatment of mood disorders: A review and meta-analysis of the evidence. *Am J Psychiatry.* 2005 Apr;162(4):656–662.

Grant W. Dietary links to Alzheimer's disease. *Alzheimer's Dis Rev.* 1997;2:42–55.

Gruzelier J, Egner T. Critical validation studies of neurofeedback. *Child Adolesc Psychiatr Clin N Am.* 2005 Jan; 14(1):83–104.

Guenther R. Role of nutritional therapy in alcoholism treatment. *Int J Biosoc Med Res.* 1983;4:15–18.

Guevara E, Menidas N, Silva C. Developing a protocol for decreasing post traumatic stress symptoms in abused women. Paper presented at the 8th Nursing Research Pan American Colloquium. Mexico City;2002.

Hammer L. Qualities as signs of psychological disharmony. In: *Chinese Pulse Diagnosis: A Contemporary Approach.* Seattle, WA: Eastland Press; 2001:539–594

Hankey A. Are we close to a theory of energy medicine? *JACM.* 2004;10(1):83–86.

Harkness R, Bratman, S. *Mosby's Handbook of Drug-Herb and Drug-Supplement Interactions.* St. Louis, MO: Mosby, Inc; 2003.

Hechun, L. Advances in clinical research on common mental disorders with computer controlled electro-acupuncture treatment. In: Tang L, Tang S, eds. *Neurochemistry in Clinical Applications.* New York, NY: Plenum Press; 1995:109–122.

Hemmeter U, Annen B, Bischof R, et al. Polysomnographic effects of adjuvant ginkgo biloba therapy in patients with major depression medicated with trimipramine. *Pharmacopsychiatry.* 2001 Mar;34(2):50–59.

Heresco-Levy U, Javitt D, Ermilov M, et al. Efficacy of high-dose glycine in the treatment of enduring negative symptoms of schizophrenia. *Arch Gen Psychiatry.* 1999;56:29–36.

Herxheimer A, Petrie KJ. Melatonin for the prevention and treatment of jet lag (Cochrane Review). In: *The Cochrane Library,* Issue 2. Chichester, UK: John Wiley & Sons, Ltd; 2004.

Heseker H, Kubler W, Pudel V, Westenhoffer J. Psychological disorders as early symptoms of a mild-moderate vitamin deficiency. *Ann N.Y. Acad Sci.* 1992;669:352–357.

Higgins C. Deficiency testing for iron, vitamin B-12 and folate. *Nurs Times.* 1995;91(22):38–39.

Holbrook A, Crowther R, Lotter A, Cheng C, King D. Meta-analysis of benzodiazepine use in the treatment of insomnia. *Canadian Medical Assn Journal.* 2000;162(2):225–233.

Holsboer-Trachsler E. Phytotherapeutics and sleep. *Schweizerische rundschau fur medizin praxis.* 2000;89:51–52, 2178–2182.

Horrobin D, Schizophrenia as a membrane lipid disorder which is expressed throughout the body. *Prostaglandins, Leukotrienes and Essential Fatty Acids.* 1996;55(2/2):3–7.

Horrobon D. The membrane phospholipid hypothesis as a biochemical basis for the neurodevelopmental concept of schizophrenia. *Schizophrenia Research.* 1998;30:193–208.

Hudson S, Tabet N. Acetyl-l-carnitine for dementia (Cochrane Review). In: *The Cochrane Library*, Issue 2. Chichester, UK: John Wiley & Sons, Ltd; 2004.

Hughes J, Roy E. Conventional and quantitative electroencephalography in psychiatry. *Journal of Neuropsychiatry and Clinical Neuroscience.* 1999;11:190–208.

Huong N, Matsumoto K, Yamasaki K, Duc N, Nham N, Watanabe H. Majonoside-R2, a major constituent of Vietnamese Ginseng, attenuates opioid-induced antinociception. *Pharmacology Biochemistry and Behavior.* 1996;57(1/2):185–291.

Ikeda H. Effects of taurine on alcohol withdrawal (letter). *Lancet.* 1977;509:ii.

Irwin MR. Human psychoneuroimmunology: 20 years of discovery. *Brain Behav Immun.* 2008 Feb;22(2):129–139.

Itil TM, Eralp E, Ahmed I, et al. The pharmacological effects of ginkgo bilboa, a plant extract, on the brain of dementia patients in comparison with tacrine. *Psychopharmacol Bull.* 1998;34:391–397.

Izzo A, Ernst E. Interactions between herbal medicines and prescribed drugs: A systematic review. *Drugs.* 2001;61(15):2163–2175.

Janakiramaiah N, Gangadhar BN, Naga Venkatesha Murthy PJ, et al. Antidepressant efficacy of Sudarshan Kriya Yoga (SKY) in melancholia: A randomized comparison with electroconvulsive therapy (ECT) and imipramine. *J Affect Disord.* 2000;57:255–259.

Jazayeri S, Tehrani-Doost M, Keshavarz SA, et al. Comparison of therapeutic effects of omega-3 fatty acid eicosapentaenoic acid and fluoxetine, separately and in combination, in major depressive disorder. *Aust N Z J Psychiatry.* 2008 Mar;42(3):192–198.

Jensen PS, Kenny DT. The effects of yoga on the attention and behavior of boys with Attention-Deficit/hyperactivity Disorder (ADHD). *J Atten Disord.* 2004;7(4):205–216.

Jia YK, Luo HC, Zhan L, Jia TZ, Yan M. A study on the treatment of schizophrenia with He-Ne laser irradiation of acupoint. *J Tradit Chin Med.* 1987 Dec;7(4):269–272.

John ER, Princhep LS. Principles of neurometric analysis of EEG and evoked potentials. In: Niedermeyer E, F. Lopes da Silva F, eds. *Electroencephalography: Basic Principles, Clinical Applications, and Related Fields.* Baltimore, MD: Williams & Wilkins; 1993:989–1003.

John ER, Prichep LS, Winterer G, et Al. Electrophysiological subtypes of psychotic states. *Acta Psychiatr Scand.* 2007 Jul;116(1):17–35.

Jordan N. Psychotherapy with expressive technics in psychotic patients. *Acta Psiquiatr Psicol Am Lat.* 1989;35(1–2):55–60.

Kahn RS, Westenberg HGM, Verhoeven WMA, et al. Effect of a serotonin precursor and uptake inhibitor in anxiety disorders: A double-blind comparison of 5-hydroxytryptophan, clomipramine, and placebo. *Int Clin Psychopharmacol.* 1987;2(1):33–45.

Kalmijn S, van Boxtel M, Ocke M, Verschuren W, Kromhout D, Launer L. Dietary intake of fatty acids and fish in relation to cognitive performance at middle age. *Neurology.* 2004 Jan 27;62(2):275–280.

Kaplan BJ, Simpson JSA, Ferre RC, et al. Effective mood stabilization with a chelated mineral supplement: An open-label trial in bipolar disorder. *J Clin Psychiatry.* 2001;62:936–944.

Kaptsan A, Yaroslavsky Y, Applebaum J, Belmaker RH, Grisaru N. Right prefrontal TMS versus sham treatment of mania: A controlled study. *Bipolar Disorders.* 2003 Feb 5;1:36–39.

Kayumov L, Brown G, Jindal R, et al. A randomized, double-blind, placebo-controlled crossover study of the effect of exogenous melatonin on delayed sleep phase syndrome. *Psychosom Med.* 2001;63:40–48.

Keefer L, Blanchard E. The effects of relaxation response meditation on the symptoms of irritable bowel syndrome: Results of a controlled treatment study. *Behavior Research and Therapy.* 2001 July;39(7)801–811.

Kelly CB, McDonnell AP, Johnston TG, et al. The MTHFR C677T polymorphism is associated with depressive episodes in patients from Northern Ireland. *J Psychopharmacol.* 2004;18:567–571.

Kendler SK, Liu XQ, Gardner CO, McCullough ME, Larson D, Prescott CA. Dimensions of religiosity and their relationship of lifetime psychiatric and substance use disorders. *American Journal of Psychiatry.* 2003;160:496–503.

Kerr T, Walsh J, Marshall A. Emotional change processes in music-assisted reframing. *Journal of Music Therapy.* 2001 Fall;38(3):193–211.

Keshavarz S, Jazayeri S, Tehrani-Doost M, et al. Effects of n-3 fatty acid EPA in the treatment of depression. *Proc Nutr Soc.* 2008 May;67(OCE):E2i10.

Kessler RC, Soukup J, Davis RB, et al. The use of complementary and alternative therapies to treat anxiety and depression in the United States. *Am J Psychiatry.* 2001;158(2):289–294.

Kim MS, Cho KS, Woo H, et al. Effects of hand massage on anxiety in cataract surgery using local anesthesia. *J Cataract Refract Surg.* 2002;27(6):884–890.

Kirsch I, Deacon BJ, Huedo-Medina TB, Scoboria A, Moore TJ, Johnson BT. Initial severity and antidepressant benefits: A meta-analysis of data submitted to the Food and Drug Administration. *PLoS Med.* 2008 Feb;5(2):e45.

Kirsch I, Moore T, Scoboria A, Nicholls S. The emperor's new drugs: An analysis of antidepressant medication data submitted to the U.S. Food and Drug Administration. *Prevention & Treatment.* 5;Article 23:2002.

Koenig H. Futterman A. 1995 religion and health outcomes: A review and synthesis of the literature presented at the Conf on Methodological Advances in the study of religion, health and aging, Mar 16–17. Sponsored by the Natl. Inst. On Aging and Fetzer Inst, Kalamazoo, MI.

Koger S, Chapin K, Brotons M. Is music therapy an effective intervention for dementia? A meta-analytic review of literature. *Jour of Music Therapy.* 1999;36(1):2–15.

Konofal E, Lecendreux M, Deron J, et al. Effects of iron supplementation on attention deficit hyperactivity disorder in children. *Pediatr Neurol.* 2008 Jan;38(1):20–26.

Konefal J, Duncan R, Clemence C. The impact of an acupuncture treatment program to an existing Metro-Dade County outpatient substance abuse treatment facility. *Journal of Addictive Diseases.* 1994;13(3):71–99.

Konefal J, Duncan R, Clemence C. Comparison of three levels of auricular acupuncture in an outpatient substance abuse treatment program. *Alt Medicine Journal.* Sept 1995;2(5).

Kris-Etherton PM, Harris WS, Appel LJ, AHA Nutrition Committee, American Heart Association. Omega—3 fatty acids and cardiovascular disease: new recommendations from the American Heart Association. *Arterioscler Thromb Vasc Biol.* 2003;23(2):151–152.

Krystal AD, Ressler I. The use of valerian in neuropsychiatry. *CNS Spectrum.* 2002;6:841–847.

Kulkarni SK, Ninan I. Inhibition of morphine tolerance and dependence by Withania somnifera in mice. *J Ethnopharmacol.* 1997;57(3):213–217.

Kulmatycki KM, Jamali F. Drug disease interactions: Role of inflammatory mediators in depression and variability in antidepressant drug response. *J Pharm Pharm Sci.* 2006;9(3):292–306.

Lane RD, McRae K, Reiman EM, Chen K, Ahern GL, Thayer JF. Neural correlates of heart rate variability during emotion. *Neuroimage.* Aug 9 2008.

Lake J. *Qigong.* In *Alternative and Complementary Therapies in Mental Health: Innovation and Integration.* Academic Press; 2001.

Langevin H, Badger G, Povolny B, et al. Yin and Yang Scores: A new method for quantitative diagnostic evaluation in traditional Chinese Medicine Research. *JACM.* 2004;10(2):389–395.

Larson D, Milano M. Religion and mental health: should they work together? *Alt. and Comp Therapies.* March/April 1996;91–98.

Larun L, Nordheim LV, Ekeland E, Hagen KB, Heian F. Exercise in prevention and treatment of anxiety and depression among children and young people. *Cochrane Database Syst Rev.* 2006 Jul 19;3:CD004691.

Lau MA, Bishop SR, Segal ZV, et al. The Toronto mindfulness scale: Development and validation. *J Clin Psychol.* 2006 Dec;62(12):1445–1467.

Lawlor D, Hopker S. The effectiveness of exercise as an intervention in the management of depression: systematic review and meta-regression analysis of randomized controlled trials. *Br Med J.* 2001;322:1–8.

Leo RJ, Ligot JS Jr. A systematic review of randomized controlled trials of acupuncture in the treatment of depression. *J Affect Disord.* 2007 Jan;97(1–3):13–22.

Levitan RD, Shen JH, Jindal R, Driver HS, Kennedy SH, Shapiro CM. Preliminary randomized double-blind placebo-controlled trial of tryptophan combined with fluoxetine to treat major depressive disorder: antidepressant and hypnotic effects. *Journal of Psychiatry & Neuroscience.* 2000 Sept 25:4; 337–346.

Li M, Chen K, Mo Z. Detoxification with qigong therapy for heroin addicts. *Altern Thera Health Med.* 2002;8:50–59.

Lieber CS. Role of oxidative stress and antioxidant therapy in alcoholic and nonalcoholic liver diseases. *Adv. Pharmacol.* 1997;38:601–628.

Lin PY, Su KP. A meta-analytic review of double-blind, placebo-controlled trials of antidepressant efficacy of omega-3 fatty acids. *J Clin Psychiatry.* 2007;68(7):1056–1061.

Linde K. How to evaluate the effectiveness of complementary therapies. *JACM.* 2000; 253–256.

Linde K, Mulrow CD. St John's wort for depression (Cochrane Review). In: The Cochrane Library, Issue 2, 2004. Chichester, UK: John Wiley & Sons, Ltd.

Linde K, Ramirez G, Mulrow, CD, Pauls A, Weidenhammer W, Melchart D. St. John's wort for depression: An overview and meta-analysis of randomized clinical trials. *BMJ.* 1996;313(7052):253–258.

Lolic MM, Fiskum G, Rosenthal RE. Neuroprotective effects of acetyl-L-carnitine after stroke in rats. *Ann Emerg Med.* 1997;29:758–765.

Lopez HH, Bracha AS, Bracha HS. Evidence based complementary intervention for insomnia. *Hawaii Med J.* 2002 Sep;61(9):192, 213.

Luo Z, Wang Y, Zhang S, He A, Chen Y, Liu X. Therapeutic effect of He-Ne laser irradiation of point erman in schizophrenic auditory hallucination—a clinical assessment. *J Tradit Chin Med.* 1986 Dec;6(4):253–256.

Mackay N, Hansen S, McFarlane O. Autonomic nervous system changes during reiki treatment: A preliminary study. *Jour Alt Comp Med.* 2004;10(6):1077–1081.

Malouf R, Areosa Sastre A. Vitamin B12 for cognition (Cochrane Review). In: The Cochrane Library, Issue 2, 2004. Chichester, UK: John Wiley & Sons, Ltd. Shang C Emerging paradigms in mind-body medicine JACM 7;1:2001, 83–91.

Manabu T, et al. Three-dimensional PET: An approach in psychology. *J International Society Life Information Science.* 1996;14(2):282–284.

Mant A, Mattick R, de Burgh S, et al. Benzodiazepine prescribing in general practice: Dispelling some myths. *Fam Pract.* 1995;12(1):37–43.

Marasco A, Ruiz R, Villagomex A, Infante C. Double-blind study of a multivitamin complex supplemented with ginseng extract. *Drugs Under Exp Clin Res.* 1996;22:323–329.

Margolin A, Avants K, Chang P, Kosten T. Acupuncture for the treatment of cocaine dependence in methadone-maintained patients. *Am J Addict.* 1993;2(3):194–201.

Martin JLR, Barbanoj MJ, Schlaepfer TE, et al. Transcranial magnetic stimulation for treating depression (Cochrane Review). In: The Cochrane Library, Issue 2, 2004. Chichester, UK: John Wiley & Sons, Ltd.

Mason O, Hargreaves I. A qualitative study of mindfulness-based cognitive therapy for depression. *Br J Med Psychol.* 2001;74(Pt 2):197–212.

Mason R. 200 mg of Zen; L-theanine boosts alpha waves, promotes alert relaxation. *Alternative & Complementary Therapies.* 2001 April; 7:91–95.

McCaffrey A, Eisenberg D, Legedza A, Davis R, Phillips R. Prayer for health concerns: Results of a national survey on prevalence and patterns of use. *Arch Intern Med.* Apr 26 2004;164:858–862.

McCauley Chapman K, Prabhudesai M, Erdman J. Vitamin status of alcoholics upon admission and after two weeks of hospitalization. *J Am Coll Nutr.* 1993;12(1):77–83.

McCleane G, Watters C. Pre-operative anxiety and serum potassium. *Anaesthesia.* 1990;45(7):583–585.

McLellan A, Metzger D, Alterman A, Cornish J, Urschel H. How effective is substance abuse treatment—compared to what? In: O'Brien C, Jaffe J, eds. *Advances in understanding the addictive states.* New York: Raven Press; 1992.

McCraty R, Atkinson M, Tomasino D. Science of the heart: Exploring the role of the heart in human performance. HeartMath Research Center, Institute of HeartMathj, Publication 01–001. Boulder Creek, CA: 2001.

McGuffin M, Hobbs C, Upton R, Goldberg A. *Botanical Safety Handbook.* Boca Raton: CRC Press; 1997.

McPherson M, Harmer C, Clark L, Sharp T, Goodwin G, Cowen P. Antidopaminergic effects of dietary tyrosine depletion in healthy subjects and patients with manic illness. *British Jour of Psychiatry.* 2001 Oct;179:356–360.

Menzano E, Carlen P. Zinc deficiency and corticosteroids in the pathogenesis of alcoholic brain dysfunction—a review. *Alcohol Clin Exp Res.* 1994;18(4):894–901.

Middleton P, Pollard H. Are chronic low back pain outcomes improved with co-management of concurrent depression? *Chiropr Osteopat.* 2005 Jun 22;13(1):-8.

Miller JJ, Fletcher K, Kabat–Zinn J. Three-year follow-up and clinical implications of a mindfulness meditation-based stress reduction intervention in the treatment of anxiety disorders. *Gen Hosp Psychiatry.* 1995;17(3):192–200.

Milligan J, Waldkoetter R. Use of hemi-sync audiotapes to reduce levels of depression for alcohol-dependent patients. *Hemi-Sync Journal.* Winter 2000;18(1):i–iii.

Mimori Y, Katsuoka H, Nakamuri S. Thiamine therapy in Alzheimer's disease. *Metab Brain Dis.* 1996;11(1):89–94.

Mischoulon D. Update and critique of natural remedies as antidepressant treatments. *Psychiatr Clin North Am.* 2007 Mar;30(1):51–68.

Mischoulon D, Best–Popescu C, Laposata M, et al. A double-blind dose-finding pilot study of docosahexaenoic acid (DHA) for major depressive disorder. *Eur Neuropsychopharmacol.* 2008 Sep;18(9):639–45.

Moncrieff J, Wessely S, Hardy R. Active placebos versus antidepressants for depression (Cochrane Review) In: The Cochrane Library, Issue 2, 2004 Chichester, U.K. John Wiley & Sons, Ltd.

Monasstra VJ, Lynn S, Linden M, Lubar JF, Gruzelier J, La Vaque TJ. Electroencephalographic biofeedback in the treatment of attention-deficit/hyperactivity disorder *Applied Psychophysiology and Biofeedback.* 2005 Jun;30(2):95–114.

Monastra VJ, Monastra DM, George S. The effects of stimulant therapy, EEG biofeedback, and parenting style on the primary symptoms of attention-deficit/hyperactivity disorder. *Appl Psychophysiol Biofeedback.* 2002;27(4):231–249.

Montgomery P, Dennis J. Physical exercise for sleep problems in adults aged 60+ (Cochrane Review). In: The Cochrane Library, Issue 2, 2004. Chichester, UK: John Wiley & Sons, Ltd.

Morin CM, Culbert J, Schwartz M. Nonpharmacological interventions for insomniaA meta-analysis of treatment efficacy. Am J Psychiatry. 1994;151:1172–1180.

Morin CM, Hauri PJ, Espie CA, Spielman AJ, Buysse DJ, Bootzin RR. Nonpharmacologic treatment of chronic insomnia. An American Academy of Sleep Medicine review. Neuroscience and Behavior Physiology. 1998;28(3):330–335.

Mukaino Y, Park J, White A, Ernst E. The effectiveness of acupuncture for depression—a systematic review of randomised controlled trials. Acupunct Med. 2005 Jun;23(2):70–76.

Murtagh DR, Greenwood KM. Identifying effective psychological treatments for insomnia: A meta-analysis. Journal of Consulting and Clinical Psychology. 1995;63(1):79–89.

Nahas Z, Kozel F, Li X, Anderson B, George M. Left prefrontal transcranial magnetic stimulation (TMS) treatment of depression in bipolar affective disorder: A pilot study of acute safety and efficacy. Bipolar Disorders. 2003 Feb;5(1):40–47.

Newcorn JH, Weiss M, Stein MA. The complexity of ADHD: Diagnosis and treatment of the adult patient with comorbidities. CNS Spect. 2007 Aug;12(8 Suppl 12):1–14.

Ng F, Dodd S, Berk M. The effects of physical activity in the acute treatment of bipolar disorder: A pilot study. J Affect Disord. 2007 Aug;101(1–3):259–62.

Nieber D, Schlegel S. Relationships between psychomotor retardation and EEG power spectrum in major depression. Neuropsychobiology. 1992;25:20–23.

Ohayon M. Epidemiology of insomnia: What we know and what we still need to learn. Sleep Med Rev. 2002;6:97–111.

Oken BS, Storzbach DM, Kaye JA. The efficacy of Ginkgo biloba on cognitive function in Alzheimer Disease. Arch Neurol. 1998;55:1409–1415.

Oner O, Alkar OY, Oner P. Relation of ferritin levels with symptom ratings and cognitive performance in children with attention deficit-hyperactivity disorder. Pediatr Int. 2008 Feb;50(1):40–44.

Orgogozo J, et al. Wine consumption and dementia in the elderly: A prospective community study in the Bordeaux area. Rev Neurol. (Paris) 1997;153(3)185–192.

Palmer J, Palmer L, Michiels K. Thigpen B effects of type of exercise on depression in recovering substance abusers. Perceptual and Motor Skills. 1995;80:523–530.

Palmer R, Katerndahl D, Morgan–Kidd J. A randomized trial of the effects of remote intercessory prayer: interactions with personal beliefs on problem-specific outcomes and functional status. JACM. 2004;10(3):438–448.

Paluska SA, Schwenk TL. Physical activity and mental health. Sports Med. 2000 Mar;29(3):167–180.

Pampallona S, Bollini P, Tibaldi G, Kupelnick B, Munizza C. Combined pharmacotherapy and psychological treatment for depression: A systematic review. *Arch Gen Psychiatry.* 2004;61:714–719.

Papakostas G, Petersen T, Mischoulon D, Ryan J, Nierenberg A, Bottiglieri T. Serum folate, vitamin B-12, and homocysteine in major depressive disorder, Part 1: Predictors of clinical response in fluoxetine-resistant depression. *J Clin Psychiatry.* 2004a;65(8):1090–1095.

Parker G, Gibson NA, Brotchie H, Heruc G, Rees AM, Hadzi–Pavlovic D. Omega-3 fatty acids and mood disorders. *Am J Psychiatry.* 2006 Jun;163(6):969–978.

Partonen T, Leppamaki S, Hurme J, Lonnqvist J. Randomized trial of physical exercise alone or combined with bright light on mood and health-related quality of life. *Psychol Med.* 1998 Nov;28(6):1359–1364.

Passeri M, Cucinotta D, Abate G, et al. Oral 5-methyltetrahydrofolic acid in senile organic mental disorders with depression: Results of a double-blind multicenter study. *Aging.* (Milano) 1993;5(1):63–71.

Patterson M, Firth J, Gardiner R. Treatment of drug, alcohol and nicotine addiction by neuroelectric therapy: Analysis of results over 7 years. *Jour of bioelectricity.* 1984;3(1&2):193–221.

Peet M, Horrobin DF, E–E Multicentre Study Group. A dose-ranging exploratory study of the effects of ethyl-eicosapentaenoate in patients with persistent schizophrenic symptoms. *J Psychiatr Res.* 2002;36(1):7–18.

Pelka RB, Jaenicke C, Gruenwald J. Impulse magnetic-field therapy for insomnia: A double-blind, placebo-controlled study. *Advances in Therapy.* 2001 Jul–Aug;18(4):174–180.

Pelka RB, Leuchtgens H. Pre-Alzheimer study: Action of a herbal yeast preparation (Bio-Strath) in a randomised double-blind trial. *Ars Neducu.* 1995;85.

Peniston E, Kulkosky P. Brainwave training and beta-endorphin levels in alcoholics. *Alcoholism: Clinical and Experimental Research.* 1989;13:272–279.

Peter H, Tabrizian S, Hand I. Serum cholesterol in patents with obsessive compulsive disorder during treatment with behavior therapy and ssri or placebo. *International Journal of Psychiatry in Medicine.* 2000;30(1):27–39.

Petersen R, Doody R, Kurz A, et al. Current concepts in mild cognitive impairment. *Arch Neurol.* 2001;58:1985–1992.

Pettegrew JW, Levine J, McClure RJ. Acetyl-L-carnitine physical-chemical, metabolic, and therapeutic properties: Relevance for its mode of action in Alzheimer's disease and geriatric depression. 2000;5:616–632.

Pilkington K, Kirkwood G, Rampes H, Cummings M, Richardson J. Complementary medicines in psychiatry: review of effectiveness and safety. Acupuncture for anxiety and anxiety disorders—a systematic literature review. *Br J Psychiatry.* 2006 Jun;188:587.

Pittler MH, Ernst E. Kava extract for treating anxiety (Cochrane Review). In: The Cochrane Library, Issue 2, 2004. Chichester, UK: John Wiley & Sons, Ltd.

Princhep L, Mas F, Hollander E, et al. Quantitative electroencephalographic (QEEG) subtyping of obsessive-compulsive disorder. *Psychiatry Res.* 1993;50:25–32.

Procter A. Enhancement of recovery From psychiatric illness by methylfolate. *Br J Psychiatry.* 1991;159:271–272.

Radin R. Event-related electroencephalographic correlations between isolated human subjects. *JACM.* 2002;10(2):315–323.

Ramu M, Venkataram B, Mukundan H, Shankara M, Leelavathy S, Janakiramaiah N. A controlled study of Ayurvedic treatment in the acutely ill patients with schizophrenia (Unmada)—rationale and results. *NIMHANS Journal.* 1992;10(1):1–16.

Rani P, Naidu M. Subjective and polysomnographic evaluation of a herbal preparation in insomnia. *Phytomedicine.* 1998;5:253–257.

Rettenbacher M, Hofer A, Eder U, et al. Compliance in schizophrenia: Psychopathology, side effects, and patients' attitudes toward the illness and medication. *J Clin Psychiatr.* 2004;65:1211–1218.

Rice KM, Blanchard EB, Purcell M. Biofeedback treatments of generalized anxiety disorder: Preliminary results. *Biofeedback & Self-Regulation.* 1993;18(2):93–105.

Richard AJ, Montoya ID, Nelson R, Spence RT. Effectiveness of adjunct therapies in crack cocaine treatment. *J Substance Abuse Treatment.* 1995;12(6):401–413.

Richardson AJ, Puri BK. The potential role of fatty acids in attention-deficit/hyperactivity disorder. *Prostaglandins Leukot Essent Fatty Acids.* 2000;63:79–87.

Richardson AJ, Puri BK. A randomized double-blind, placebo-controlled study of the effects of supplementation with highly unsaturated fatty acids on ADHD-related symptoms in children with specific learning difficulties. *Prog Neuropsychopharmacol Biol Psychiatry.* 2002;26:233–239.

Riemann D, Volderholzer U, Cohrs S, et al. Trimipramine in primary insomnia: Results of a polysomnographic double-blind controlled study. *Pharmacopsychiatry.* 2002;35:165–174.

Ritter M, Low K. Effects of dance/movement therapy: A meta-analysis. *The Arts in Psychotherapy.* 1996;23(3):249–260.

Riva G, Alcaniz A, Anolli L, et al. The VESPY updated project: Virtual environments in clinical psychology. *Cyberpsychology and Behav.* 2001;4(4):449–455.

Rizzo A, Wiederhold B. Applications and issues for the use of virtual reality technology for cognitive-behavioral/neuropsychological assessment and intervention. A workshop at the 34th annual convention of the Assoc. for Advancement of behavior therapy New Orleans, Louisiana U.S. Nov 16–20, 2000.

Robinson, L. *The effects of Therapeutic Touch on the Grief Experience.* doctoral dissertation, Univ of Alabama Birmingham, 1996.

Rojas NL, Chan E. Old and new controversies in the alternative treatment of attention-deficit hyperactivity disorder. *Ment Retard Dev Disabil Res Rev.* 2005;11(2):116–130.

Ross BM, Seguin J, Sieswerda LE. Omega-3 fatty acids as treatments for mental illness: Which disorder and which fatty acid? *Lipids Health Dis.* 2007 Sep 18;6:21.

Sackett DL, Rosenberg WM, Gray JA, Haynes RB, Richardson WS. Evidence based medicine: What it is and what it isn't. *BMJ.* 1996;312(7023):71–72.

Sacks W, et al. Acetazolamide and thiamine: An ancillary therapy for chronic mental illness. *Psych Res.* 1989;28:279–288.

Sageman S. Breaking through the despair: Spiritually oriented group therapy as a means of healing women with severe mental illness. *J Am Acad Psychoanal Dyn Psychiatry.* 2004;32(1):125–141.

Saladin ME, Brady KT, Graap K, Rothbaum BO. A preliminary report on the use of virtual reality technology to elicit craving and cue reactivity in cocaine dependent individuals. *Addict Behav.* 2006 Oct;31(10):1881–1894.

Sancier KM. Electrodermal measurements for monitoring the effects of a qigong workshop. *J Altern Complement Med.* 2003 Apr;9(2):235–241.

Sargent PA, Williamson DJ, Cowen PJ. Brain 5-HT neurotransmission during paroxetine treatment. *Br J Psychiatry.* 1998 Jan;172:49–52.

Sarkar P, Rathee SP, Neera N. Comparative efficacy of pharmacotherapy and biofeedback among cases of generalized anxiety disorder. *Journal of Projective Psychology & Mental Health.* 1999;6(1):69–77.

Sarris J. Herbal medicines in the treatment of psychiatric disorders: A systematic review. *Phytother Res.* 2007 Aug;21(8):703–716.

Schachter HM, Pham B, King J, et al., How efficacious and safe is short-acting methylphenidate for the treatment of attention-deficit disorder in children and adolescents? A meta-analysis. *CMAJ.* 2001;165(11):1475–1488.

Schmidt P, Daly R, Bloch M, et al. Dehydroepiandrosterone monotherapy in midlife-onset major and minor depression. *Arch Gen Psychiatry.* 2005;62:154–162.

Schneider-Helmert D, Spinweber C. Evaluation of L-tryptophan for treatment of insomnia: A review. *Psychopharmacology.* (Berlin) 1986;89(1)1–7..

Shore, A. *Long-term effects of energetic healing on symptoms of psychological depression and self-perceived stress. Alt Therapies* May/June 2004; 10:3: 42–48.

Schwabl H, Klima H. Spontaneous ultraweak photon emission from biological systems and the endogenous light field. *Forsch Komplementarmed Klass Naturheilkd.* 2005 Apr;12(2):84–89.

Schwartz G, Russek L. Neurotherapy and the heart: The challenge of energy cardiology. *Jour of Neurotherapy.* 1996 Spring/Summer;1–8.

Semlitsch HV, Anderer P, Saletu B, et al. Cognitive psychophysiology in nootropic drug research: Effects of Ginkgo bilboa on event-related potentials (P300) in age-associated memory impairment. *Pharmacopsychiatry.* 1995;28(4):134–142.

Shaffer HJ, LaSalvia TA, Stein JP. Comparing Hatha yoga with dynamic group psychotherapy for enhancing methadone maintenance treatment: A randomized clinical trial. *Altern Ther Health Med.* 1997;3(4):57–66.

Shannahoff–Khalsa D. Kundalini Yoga meditation techniques in the treatment of obsessive compulsive and OC spectrum disorders. *Brief treatment crisis intervention.* 2003;3:369–382.

Shannahoff–Khalsa DS, Ray LE, Levine S, et al. Randomized controlled trial of yogic meditation techniques for patients with obsessive–compulsive disorder. *CNS Spectrums.* 1999 Dec;4(12):34–47.

Sharp C, Hurford DP, Allison J, Sparks R, Cameron BP. Facilitation of internal locus of control in adolescent alcoholics through a brief biofeedback-assisted autogenic relaxation training procedure. *Journal of Substance Abuse Treatment.* 1997;14(1):55–60.

Shaw K, Turner J, Del Mar C. Tryptophan and 5-Hydroxytryptophan for depression (Cochrane Review). In: The Cochrane Library, Issue 2, 2004. Chichester, UK: John Wiley & Sons, Ltd.

Shi Z, Tan M. An analysis of the therapeutic effect of acupuncture in 500 cases of schizophrenia. *J Trad Chin Med.* 1986; Jun 6(2):99–104.

Shore A. Long-term effects of energetic healing on symptoms of psychological depression and self-perceived stress. *Alt Therapies.* May/June 2004;10(3):42–48.

Simmons M. Nutritional approach to bipolar disorder [Letter to the editor]. *Jour Clin Psychiatry.* 2002;64:338.

Simmons M. Nutritional approach to bipolar disorder. *The Journal of Clinical Psychiatry.* 2003 Mar;64(3):338.

Simon GE, Cherkin DC, Sherman KJ, Eisenberg DM, Deyo RA, Davis RB. Mental health visits to complementary and alternative medicine providers. *Gen Hosp Psychiatry.* 2004;26(3):171–177.

Sinn N, Bryan J. Effect of supplementation with polyunsaturated fatty acids and micronutrients on learning and behavior problems associated with child ADHD. *J Dev Behav Pediatr.* 2007;28(2):82–91.

Small J. Psychiatric disorders and EEG. In E. Niedermeyer & F. Lopes da Silva, eds. *Electroencephalography: Basic principles, clinical applications, and related fields.* Baltimore: Williams & Wilkins; 1993: 581–596.

Small JG, Milstein V, Malloy FW, Medlock CE, Klapper MH. Clinical and quantitative EEG studies of mania. *J Affect Disord.* 1999 Jun;53(3):217–224.

Smidt L, Cremin F, Grivetti L, Clifford A. Influence of thiamin supplementation on the health and general well-being of an elderly Irish population with marginal thiamin deficiency. *J Gerontol.* 1991;46(1):M16–M22.

Smith C. Quanta and coherence effects in water and living systems. *JACM.* 2004;10(1):69–78.

Smith CA, Hay PP. Acupuncture for depression. *Cochrane Database Syst Rev.* 2005 Apr 18;(2):CD004046.

Smith LA, Cornelius V, Warnock A, Bell A, Young AH. Effectiveness of mood stabilizers and antipsychotics in the maintenance phase of bipolar disorder: A systematic review of randomized controlled trials. *Bipolar Disord.* 2007 Jun;9(4):394–412.

Snow A, Hovane, L, Brandt J. A controlled trial of aromatherapy for agitation in nursing home patients with dementia. *The Jour. Of Alt. and Comp Medicine.* 2004;10(3):431–437.

Soderpalm B, Engel JA. Serotonergic involvement in conflict behavior. *Eur Neuropsychopharmacol.* 1990;1(1):7–13.

Sok SR, Erlen JA, Kim KB. Effects of acupuncture therapy on insomnia. *J Adv Nurs.* 2003 Nov;44(4):375–384.

Sorgi PJ, Hallowell EM, Hutchins HL, Sears B. Effects of an open-label pilot study with high-dose EPA/DHA concentrates on plasma phospholipids and behavior in children with attention deficit hyperactivity disorder. *Nutrition Journal.* 2007;6(16).

Sperner-Unterweger B. Immunological aetiology of major psychiatric disorders: Evidence and therapeutic implications. *Drugs.* 2005;65(11):1493–1520. Review.

Standish LJ, Johnson LC, Kozak L, Richards T. Evidence of correlated functional magnetic resonance imaging signals between distant human brains. *Alternative Therapies in Health and Medicine.* 2003;9(1):128.

Stevens LJ, Zentall SS, Deck JL, et al. Essential fatty acid metabolism in boys with attention-deficit hyperactivity disorder. *Am J Clin Nutr.* 1995;62(4):761–768.

Stouffer D, Kaiser D, Pitman G, Rolf W. Electrodermal testing to measure the effect of a Healing Touch treatment. *Journal of Holistic Nursing.* 2003.

Ströhle A. Physical activity, exercise, depression and anxiety disorders. *J Neural Transm.* 2008 Aug 23.

Strous RD. Dehydroepiandrosterone (DHEA) augmentation in the management of schizophrenia symptomatology. *Essent Psychopharmacol.* 2005;6(3):141–147.

Strous RD, Maayan R, Lapidus R, Stryjer R, Lustig M, Kotler M, Weizman A. Dehydroepiandrosterone augmentation in the management of negative, depressive, and anxiety symptoms in schizophrenia. *Archives of General Psychiatry.* 2003 Feb;60(2):133–141.

Strous RD, Shoenfeld Y. Schizophrenia, autoimmunity and immune system dysregulation: A comprehensive model updated and revisited. *J Autoimmun.* 2006 Sep;27(2):71–80.

Suen LK, Wong TK, Leung AW, Ip WC. The long-term effects of auricular therapy using magnetic pearls on elderly with insomnia. *Complementary Therapies in Medicine.* 2003 June;11(2):85–92.

Sussman N. The "file-drawer" effect: Assessing efficacy and safety of antidepressants. *Primary Psychiatry.* 2004 July;12.

Swanson JM, Kinsbourne M, Nigg J, et al. Etiologic subtypes of attention-deficit/hyperactivity disorder: brain imaging, molecular genetic and environmental factors and the dopamine hypothesis. *Neuropsychol Rev.* 2007 Mar;17(1):39–59.

Szegedi A, Kohnen R, Dienel A, Kieser M. Acute treatment of moderate to severe depression with hypericum extract WS 5570 (St John's wort): Randomised controlled double blind non-inferiority trial versus paroxetine. *BMJ.* 2005 Mar 5;330(7490):503. Erratum in: *BMJ.* 2005 Apr 2;330(7494):759. Dosage error in text.

Tahiliani A, Beinlich C. Pantothenic acid in health and disease. *Vitam Horm.* 1991;46:165–228.

Taylor MJ, Wilder H, Bhagwagar Z, Geddes J Inositol for depressive disorders (Cochrane Review). In: The Cochrane Library, Issue 2, 2004. Chichester, UK: John Wiley & Sons, Ltd.

Tempesta E, Troncon R, Janiri L, et al. Role of acetyl-L-carnitine in the treatment of cognitive deficit in chronic alcoholism. *Int J Clin Pharmacol Res.* 1990;10(1–2):101–107.

Terman M, Terman J. Treatment of seasonal affective disorder with a high-output negative ionizer. *J Altern Complement Med.* 1995 Jan;1(1):87–92.

Terman M, Terman J, Ross D. A controlled trial of timed bright light and negative air ionization for treatment of winter depression. *Arch Gen Psychiatry.* 1998 Oct;55(10):861–862.

Thachil AF, Mohan R, Bhugra D. The evidence base of complementary and alternative therapies in depression. *J Affect Disord.* 2007 Jan;97(1–3):23–35.

Thase M. Antidepressant effects: The suit may be small, but the fabric is real. *Prevention & Treatment.* 2002;5:Article 32.

Thatcher R. Normative EEG databases and EEG biofeedback. *Jour of Neurotherapy.* 1998 Spring;8–36.

Thomson AD, Pratt OE, Jeyasingham M, Shaw GK. Alcohol and brain damage. *Hum. Toxicol.* 1988 Sep;7(5):455–463.

Tiemeier H, Van Tuijl H, Hofman A, Kiliaan A, Breteler M. Plasma fatty acid composition and depression are associated in the elderly: The Rotterdam study. *Am J Clin Nutr.* 2003 Jul;78:1;40–46.

Tindle HA, Davis RB, Phillips RS, Eisenberg, DM. Trends in use of complementary and alternative medicine by US adults: 1997–2002. *Altern Ther Health Med.* 2005;11(1):42–49.

Tkachuk G, Martin G. Exercise therapy for patients with psychiatric disorders: research and clinical implications. *Prof Psychol Res Pract.* 1999;30:275–282.

Torrioli MG, Vernacotola S, Peruzzi L, et al. A double-blind, parallel, multicenter comparison of L-acetylcarnitine with placebo on the attention deficit hyperactivity disorder in fragile X syndrome boys. *Am J Med Genet A.* 2008 Apr 1;146(7):803–812.

Traylor AC, Bordnick PS, Carter BL. Assessing craving in young adult smokers using virtual reality. *Am J Addict.* 2008 Sep–Oct;17(5):436–440.

Trebaticka J, Kopasova S, Hradecna Z, et al. Treatment of ADHD with French maritime pine bark extract Pycnogenol. *Eur Child Adolesc Psychiatry.* 2006;15(6):329–335.

Tsuang M, Williams W, Simpson J, Lyons M. Pilot study of spirituality and mental health in twins. *Am J Psychiatry.* 2002;159(3):486–488.

Tully AM, Roche HM, Doyle R, et al. Low serum cholesteryl ester-docosahexaenoic acid levels in Alzheimer's disease: A case-control study. *Br J Nutr.* 2003;89(4):483–489.

Tuunainen A, Kripke DF, Endo T. Light therapy for non-seasonal depression. Cochrane Database Syst Rev. 2004;(2):CD004050.

Unutzer J, Klap R, Sturm R, et al. Mental disorders and the use of alternative medicine: Results from a national survey. *Am J Psychiatry.* 2000;157(11):1851–1857.

Vaidya ADB. The status and scope of Indian medicinal plants acting on central nervous system. *Indian J Pharmacol.* 1997;29(5):S340–S343.

Vedamurthachar A. Biological effects of Sudarshan Kriya on alcoholics [dissertation]. Bangalore, India: National Institute of Mental Health and Neurosciences and Mangalore University; 2002.

Venneman S, Leuchter A, Bartzokis G, et al. Variation in neurophysiological function and evidence of quantitative electroencephalogram discordance: predicting cocaine-dependent treatment attrition. *J Neuropsychiatry Clin Neurosci.* 2006 Spring;18(2):208–216.

Verhoef MI, Casebeer AL, Hilsdew RJ. Assessing efficacy of complementary medicine: Adding qualitative research methods to the "gold standard." *JACM.* 2000;8(3):275–281.

Vgontzas AN, Zoumakis M, Papanicolaou DA, et al. Chronic insomnia is associated with a shift of interleukin-6 and tumor necrosis factor secretion from nighttime to daytime. *Metabolism: Clinical & Experimental.* 2002 July;51(7):887–892.

Vincelli F, Anolli L, Bouchard S, Wiederhold B, Zurloni V, Riva G. Experiential cognitive therapy in the treatment of panic disorders with agoraphobia: A controlled study. *CyberPsychology & Behavior.* 2003;6(3):321–328.

Voigt RG, Llorente AM, Jensen CL, et al. A randomized, double-blind, placebo-controlled trial of docosahexaenoic acid supplementation in children with attention-deficit/hyperactivity disorder. *J Pediatr.* 2001;139(2):189–196.

Wang H, Qi H, Wang BS, et al. Is acupuncture beneficial in depression: A meta-analysis of 8 randomized controlled trials. *J Affect Disord.* 2008 Jun 10.

Wang Z, Ren Q, Shen Y. A double-blind controlled study of Huperzine A and Piracetam in patients with age-associated memory impairment and Alzheimer's disease (abstract S–181–770). *Neuropsychopharmacology.* 1994 May;10(3S/Part 1):763S.

Wardell W. The trauma release technique: How it is taught and experienced in Healing Touch. *Alternative and Complementary Therapies.* 2000;6(1):20–27.

Weber W, Newmark S. Complementary and alternative medical therapies for attention-deficit/hyperactivity disorder and autism. *Pediatr Clin North Am.* 2007 Dec;54(6):983–1006;xii.

Wender EH. The food additive-free diet in the treatment of behavior disorders: A review. *J Dev Behav Pediatr.* 1986;7(1):35–42.

Werbach MR. *Nutritional Influences on Mental Illness: A Sourcebook of Clinical Research.* Tarzana, California: Third Line Press; 1999.

Westen D, Morrison K. A multidimensional meta-analysis of treatments for depression, panic and generalized anxiety disorder: An empirical examination of the status of empirically supported therapies. *Jour Consulting and Clinical Psychology.* 2001 Dec;69(6):875–899.

Weuve J, Kang J, Manson J, Breteler M, Ware J, Grodstein F. Physical activity, including walking, and cognitive function in older women. *JAMA.* 2004;292(12):1454–1461.

White AR, Rampes H, Ernst E. Acupuncture for smoking cessation (Cochrane Review). In: The Cochrane Library, Issue 2, 2004. Chichester, UK: John Wiley & Sons, Ltd.

White AR, Resch K. Ernst E. Randomized trial of acupuncture for nicotine withdrawal symptoms. *Arch Intern Med.* 1998;158:2251–2255.

Wiederhold B, Jang D, Gevirtz R, Kim S, Kim Y, Wiederhold M. The treatment of fear of flying: A controlled study of imaginal and virtual reality graded exposure therapy. *IEEE: Transactions on Information Technology in Biomedicine.* 2002 Sept;6(3):218–223.

Wiederhold B, Wiederhold M. Lessons learned from 600 virtual reality sessions. *CyberPsychology & Behavior.* 2000;3(3):393–400.

Wijk EP, Wijk RV. Multi-site recording and spectral analysis of spontaneous photon emission from human body. *Forsch Komplementarmed Klass Naturheilkd.* 2005 Apr;12(2):96–106.

Wileman SM, Eagles JM, Andrew JE, et al. Light therapy for seasonal affective disorder in primary care: Randomized controlled trial. *British Jour Psychiatr.* 2001;178:311–316.

Wittenborn J. A search for responders to niacin supplementation. *Arch Gen Psychiatry.* 1974;31:547–552.

Wong AH, Smith M, Boon HS. Herbal remedies in psychiatric practice. *Arch Gen Psychiatry.* 1998;55:1033–1043.

Woods D, Craven R, Whitney J. The effect of therapeutic touch on behavioral symptoms of persons with dementia. *Alt Ther Health Med.* 2005;11:66–74.

Woolery A, Meyers H, Sternlieb B, Zeltzer L. A yoga intervention for young adults with elevated symptoms of depression. *Alternative Therapies.* 2004;10(1):60–63.

Xu G. 45 cases of insomnia treated by acupuncture. *Shanghai Journal of Acupuncture and Moxibustion.* 1997;16(6):10.

Yang JM, Choi C, Woo WM, et al. Left-right and Yin-Yang balance of biophoton emission from hands. *Acupunct Electrother Res.* 2004;29(3–4):197–211.

Yankovskis G, Beldava I, Livina B. Osteoreflectory treatment of alcohol abstinence syndrome and craving for alcohol in patients with alcoholism. *Acupunct Electrother Res.* 2000;25(1):9–16.

Yorbik O, Ozdag MF, Olgun A, Senol MG, Bek S, Akman S. Potential effects of zinc on information processing in boys with attention deficit hyperactivity disorder. *Prog Neuropsychopharmacol Biol Psychiatry.* 2008 Apr 1;32(3):662–667.

Zahourek R. Intentionality forms the matrix of healing: A theory. *Alt Therapies.* 2004;10(6):40–49.

Zhang B. A controlled study of clinical therapeutic effects of laser acupuncture for schizophrenia. *Zhonghua Shen Jing Jing Shen Ke Za Zhi.* 1991 Apr;24(2):81–83, 124.

Zhang, C. Skin resistance vs body conductivity: On the background of electronic measurement on skin. *Frontier Perspectives.* 2002;11(2):15–25.

Zhang XY, Zhou DF, Zhang P, et al. A double-blind, placebo-controlled trial of extract of Ginkgo biloba added to haloperidol in treatment-resistant patients with schizophrenia. *J Clin Psychiatry.* 2001;62:878–883.

Zhao HW, Li XY. Ginkgolide A, B, and huperzine A inhibit nitric oxide-induced neurotoxicity. *Int Immunopharmacol.* 2002 Oct;2(11):1551–1556.

Ziegler G, Ploch M, Miettinen-Baumann A, Collet W. Efficacy and tolerability of valerian extract LI 156 compared with oxazepam in the treatment of nonorganic insomnia—a randomized, double-blind, comparative clinical study. *European Journal of Medical Research.* 2002 Nov 25;7(11):480–486.

Zucker M. Huperzine-A: The newest brain nutrient. *Let's Live.* 1999 May;47–48.

Zylowska L, Ackerman DL, Yang MH, et al. Mindfulness meditation training in adults and adolescents with ADHD: A feasibility study. *J Atten Disord.* 2008 May;11(6):737–746.

Index